Assessment of Environmental Radioactivity and Radiation for Human Health Risk

Assessment of Environmental Radioactivity and Radiation for Human Health Risk

Editors

Shinji Tokonami
Ikuo Kashiwakura

MDPI • Basel • Beijing • Wuhan • Barcelona • Belgrade • Manchester • Tokyo • Cluj • Tianjin

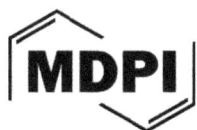

Editors
Shinji Tokonami
Institute of Radiation Emergency Medicine
Hirosaki University
Aomori
Japan

Ikuo Kashiwakura
Vice president
Hirosaki University
Aomori
Japan

Editorial Office
MDPI
St. Alban-Anlage 66
4052 Basel, Switzerland

This is a reprint of articles from the Special Issue published online in the open access journal *International Journal of Environmental Research and Public Health* (ISSN 1660-4601) (available at: https://www.mdpi.com/journal/ijerph/special_issues/radioactivity_radiation).

For citation purposes, cite each article independently as indicated on the article page online and as indicated below:

LastName, A.A.; LastName, B.B.; LastName, C.C. Article Title. *Journal Name* **Year**, *Volume Number*, Page Range.

ISBN 978-3-0365-1225-9 (Hbk)
ISBN 978-3-0365-1224-2 (PDF)

© 2021 by the authors. Articles in this book are Open Access and distributed under the Creative Commons Attribution (CC BY) license, which allows users to download, copy and build upon published articles, as long as the author and publisher are properly credited, which ensures maximum dissemination and a wider impact of our publications.

The book as a whole is distributed by MDPI under the terms and conditions of the Creative Commons license CC BY-NC-ND.

Contents

About the Editors vii

Preface to "Assessment of Environmental Radioactivity and Radiation for Human Health Risk" ix

Shinji Tokonami
Characteristics of Thoron (^{220}Rn) and Its Progeny in the Indoor Environment
Reprinted from: *Int. J. Environ. Res. Public Health* **2020**, *17*, 8769, doi:10.3390/ijerph17238769 ... 1

Yohei Fujishima, Yasushi Kino, Takumi Ono, Valerie Swee Ting Goh, Akifumi Nakata, Kentaro Ariyoshi, Kosuke Kasai, Tadashi Toyoda, Toru Akama, Hirofumi Tazoe, Masatoshi Yamada, Mitsuaki A. Yoshida and Tomisato Miura
Transition of Radioactive Cesium Deposition in Reproductive Organs of Free-Roaming Cats in Namie Town, Fukushima
Reprinted from: *Int. J. Environ. Res. Public Health* **2021**, *18*, 1772, doi:10.3390/ijerph18041772 ... 21

Oumar Bobbo Modibo, Yuki Tamakuma, Takahito Suzuki, Ryohei Yamada, Weihai Zhuo, Chutima Kranrod, Kazuki Iwaoka, Naofumi Akata, Masahiro Hosoda and Shinji Tokonami
Long-Term Measurements of Radon and Thoron Exhalation Rates from the Ground Using the Vertical Distributions of Their Activity Concentrations
Reprinted from: *Int. J. Environ. Res. Public Health* **2021**, *18*, 1489, doi:10.3390/ijerph18041489 ... 35

Alicia Fernández, Carlos Sainz, Santiago Celaya, Luis Quindós, Daniel Rábago and Ismael Fuente
A New Methodology for Defining Radon Priority Areas in Spain
Reprinted from: *Int. J. Environ. Res. Public Health* **2021**, *18*, 1352, doi:10.3390/ijerph18031352 ... 47

Tetsuya Sanada
Measurement of Indoor Thoron Gas Concentrations Using a Radon-Thoron Discriminative Passive Type Monitor: Nationwide Survey in Japan
Reprinted from: *Int. J. Environ. Res. Public Health* **2021**, *18*, 1299, doi:10.3390/ijerph18031299 ... 63

Shunya Nakasone, Akinobu Ishimine, Shuhei Shiroma, Natsumi Masuda, Kaori Nakamura, Yoshitaka Shiroma, Sohei Ooka, Masahiro Tanaka, Akemi Kato, Masahiro Hosoda, Naofumi Akata, Yumi Yasuoka and Masahide Furukawa
Temporal and Spatial Variation of Radon Concentrations in Environmental Water from Okinawa Island, Southwestern Part of Japan
Reprinted from: *Int. J. Environ. Res. Public Health* **2021**, *18*, 998, doi:10.3390/ijerph18030998 ... 71

Koya Ogura, Masahiro Hosoda, Yuki Tamakuma, Takahito Suzuki, Ryohei Yamada, Ryoju Negami, Takakiyo Tsujiguchi, Masaru Yamaguchi, Yoshitaka Shiroma, Kazuki Iwaoka, Naofumi Akata, Mayumi Shimizu, Ikuo Kashiwakura and Shinji Tokonami
Discriminative Measurement of Absorbed Dose Rates in Air from Natural and Artificial Radionuclides in Namie Town, Fukushima Prefecture
Reprinted from: *Int. J. Environ. Res. Public Health* **2021**, *18*, 978, doi:10.3390/ijerph18030978 ... 83

Eka Djatnika Nugraha, Masahiro Hosoda, June Mellawati, Untara Untara, Ilsa Rosianna, Yuki Tamakuma, Oumar Bobbo Modibo, Chutima Kranrod, Kusdiana Kusdiana and Shinji Tokonami
Radon Activity Concentrations in Natural Hot Spring Water: Dose Assessment and Health Perspective
Reprinted from: *Int. J. Environ. Res. Public Health* **2021**, *18*, 920, doi:10.3390/ijerph18030920 ... 99

Mohammademad Adelikhah, Amin Shahrokhi, Morteza Imani, Stanislaw Chalupnik and Tibor Kovács
Radiological Assessment of Indoor Radon and Thoron Concentrations and Indoor Radon Map of Dwellings in Mashhad, Iran
Reprinted from: *Int. J. Environ. Res. Public Health* **2020**, *18*, 141, doi:10.3390/ijerph18010141 . . . 107

Jun Hu, Guosheng Yang, Chutima Kranrod, Kazuki Iwaoka, Masahiro Hosoda and Shinji Tokonami
An Improved Passive CR-39-Based Direct ^{222}Rn/^{220}Rn Progeny Detector
Reprinted from: *Int. J. Environ. Res. Public Health* **2020**, *17*, 8569, doi:10.3390/ijerph17228569 . . . 123

Hiroshi Terada, Ikuyo Iijima, Sadaaki Miyake, Kimio Isomura and Hideo Sugiyama
Total Diet Study to Assess Radioactive Cs and ^{40}K Levels in the Japanese Population before and after the Fukushima Daiichi Nuclear Power Plant Accident
Reprinted from: *Int. J. Environ. Res. Public Health* **2020**, *17*, 8131, doi:10.3390/ijerph17218131 . . . 137

Yuki Tamakuma, Chutima Kranrod, Takahito Suzuki, Yuki Watanabe, Thamaborn Ploykrathok, Ryoju Negami, Eka Djatnika Nugraha, Kazuki Iwaoka, Mirosław Janik, Masahiro Hosoda and Shinji Tokonami
Passive-Type Radon Monitor Constructed Using a Small Container for Personal Dosimetry
Reprinted from: *Int. J. Environ. Res. Public Health* **2020**, *17*, 5660, doi:10.3390/ijerph17165660 . . . 155

Aoife Kinahan, Masahiro Hosoda, Kevin Kelleher, Takakiyo Tsujiguchi, Naofumi Akata, Shinji Tokonami, Lorraine Currivan and Luis León Vintró
Assessment of Radiation Dose from the Consumption of Bottled Drinking Water in Japan
Reprinted from: *Int. J. Environ. Res. Public Health* **2020**, *17*, 4992, doi:10.3390/ijerph17144992 . . . 165

Hirofumi Tazoe, Takeyasu Yamagata, Kazuki Tsujita, Hisao Nagai, Hajime Obata, Daisuke Tsumune, Jota Kanda and Masatoshi Yamada
Observation of Dispersion in the Japanese Coastal Area of Released ^{90}Sr, ^{134}Cs, and ^{137}Cs from the Fukushima Daiichi Nuclear Power Plant to the Sea in 2013
Reprinted from: *Int. J. Environ. Res. Public Health* **2019**, *16*, 4094, doi:10.3390/ijerph16214094 . . . 177

Naofumi Akata, Masahiro Tanaka, Chie Iwata, Akemi Kato, Miki Nakada, Tibor Kovács and Hideki Kakiuchi
Isotope Composition and Chemical Species of Monthly Precipitation Collected at the Site of a Fusion Test Facility in Japan
Reprinted from: *Int. J. Environ. Res. Public Health* **2019**, *16*, 3883, doi:10.3390/ijerph16203883 . . . 193

Masahiko Matsuo, Yasuyuki Taira, Makiko Orita, Yumiko Yamada, Juichi Ide, Shunichi Yamashita and Noboru Takamura
Evaluation of Environmental Contamination and Estimated Radiation Exposure Dose Rates among Residents Immediately after Returning Home to Tomioka Town, Fukushima Prefecture
Reprinted from: *Int. J. Environ. Res. Public Health* **2019**, *16*, 1481, doi:10.3390/ijerph16091481 . . . 205

Van-Hao Duong, Thanh-Duong Nguyen, Miklos Hegedus, Erika Kocsis and Tibor Kovacs
Study of Well Waters from High-Level Natural Radiation Areas in Northern Vietnam
Reprinted from: *Int. J. Environ. Res. Public Health* **2021**, *18*, 469, doi:10.3390/ijerph18020469 . . . 217

About the Editors

Shinji Tokonami

Professor Shinji Tokonami is director of the Institute of Radiation Emergency Medicine, Hirosaki University, Japan. He specializes in radiation measurement and dose assessment. In 1995, Dr. Tokonami earned his Ph.D. in engineering from Waseda University. Throughout his career he has been involved with radiation research at Waseda University, the National Institute of Radiological Sciences, and Hirosaki University. In addition, he is a member of several International Organizations for Standards'committees regarding radon and radiation measurements. Dr. Tokonami also developed multiple measurement techniques and equipment related to his field. In particular, he established a passive measurement technique for detecting radon-222 and radon-220. This discriminative measurement technique for radon isotopes was published as ISO 16641.

Ikuo Kashiwakura

Professor Ikuo Kashiwakrua is the Vice President of Hirosaki University, Japan and is in charge of radiation emergency medicine-related activities. In addition, his specialty is radiation biology, especially on radiation's effects on the differentiation and proliferation of hematopoietic stem cells and the development of radiomitigative protocols. Dr. Kashiwakura earned his Ph.D. in Pharmacology from Hokkaido Pharmaceutical University School of Pharmacy. Throughout his career he has been involved with radiation education and research at Hokkaido Pharmaceutical University School of Pharmacy and Hirosaki University for about 40 years. Meanwhile, he served as a program officer of the Science Center for Science Systems established within JSPS for three years (2009–2011). Currently, his research is focusing on the development of radiomitigative protocols utilizing domestically approved pharmaceutical drugs.

Preface to "Assessment of Environmental Radioactivity and Radiation for Human Health Risk"

In 2010, the Institute of Radiation Emergency Medicine (IREM) was established as a strategic research institute at Hirosaki University, Japan. Subsequently, the Great East Japan Earthquake occurred on 11 March 2011, and consequently a nuclear accident occurred at Tokyo Electric Power's Fukushima Daiichi Nuclear Power Plant. We played an important role in the response to the disaster and transmitted a wide range of academic information. This achievement has been highly rated, not only in Japan but also internationally. In parallel, we have started a human resources development project for the Nuclear Regulation Authority and other projects that aim to create a hub institution for domestic utilization and collaborative research.

This Special Issue book of the *International Journal of Environmental Research and Public Health*, titled "Assessment of Environmental Radioactivity and Radiation for Human Health Risk", is the one of IREM's accomplishments and is published to commemorate the 10th anniversary of the Institute of Radiation Emergency Medicine. This book provides a collection of high-quality research papers in radiation-related fields, such as environmental radioactivity, environmental radiation, measurement data, methodology, monitoring, and risk assessment. Finally, we thank all the reviewers, editors and authors for their important anonymous contributions under a very strict time constraint, and we would like to acknowledge all of the authors for their excellent research.

Shinji Tokonami, Ikuo Kashiwakura
Editors

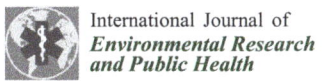

Review

Characteristics of Thoron (^{220}Rn) and Its Progeny in the Indoor Environment

Shinji Tokonami

Institute of Radiation Emergency Medicine, Hirosaki University, Hirosaki 036-8564, Aomori, Japan; tokonami@hirosaki-u.ac.jp; Tel.: +81-172-39-5404

Received: 19 October 2020; Accepted: 23 November 2020; Published: 25 November 2020

Abstract: The present paper outlines characteristics of thoron and its progeny in the indoor environment. Since the half-life of thoron (^{220}Rn) is very short (55.6 s), its behavior is quite different from the isotope radon (^{222}Rn, half-life 3.8 days) in the environment. Analyses of radon and lung cancer risk have revealed a clearly positive relationship in epidemiological studies among miners and residents. However, there is no epidemiological evidence for thoron exposure causing lung cancer risk. In contrast to this, a dosimetric approach has been approved in the International Commission on Radiological Protection (ICRP) Publication 137, from which new dose conversion factors for radon and thoron progenies can be obtained. They are given as 16.8 and 107 nSv (Bq m^{-3} h)$^{-1}$, respectively. It implies that even a small quantity of thoron progeny will induce higher radiation exposure compared to radon. Thus, an interest in thoron exposure is increasing among the relevant scientific communities. As measurement technologies for thoron and its progeny have been developed, they are now readily available. This paper reviews measurement technologies, activity levels, dosimetry and resulting doses. Although thoron has been underestimated in the past, recent findings have revealed that reassessment of risks due to radon exposure may need to take the presence of thoron and its progeny into account.

Keywords: thoron; thoron progeny; indoor environment; measurement technique; radioactivity; dose assessment

1. Introduction

Radon (^{222}Rn), thoron (^{220}Rn) and their progeny can be regarded as the largest contributor annually to an effective dose for the public globally [1,2]. According to the United Nations Scientific Committee on the Effects of Atomic Radiation (UNSCEAR) 2008 report, an annual effective dose from natural radiation sources is calculated to be 2.4 mSv as the worldwide average, whereas radon and thoron contribute 1.2 and 0.1 mSv, respectively. When they are inhaled, although radon and thoron gases are not significant, their progeny particularly affect the lung tissue due to alpha particles emitted in their decay chains deposited in the airways. In the past, lung cancer incidence had been found only among miners as shown in many epidemiological studies, whereas recent investigations have revealed that even indoor radon resulted in lung cancer among residents [3]. These surveys were carried out in Europe, North America and China. Therefore, the World Health Organization (WHO) issued a handbook where special attention was paid to indoor radon [3]. Subsequently, the International Commission on Radiological Protection (ICRP) has recently published two publications and one statement related to radon. In these documents, the upper value of the reference level for radon gas in homes was revised downward from the value in the 2007 Recommendations of 600 Bq m^{-3} to 300 Bq m^{-3} [4,5]. The International Atomic Energy Agency (IAEA) revised the previous Basic Safety Standard (BSS) in the same manner as the ICRP and a related guide was issued [6,7]. The WHO further advised a reference level of 100 Bq m^{-3} though it may be impossible to achieve such a low radon gas concentration in many countries. Such recommendations depend on results of an indoor radon survey.

In most cases, these surveys were carried out using passive radon monitors so as to obtain an annual indoor radon concentration. Even in epidemiological surveys, the same type of radon monitor was used, because lung cancer incidence was closely related to long-term exposure to radon. Previous recommendations were given based on not the dosimetric, but on the epidemiological approach. It had been previously believed that the epidemiological approach was more reliable than the dosimetric. In ICRP Publication 65, the risk estimate was given based on the epidemiological approach [8]. As was concluded according to studies of miners, however, the conversion convention, though scientifically vague, needed to be used when applied to indoor radon studies. There was a large difference between the two approaches by a factor of more than three and many technical issues to be solved. After the data analyses on the indoor radon and lung cancer study were vigorously carried out, the risk estimates in residential radon studies were eventually concluded without using the conversion convention and came close to those given by the dosimetric approach. This is why many authoritative publications were issued and revised. However, they still state that the effect of thoron is negligible compared to that of radon, though the amount of related data is limited. It should be noted that measurement techniques for thoron are not so easy as those for radon. As the half-life of thoron atoms is much shorter than that of radon, they immediately decay, followed by ^{216}Po with a half-life much shorter than thoron. A question arises here. Many passive radon monitors have been used in both national and epidemiological surveys. If thoron is present together with radon, are these well designed so as to effectively detect radon only? If high diffusion barriers are used, they depress the detection of thoron. Otherwise they may mislead and lead to wrong calculation of radon concentrations. In epidemiological surveys, this will result in incorrect lung cancer risk estimates. Most passive radon monitors have never been examined from the viewpoint of thoron interference on radon measurements. Limited data on thoron is given in UNSCEAR reports and indoor thoron surveys have never been systematically conducted. It is well known that there is no epidemiological evidence for thoron risk related to lung cancer. The risk can be estimated based only on the dosimetric approach. Under the current situation in which the dosimetric approach has become more reliable, it is important to know how large the total lung cancer risk is when influenced by thoron and its progeny. This paper comprehensively describes characteristics of thoron and its progeny in the indoor environment from the viewpoint of measurements, dose assessment and health risk.

2. Physical Property and Behavior

Figure 1 illustrates the radioactive decay series for thorium-232 [9] where the half-life and emitted energies are given. After Ra-224 decays, Rn-220 is formed. It is commonly called thoron, an inert gas. In the uranium-238 decay series, on the other hand, radon-222 is formed as an inert gas. There is a great deal of difference in the half-life between radon-220 and radon-222. Although Po-216 is formed with alpha decay of Rn-220, it can almost be regarded as a gas because its half-life is very short. Subsequently Pb-212 and Bi-212 are formed, which need mainly to be considered for dose assessment when they are inhaled. These concentrations are collectively expressed in the equilibrium equivalent concentration (EEC). The EEC for thoron progeny (Equilibrium Equivalent Thoron Concentration: EETC [Bq m^{-3}]) can be approximately calculated by the Equation (1) after considering the contribution of Po-216:

$$\text{EETC} = 0.913 \times C_B + 0.087 \times C_C \tag{1}$$

where C_B: Pb-212 is activity concentration [Bq m^{-3}]; C_C: Bi-212 is activity concentration [Bq m^{-3}]. If the equilibrium factor for thoron (F_{Tn}) is defined in the same manner for radon, it can be expressed as the Equation (2):

$$wF_{Tn} = \frac{\text{EETC}}{C_{Tn}} \tag{2}$$

where C_{Tn} is thoron concentration [Bq m^{-3}]. The significance of the equilibrium factor for thoron is discussed in this paper from the viewpoint of dose assessment.

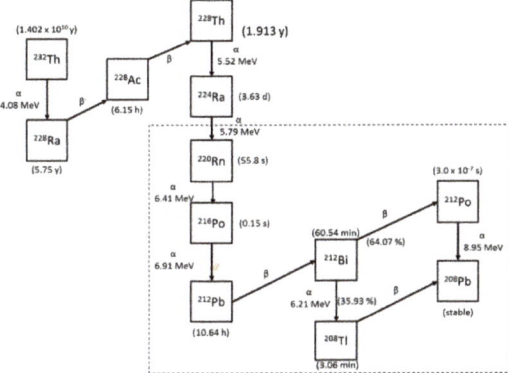

Figure 1. Radioactive decay series for thorium-232.

Figure 2 exemplifies the exhalation process of thoron from macro surfaces such as walls containing its parent nuclide ^{224}Ra. The exhalation and diffusion of thoron is approximately described as a one-dimensional phenomenon. When the exhalation rate of thoron from the wall is considered, for instance, the indoor thoron concentration ($C_{Tn}(x)$ [Bq m^{-3}]) at distance x from the wall can be expressed by the Equation (3) [10,11]:

$$C_{Tn}(x) = \frac{E_{Tn}}{\sqrt{\lambda_{Tn} D}} e^{(-\sqrt{\lambda_{Tn}/D} x)} \tag{3}$$

where E_{Tn} is surface exhalation rate of thoron from the wall [Bq m^{-2} s^{-1}]; λ_{Tn} is decay constant of thoron [s^{-1}]; and D is diffusion coefficient of thoron [m^2 s^{-1}]. If the thoron concentrations are measured at two different locations, respectively, the exhalation rate of thoron can be estimated. As the half-life of Po-216 is much shorter than that of the parent nuclide thoron, there is a radioactive equilibrium between the two isotopes.

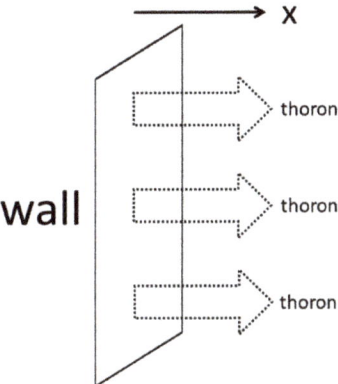

Figure 2. Exhalation process of thoron from macro surface.

Figure 3 illustrates the behavior of radon/thoron and their progeny in indoor air. After radon and thoron decay, their progenies are formed. Most of these are positively charged and they rapidly capture water molecules, thus forming clusters. They move so quickly in air that some of them attach to ambient aerosols and the others deposit on the wall, ceiling, floor and macro-surfaces. Therefore radon/thoron progeny are generally classified into two fractions: unattached and attached fractions. As unattached progenies have a high diffusive velocity, they deposit on available surfaces very quickly. Even progeny attached to ambient aerosols may eventually deposit on the surface. Before Po-216 atoms are captured by ambient aerosols, they decay to Pb-212 atoms. After considering the half-life of Pb-212, the negligible outdoor Pb-212 activity concentration, and the attachment process to aerosols, Pb-212 activity concentration (C_B [Bq m^{-3}]) in a room can be obtained by the Equation (4):

$$C_B = \frac{\lambda_a \lambda_B E_{Tn}}{\lambda_{Tn}(\lambda_B + \lambda_v + \lambda_d^a)\{\lambda_B + \lambda_a + \sqrt{\lambda_{Tn}(\lambda_B + \lambda_a)}\}} \cdot \frac{S}{V} \quad (4)$$

where λ_B is decay constant of Pb-212 [s^{-1}]; λ_a is attachment rate of unattached thoron progeny onto ambient aerosols [s^{-1}]; λ_v is ventilation rate of the room [s^{-1}]; λ_d^a is deposition rate of attached thoron progeny [s^{-1}]; S is surface area where thoron atoms are emitted [m^2]; and V is inner volume of the room [m^3]. Based on the same manner, Bi-212 activity concentration (C_C) is subsequently given by the Equation (5):

$$C_C = \frac{\lambda_C C_B}{\lambda_C + \lambda_v + \lambda_d^a} \quad (5)$$

where λ_C is decay constant of Bi-212 [s^{-1}]. When the typical parameters are given in Table 1 [10,12,13], EETC can be estimated with the exhalation rate of thoron as shown in Figure 4. De With et al. [14] reported the thoron exhalation rate from the wall against the EETC value in the room. As the physical parameters except Surface-to-Volume (S-V) ratio are not expected to be much different in any indoor environment, EETC can be simply expressed along with the exhalation rate of thoron and S-V ratio as the Equation (6):

$$\text{EETC} = 3.36 E_{Tn} \frac{S}{V} \quad (6)$$

Note that the EETC may change if another value of each parameter is adopted from the range.

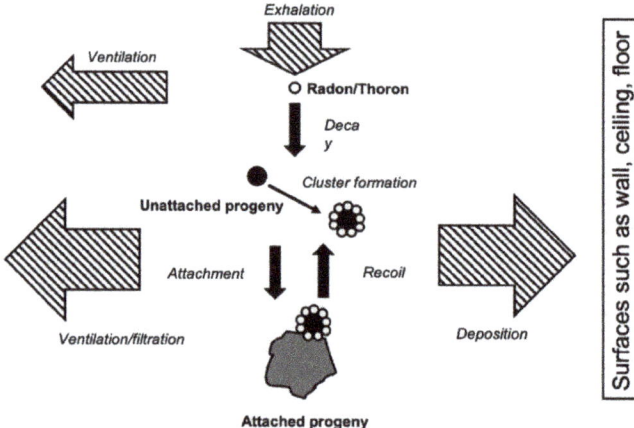

Figure 3. Behavior of radon/thoron and their progeny in indoor air.

Table 1. Physical parameters for indoor model [10,12,13].

Parameter [1]	Range	Typical
Decay constant of thoron [h^{-1}]	-	44.74
Decay constant of Pb-212 [h^{-1}]	-	0.065
Attachment rate of unattached thoron progeny onto ambient aerosols [h^{-1}]	3–110	50
Ventilation rate of the room [h^{-1}]	0.1–1	0.5
Deposition rate of attached thoron progeny [h^{-1}]	0.015–0.35	0.2
Surface-to-Volume ratio [m^{-1}]	-	0.36

[1] Unit is expressed in h^{-1} so as to easily compare with previous studies.

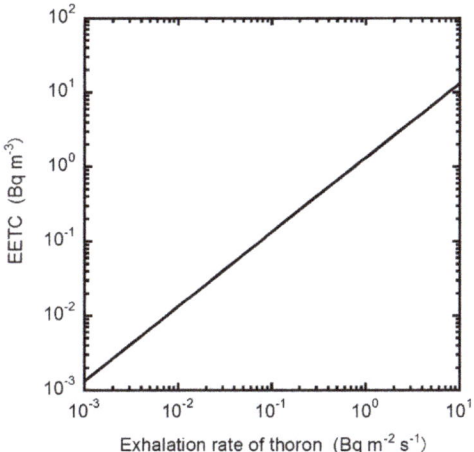

Figure 4. The relationship between Equilibrium Equivalent Thoron Concentration (EETC) and exhalation rate of thoron.

3. Measurement Techniques

3.1. Spot Measurement

3.1.1. Thoron

As the half-life of thoron is shorter than 1 min, thoron gas measurement needs to start immediately after sampling. In this section, the measurement method using one scintillation cell is briefly introduced. Tokonami et al. [15] developed a discriminative measurement technique for radon and thoron concentrations with time-sequential counting. Prior to the measurement, alpha counting efficiencies for radon, ^{218}Po, ^{214}Po, thoron and ^{216}Po were estimated by a Monte Carlo Calculation after taking their range into account based on their emitted energies as well as the size of the cell. In their study, Pylon scintillation cells of 300A and 110A were used. Their inner volumes are 270 [mL] and 151 [mL], respectively. As this technique can be completed within 15 min, contribution from any other alpha emitters of the remaining thoron progeny, such as ^{212}Bi and ^{212}Po, can be ignored for the determination of thoron concentration. In order to validate justification of the alpha counting efficiencies by the Monte Carlo simulation, the conversion factor theoretically drawn was compared with that experimentally given by the manufacturer. The large cell conversion factor (300A) provided by the manufacturer is the value at radioactive equilibrium, which is given as 27.9 [Bq m^{-3} cpm^{-1}]. After radon gas is drawn into the cell, it takes 3.5 h to reach the equilibrium between radon and its progeny. With the latest nuclear data, the theoretical conversion factor is eventually estimated to be 28.3 [Bq m^{-3} cpm^{-1}], where there is only a small difference between the two approaches. Zhang et al.

made a similar approach in the conversion factor of the same scintillation cell [16]. The alpha counting efficiencies for thoron and its progeny are close to those given by Tokonami et al. [17]. As the theoretical approach has been justified, it can be also applicable to the determination of thoron concentration with the alpha counting efficiencies of thoron and ^{216}Po. Furthermore, it can be regarded that ^{216}Po atoms behave like a gas in the cell and that thoron and ^{216}Po are at equilibrium because its half-life is very short. The thoron concentration (C_{Tn} [Bq m^{-3}]) is given by the Equation (7):

$$C_{Tn} = \frac{N_{Tn}}{V_c \times (\eta_{Tn} + \eta_{ThA}) \int_{t_0}^{t_0+t_m} e^{-\lambda_{Tn} t} dt} \quad (7)$$

where N_{Tn} is counts during the period; V_c is inner volume of the cell [m^{-3}]; η_{Tn} is counting efficiency of thoron; η_{ThA} is counting efficiency of ^{216}Po; t_0 is beginning of the measurement [s]; and t_m is measurement period [s]. If radon is present together with thoron, however, counts derived from radon and its progeny need to be subtracted from N_{Tn}. In order to obtain net counts derived from thoron and its progeny, another measurement is therefore necessary after thoron and ^{216}Po completely decay. N_{Tn} can be expressed as the Equation (8):

$$N_{Tn} = N_1 - k N_2 \quad (8)$$

where N_1 is counts during the first period; N_2 is counts during the second period. The constant k depends on the existing ratio of radon and its progeny in the cell and the measurement timetable. In the previous study, an optimal timetable with a 15 min time interval was discussed. The following timetable was proposed: twenty seconds after sampling, the first measurement is made over 100 s. Ten minutes after sampling, a 5 min counting, as the second measurement, is made.

3.1.2. Thoron Progeny

The measurement technique for thoron progeny is similar to that for radon progeny. In general, an alpha counting method is preferable. As ^{212}Pb and ^{212}Bi concentrations are assigned to the subject of dose assessment in thoron progeny measurement, the counting method is simpler than that for radon progeny. Two time-sequential counts are necessary to measure two kinds of thoron progeny concentration in both gross alpha counting and alpha spectroscopic methods. As the half-life of ^{212}Pb is as long as 10 h, however, it takes a significant amount of time to measure thoron progeny concentrations precisely. In the gross counting method, a ZnS(Ag) (silver-activated zinc sulfide) scintillation counting system is commonly used. As this technique has no alpha energy discrimination, however, it will be impossible to complete the determination of thoron progeny concentration in a natural environment because radon will also be present together with thoron. Therefore, the measurement timetable needs to be optimized so as to determine thoron progeny concentrations. Unless radon progeny concentrations are the subject of measurement, the measurement can begin after radon progeny completely decay (practically after 6 h). Note that accuracy of ^{212}Bi activity concentration will be diminished when considering the half-life of ^{212}Bi (60 min). In order to overcome such practical problems, the least-square method will be suitable. This can give any activity concentrations regardless of the number of unknown concentrations. In contrast, the alpha spectroscopic method can quickly terminate the measurement for both radon and thoron progeny, because the alpha particles emitted from them can be identified due to the high resolution of the alpha spectrum. Information on the highest alpha particle energy emitted from ^{212}Po is available via this technique without any interference from any other alpha emitters. When the dose assessment is referred, determination of ^{212}Pb will be emphasized because the contribution from ^{212}Bi is much smaller than that from ^{212}Pb as shown in the Equation (1). Tokonami et al. [17] developed a simple measurement technique for the equilibrium equivalent thoron concentration with a solid-state nuclear track detector. A poly allyl diglycol carbonate (PADC), commercially named CR-39, is used as the detecting material [17]. This passive technique is applicable to determine the radioactivity level anywhere without electricity supply. The following procedure, before chemical etching and track reading, can be introduced for the determination of thoron progeny:

1. Air samples are taken over several hours with a membrane filter (Millipore AA) or glass microfiber filter (Whatman GF/F) installed in an open-faced filter holder and a DC powered air pump;
2. The filter is left until radon progeny completely decay (more than 6 h);
3. An aluminum foil (4.0 mg cm^{-2}) as the energy absorber is directly placed on the filter so as to detect alpha energy emitted from thoron progeny, and then a CR-39 plate is attached for alpha track registration;
4. The time is recorded when the CR-39 plate is removed. This is the end of the measurement process.

3.2. Continuous Measurement

3.2.1. Thoron

There are two main ways to continuously identify thoron even though radon is present as well. Falk et al. [18] developed a delayed coincidence method. The method separates the fraction of alpha counts emitted from ^{216}Po from all the other alpha counts. This method is based on the short half-life of 150 ms of ^{216}Po. Bigu and Elliot [19] developed a continuous monitor based on their concept. Although similar monitors were also developed, a flow-through scintillation cell is used in any measurement system. Alternatively, alpha spectrometry is used. A RAD7 monitor, commercially available, is based on an electrostatic collection method (for instance, Takeuchi et al., 1999) [20]. In this monitor, air is drawn into the decay chamber through the drying column. As radon and thoron progeny are positively charged, they will be neutralized by vapor and subsequently will not be collected on the surface of the silicon semiconductor detector as the electrode unless air is dried. In addition, the half-life of ^{216}Po is so short that a large mobility will be required by high voltage to obtain a sufficient sensitivity to thoron. The voltage cannot be changed in the above monitor. Therefore, a sampling flow rate is one of the important parameters for thoron sensitivity due to its short half-life. Special attention must be paid to the flow rate when determining thoron concentrations with this monitor.

3.2.2. Thoron Progeny

There are several commercial products for continuous working level monitoring. Note that any signals derived from thoron progeny cannot be separated from those of radon progeny unless alpha spectroscopy is used. In principle, the alpha spectroscopic method can specify information regarding thoron progeny though it cannot determine the concentration. In a specific continuous monitor, the EETC can be simply determined using the count rate (*CPM*) and an experimentally obtained conversion factor (*CF*) as in the Equation (9):

$$\text{EETC} = \frac{CPM}{CF} \qquad (9)$$

As the conversion factor is obtained under the condition where the EETC is constant, however, the EETC does not always correspond to an actual variation. On the contrary, a special algorithm for potential alpha energy concentrations (PAEC) developed by Tokonami et al. [21] would be applicable in this case.

3.3. Time-Integrated Measurement

3.3.1. Thoron

Passive monitors are available for long-term measurement for both radon and thoron. This technique is commonly used in nation-wide or regional surveys. Solid state nuclear track detectors and electrets are installed in such a passive system. As they cannot separate radon and thoron signals, however, a dual measurement system needs to be chosen. This dual system is derived from the large difference of the half-life between two radioisotopes. For this purpose, the system accommodates two different diffusion chambers where detectors are installed and in each the entry rate of gas is well controlled by a gap or filter. In this section, two types of monitor are introduced.

Eappen and Mayya developed a twin cup radon-thoron dosimeter [22] (Figure 5). Three pieces of LR-115 Type II detector are fixed in the twin chamber radon dosimeter having three different mode holders. The exposure of the detector is termed as the cup mode whereas the one exposed as open is termed the bare mode. The right chamber is covered with a glass fiber filter and therefore both radon and thoron gases can easily enter the chamber. The left chamber is covered with a membrane filter so as to reduce the entry of thoron. Thus, there is less sensitivity for thoron in the left chamber than the right chamber. The third detector film exposed in the bare mode registers alpha tracks contributed by concentrations of radon, thoron and their progeny. Thereafter another type of passive monitor (Figure 6) was developed by Sahoo et al. [23]. A pin-hole based ^{222}Rn/^{220}Rn discriminator was installed in the monitor. For discriminative measurement of two radon isotopes, a pin-hole diffusion barrier was used [24,25]. This is because different entry rates of ^{222}Rn were pointed out through two entrances of the dosimeter which might arise from turbulence or air flow in one direction. The new device was designed to overcome the limitation of the conventional twin cup dosimeter. Currently this pin-hope monitor has been widely used in India.

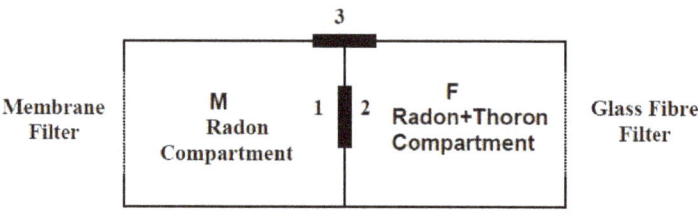

1. Radon cup mode SSNTD Film
2. Radon + Thoron Cup mode SSNTD Film
3. Bare mode SSNTD Film

Figure 5. A twin cup radon-thoron discriminative monitor [22].

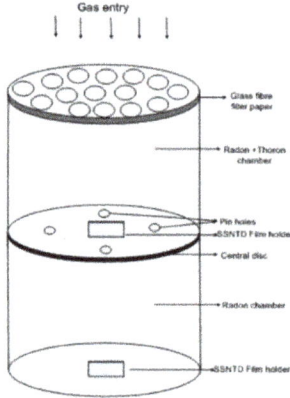

Figure 6. A pin-hole based radon-thoron measurement device [23].

Tokonami et al. [26] also developed a passive ^{222}Rn and ^{220}Rn discriminative monitor for a large-scale survey (Figure 7). The measurement principle is almost the same as the Indian monitor except for their bare mode. PADC, commercially CR-39, is used as the detecting material. This monitor and its prototype have been widely used in various countries [27–30]. The above two monitors can be calibrated in the calibration chamber at Hirosaki University Institute of Radiation Emergency Medicine, Japan [31]. For determination of radon and thoron activity concentrations with passive solid-state nuclear track detectors, ISO 16,641 [32] is currently available. The detection threshold, detection limit and confidence lower/upper limits in this technique are calculated based on ISO 11,929 [33]. A comparative performance test of Indian and Japanese-Hungarian monitors was carried out in the environment [34].

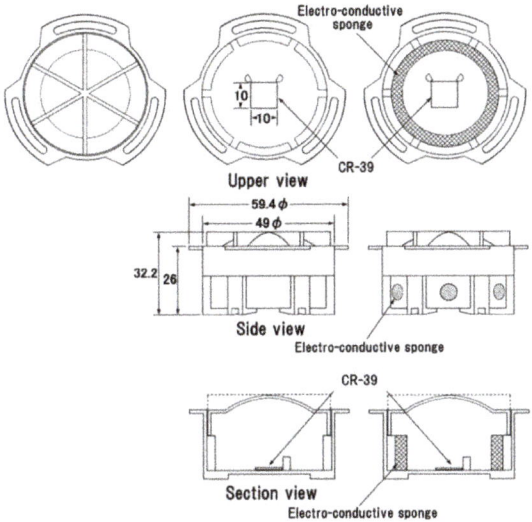

Figure 7. A passive type radon (^{222}Rn) and thoron (^{220}Rn) discriminative monitor [26].

3.3.2. Thoron Progeny

A prototype of the passive type thoron progeny monitor was developed by Zhuo and Iida based on diffusive deposition on the surface [35]. Among thoron progeny, ^{212}Po atoms emit alpha energy of 8.8 MeV, which is the highest alpha energy of all the natural radionuclides. It is, hence, obvious that it will be easy to detect this high energy by separating different energies emitted from other radionuclides if an alpha energy absorber with a proper thickness is prepared. Figure 8 shows an overview of a thoron progeny monitor. For radiation detection, CR-39, one of the solid-state nuclear track detectors, is mounted in the monitor. The body is made of stainless steel. As shown in Figure 8, four pieces are installed in the monitor and they are covered with an aluminized Mylar film and a polypropylene film in this order (thickness: 7.1 mg cm^{-2}; air-equivalent thickness: 71 mm). By adjusting the thickness properly, only alpha energy of 8.8 MeV can be detected. Figure 9 exemplifies the detecting principle of alpha energy emitted from ^{212}Po [36].

The monitor is hung on the wall for a certain period. In a usual survey, it is exposed for a few months. Radon and thoron progeny in indoor air deposit on the wall over the time period. After they are deposited, tracks of alpha particles are recorded in the CR-39. After retrieving the monitors, they are chemically etched to identify alpha tracks with a track reading system. The etching condition for CR-39 (Baryotrak; Nagase Landauer Ltd., Japan) is as follows: solution: 6.0 M NaOH; temperature: 60 °C; time: 24 h. Using a track reading system such as a microscope, track density is determined. The relationship between track density (D) and thoron progeny concentration, i.e., equilibrium equivalent thoron concentration, is expressed as the Equation (10):

$$\text{EETC} = \frac{D}{C \times T} \tag{10}$$

where D is track density (tracks mm^{-2}); C is conversion factor experimentally obtained (0.017 tracks mm^{-2} (Bq m^{-3} day)$^{-1}$ in our monitor); T is exposure period (day); and EETC: equilibrium equivalent thoron concentration (Bq m^{-3}).

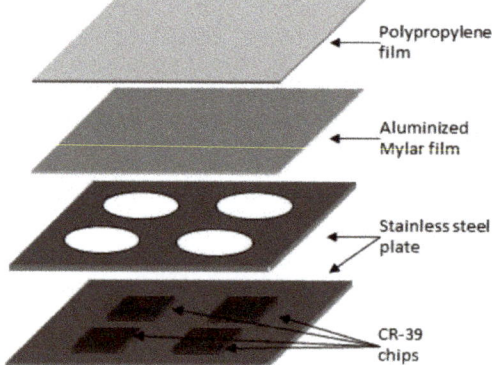

Figure 8. An overview of a thoron progeny monitor [11].

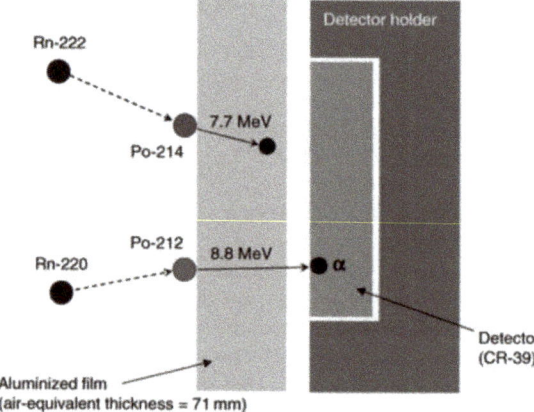

Figure 9. A detecting principle of alpha energy emitted from ^{212}Po [36].

The conversion factor was experimentally obtained by the comparison between the monitor and intermittent thoron progeny measurement. The experiment was carried out in actual dwellings. Using the proposed technique, the lowest detection limit of the EETC is estimated to be 0.005 Bq m^{-3} with 90-day exposure.

Similar techniques were found in Indian studies [37–43]. Instead of CR-39, LR-115 nuclear track detectors are used in their monitors. Not only thoron progeny sensors but also radon progeny sensors are installed by differentiating the thickness of energy absorbers. Furthermore, metal wire screens are introduced to detect fine and coarse progeny aerosols separately [44].

4. Dosimetry

When assessing the annual effective dose due to radon/thoron progeny inhalation, dose conversion factors are used. International bodies such as UNSCEAR and ICRP have their own values. The dose conversion factors (DCF) for radon are derived from both epidemiological evidence and dosimetric models, whereas the DCF for thoron is given only by the dosimetric model because there is no epidemiological evidence of lung cancer incidence due to thoron progeny inhalation. Table 2 summarizes effective dose conversion factors (mSv WLM^{-1}) (WLM: Working Level Month) for thoron. The DCF for thoron is about two–three times smaller than that for radon [1,45–51]. When rewriting the DCF, expressed in dose per unit equilibrium equivalent activity concentration of thoron/radon exposures, however, the DCF for thoron is more than two times larger than that for radon. According to the latest DCF for thoron and radon in ICRP Publ. 137 [51], they can be given as 107 nSv (Bq h m^{-3})$^{-1}$ and 16.8 nSv (Bq h m^{-3})$^{-1}$, respectively. On the contrary, UNSCEAR has recently decided to use the conventional values of 40 nSv (Bq h m^{-3})$^{-1}$ and 9 nSv (Bq h m^{-3})$^{-1}$, respectively, despite the inconsistency. This needs more consideration in order for them to correspond each other.

Table 2. Summary of effective dose conversion factors for thoron.

References	Effective Dose Conversion Factors (mSv WLM^{-1}) [1]
Marsh and Birchall [45,46]	3.8
UNSCEAR [1]	1.9
Porstendoerfer [47]	2.4
Ishikawa et al. [48]	5.4
Kendall and Phipps [49]	5.7
Hofmann et al. [50]	4.6
International Commission on Radiological Protection (ICRP) Publ. 137 [51]	5.6 (Indoor workplace) 4.8 (Mine)

[1] Working Level Month (WLM) is a historical unit of alpha potential energy exposure. 1 WLM = 3.45 mJ h m^{-3}.

5. Radioactivity and Resulting Dose

As mentioned above, thoron activity concentration is not uniformly distributed in the environment, which is far from the case for radon. It is considered that thoron concentration in air exponentially decreases with distance from the source. This behavior is derived from the very short half-life of thoron (55.6 s). The exponential change of thoron concentration is defined via the diffusion coefficient, strongly affected by the air turbulence condition.

Table 3 summarizes thoron and thoron progeny concentrations (EETC) in various countries. As can be seen from the presented data, their number is more restricted than that of radon [27,39,41,42,52–67].

In Cameroon, radon, thoron and its progeny concentrations were measured in residential areas in uranium and thorium bearing regions [52]. UNSCEAR presents the typical value of the equilibrium factor of thoron as 0.02 and this equilibrium factor of thoron is often used to estimate the annual effective dose due to thoron, in the same manner as in the case of radon. In the present study, the authors estimated a total annual effective dose derived from radon and thoron using actual measurement data on thoron progeny and compared it with that given by the UNSCEAR method. Consequently, the result based on the direct measurement was 1.5 times larger than the indirect one. They concluded that the direct measurement of thoron progeny is important for dose assessment.

The results of two surveys in Canada were tabulated. In one survey, long-term thoron and progeny measurements were simultaneously carried out for three months in two cities [53]. The simultaneous measurement of thoron and thoron progeny concentrations yielded a thoron equilibrium factor of 0.002 and therefore the authors concluded that the typical value given by UNSCEAR is reasonable for dose assessment. In contrast to a Cameroonian study, the Canadian study justified the consistency of the thoron equilibrium factor via the UNSCEAR method. In the other survey, results of simultaneous radon and thoron measurements were shown in 33 metropolitan areas [54]. The study demonstrates that thoron contributes around 3% of the effective dose due to indoor radon and thoron exposure in Canada.

Table 3. Thoron and thoron progeny concentration (EETC) in various countries.

Country		Thoron (Bq m^{-3})	EETC (Bq m^{-3})	Remarks	Reference
Cameroon	AM [1]	173 (13)	10.7 (0.9)		[52]
	GM [2]	118 (6)	7.4 (4.8)		
	Range	23–724	0.4–37.6		
Canada	AM [1]	114 (303)	1.23 (1.51)	Halifax and Fredericton	[53]
	GM [2]	51 (2.93)	0.75 (2.64)		
	Range	6–1977	0.11–7.45		
Canada (33 metropolitans)	AM [1]	9 (11)	-		[54]
	Range	ND–164	-		
China (Yangjiang)	AM [1]	1247 (1189)	7.8 (9.1)		[55]
	Median	859	4.2		
	Range	65–3957	0.6–36.2		
China (Gansu)	AM [1]	433 (210)	-		[56]
	GM [2]	347 (2.29)	-		
	Range	19–820	-		
China (Shanxi)	AM [1]	160	1.4		[57]
	GM [2]	130 (2.0)	1.2 (1.8)		
China (Shaanxi)	AM [1]	202	2.3		[57]
	GM [2]	181 (1.6)	2.1 (1.6)		
Hungary	GM [2]	341 (2.59)	-	Bauxite mine	[58]
	Range	40–2514	-		
India (Kerala)	GM [2]	41	1.81 (1.9)		[59]
	Range	11–212	0.36–8.00		
India (Odisha)	AM [1]	123 (105)	3.19 (2.75)		[27]
	GM [2]	95 (1.95)	2.37 (2.15)		
	Range	15–585	0.44–15.40		
Ireland	AM [1]	22	0.47		[60]
	Range	<1–174	<0.05–3.8		
Kenya	AM [1]	195 (36)	11.5 (2.1)		[61]
	Range	BDL–973	0.8–29.1		
Korea	AM [1]	40 (56)	0.89 (0.70)		[62]
	GM [2]	11 (2.9)	0.6 (0.41–0.78)		
	Max	731	-		
Macedonia	AM [1]	37 (36)	-		[63]
	GM [2]	28 (2.12)	-		
	Range	3–272	-		
Mexico	AM [1]	82 (75)			[64]
	GM [2]	55			
	Range	8–234			
Netherlands	AM [1]	-	0.64		[65]
	95-Percentile	-	1.37		
	Max	-	13.3		
Slovenia	AM [1]	87	-	Elementary School	[66]
	Range	21–368	-		
Srpska	AM [1]	63 (40)	0.52–0.34		[41]
	GM [2]	51 (2.07)	0.40 (2.20)		
	Range	7–198	0.09–1.16		
Kosovo	AM [1]	136	2.06		[39]
	GM [2]	90	1.90		
	Range	18–1313	0.87–4.38		
Serbia	AM [1]	116	1.1		[42]
	GM [2]	89	0.86		
	Range	10–412	0.1–3.4		
Indonesia	AM [1]	152 (indoor) 139 (outdoor)	13 (indoor) 15 (outdoor)	West Sulawesi (HNBR) Number of dwellings Indoor: 45 Outdoor: 18	[67]
	GM [2]	141 (indoor) 121 (outdoor)	13 (indoor) 15 (outdoor)		
	Range	20–618 (indoor) 23–457 (outdoor)	4–40 (indoor) 4–37 (outdoor)		

[1] AM: Arithmetic mean, [2] GM: Geometric mean.

The US National Cancer Institute and the China Ministry of Health conducted an epidemiological survey for residential radon and lung cancer in Gansu Province, China [68]. This study can be recognized as one of the main studies of residential radon by pooling the analyses of European [69,70], North American [71,72] and Chinese [73] residential case-control studies. They used alpha track detectors, but the monitors were proved to be influenced by thoron and overestimated radon concentrations [74]. Thereafter radon measurements were made with the above mentioned improved detectors, discriminating two radon isotopes [56]. Remarkably high thoron levels were observed in these areas. This finding suggests two key points, as follows: (1) their previous radon data and the lung cancer risk were incorrect; (2) the thoron contribution to radiation exposure will be important in those areas. Another Gansu survey was conducted with simultaneous measurements of radon, thoron and thoron progeny [75]. Correlation analyses were made among three activity concentrations. There was no correlation whenever any two concentrations were chosen. This means that these three concentrations are so independent that it is difficult to estimate one concentration from the other. If the thoron dose needs to be considered, direct measurement of thoron progeny is required. This further implies that thoron progeny concentration cannot be accurately obtained with a fixed thoron equilibrium factor.

Simultaneous measurements of radon, thoron and thoron progeny were made in other provinces close to Gansu province, namely Shanxi and Shaanxi provinces [57]. From the topographical and geological points of view, the same radiological features were obtained. Compared to thoron concentrations, thoron progeny concentrations were so low that it resulted in small thoron equilibrium factors (arithmetic mean = 0.01). Tokonami [36] evaluated the influence on the risk estimate of misleading radon data. Annual effective doses due to radon and thoron were estimated in the UNSCEAR manner. Comparison of the annual effective dose was made between misleading radon concentrations and modified, i.e., to achieve correct radon concentrations. Misleading radon concentrations resulted in an arithmetic mean of 6.4 mSv, whereas correct ones gave 1.7 mSv. When the contribution of thoron was included, the total dose was calculated to be 2.4 mSv. A series of these findings revealed that the Gansu study gave incorrect or misleading lung cancer risk estimates.

Yangjiang, Guangdong province, is famous for being one of the areas with the highest background radiation in the world. Kudo et al. [55] demonstrated how residents there are being exposed to natural radiation. As monazite sands are widely distributed in this area, high gamma dose rates are often observed. However, there is less information on internal exposure, particularly due to radon and thoron. Based on collected data on these activity concentrations using the UNSCEAR method, annual effective doses due to radon and thoron progenies were estimated to be 3.1 (SD = 2.0) mSv and 2.2 (SD = 2.5) mSv, respectively. This revealed that indoor thoron and its progeny levels were fairly high and even thoron exposures are not negligible compared to radon exposures.

Kovacs [58] summarized radon and thoron surveys in Hungary. Dwellings and workplaces were surveyed with passive radon-thoron discriminative monitors. The monitors were placed 15–30 cm from the wall. Table 2 gives examples of thoron concentrations observed in underground bauxite mines. It was concluded that the dose contribution from thoron progeny was not negligible considering all the data and consequently further surveys of thoron progeny would be required for accurate dose assessment.

Omori et al. [59] presented radon, thoron and progeny concentrations for dwellings in Kerala, India. Their study area was classified into high (3–5 mGy y^{-1}) and low (1 mGy y^{-1}) background radiation areas, respectively. In a six-month measurement, it was found that there was no major difference between the two areas. The geometric mean of the annual effective dose due to radon and thoron was estimated to be 0.10 and 0.44 mSv, respectively. The internal dose derived from thoron progeny is more significant than that from radon. However, the doses were quite small and the external dose can be regarded as the major contributor in Kerala.

Omori et al. [27] also conducted long-term measurements of indoor radon, thoron and thoron progeny concentrations in Odisha, India. They revealed that radon and thoron concentrations differ by one order of magnitude whereas thoron progeny concentrations were nearly constant throughout the whole year. Thoron and its progeny concentrations were higher than those in Kerala. Exposure to thoron is equal to or exceeds exposure to radon in internal doses. The internal dose from radon and thoron was comparable to the external dose.

In Ireland, indoor concentrations of radon, thoron and its progeny were measured in 205 dwellings during the period 2007–2009 [60]. Radon activity concentration ranged from 4 to 767 Bq m^{-3} with an arithmetic mean of 75 Bq m^{-3}. Based on these concentrations and the UNSCEAR approach, the corresponding estimated annual effective doses are 0.1 (min), 19.2 (max) and 1.9 (mean) mSv. On the other hand, the estimated annual effective doses corresponding to thoron progeny concentrations are 2.9 (max) and 0.35 (mean) mSv with the dose conversion factor based on the two dosimetric models [39,40]. Although the dose from thoron tends to be negligible in most cases worldwide, it should be noted that in some dwellings in this study the annual dose from thoron progeny exceeded that from radon. This result is the first case where two annual effective doses from radon and thoron were measured on a nationwide scale in Europe.

Nyambura et al. [61] carried out indoor radon, thoron and thoron progeny surveys in several different types of houses in Kilimambogo, Kenya, and thereafter assessed the annual effective dose attributed to inhalation of their progeny. Housing structure was classified into three categories, i.e., mud, metal and stone-walled houses. The highest mean thoron and its progeny concentrations were observed in mud-walled houses with 195 and 11.5 Bq m^{-3}, respectively, whereas the highest radon concentration was found in stone-walled ones with 75 Bq m^{-3}. Assessing the annual effective dose, the highest was given by mud-walled houses with 0.9 (min), 8.5 (max) and 3.7 (mean) mSv, respectively.

Activity concentrations of thoron and its progeny were measured in 450 houses from 2002 to 2004 in Korea [62]. The annual arithmetic and geometric means of thoron concentration were 40.4 and 10.7 Bq m^{-3}, respectively. The annual arithmetic and geometric mean were 0.89 and 0.60 Bq m^{-3}, respectively. High thoron concentrations were observed in Korean-style houses built with mud block. The average annual effective dose due to inhalation exposure to thoron and its progeny was estimated to be 0.25 mSv.

Indoor thoron concentrations were measured in 300 houses for one year, from December 2008 to December 2009 in Macedonia. using passive radon-thoron discriminative monitors [63]. They were deployed at a distance of more than 50 cm from walls. The geometric means of indoor thoron concentration in winter, spring, summer and autumn were obtained as 39 (3.4), 32 (2.8), 18 (2.8) and 31 Bq m^{-3} (2.9), respectively. Seasonal variations of thoron appear to be smaller than those of radon.

Indoor thoron concentrations in 50 houses were measured in the Metropolitan Zone of Mexico City using a passive electret system [64]. The annual arithmetic and geometric means of indoor thoron concentration were estimated to be 82 and 55 Bq m^{-3}, respectively, ranging from 8 to 234 Bq m^{-3}. As to the seasonal variation, the lowest value was found in summer.

Thoron progeny concentrations, namely equilibrium equivalent thoron concentrations (EETCs), were measured in 2900 houses, Netherlands [65]. The arithmetic mean of EETC was 0.64 Bq m^{-3}. Thoron progeny concentrations show correlations with year of construction and smoking behavior. A pilot study was also conducted to determine the relationship between the exhalation of thoron and the concentration of thoron progeny in the room. The authors pointed out that thoron might be a more important contributor to the population dose in other regions with low radon levels.

A limited number of measurements were carried out about 1 m away from any wall and 1.5 m above the floor in various environments in Slovenia using passive radon-thoron discriminative monitors [66]. Thoron and radon concentrations in 35 elementary schools ranged from 21 to 368 and 40 to 4609 Bq m^{-3}, respectively. The authors pointed out that there was a weak correlation between the two activity concentrations though both of them followed a lognormal distribution.

Results of the first investigation on indoor radon, thoron and their progeny concentrations were given in 25 primary schools of Republic Srpska [41]. For their measurements, Japanese and Indian techniques were introduced in the survey. The monitors were deployed at 10 cm distance from the wall. A weak correlation was found between radon and thoron concentrations as well as thoron and thoron progeny concentrations.

Gulan et al. [39] carried out indoor radon, thoron and their progeny survey in scattered locations around Kosovo. Estimated arithmetic mean values of concentrations in 48 houses are 122 Bq m^{-3} for radon and 136 Bq m^{-3} for thoron. This might be attributed to building materials involving bricks, sand and stones from the local area where ^{232}Th concentration in soil is higher than that of ^{226}Ra.

Simultaneous long-term measurements of radon, thoron and their progeny were conducted in 40 rural houses in Serbia [42]. The EETC was found to be relatively higher than the worldwide average value. Significant positive correlation between thoron and EETC was found, whereas there was no significant correlation between radon and EERC.

Recently, a high natural background radiation area (HNBR) due to terrestrial radiation has been reported in West Sulawesi, Indonesia [76]. EETC was measured using the thoron progeny monitor shown in Figure 4 in a total of 45 dwellings [67]. The EETC ranged from 4 to 40 Bq m^{-3} and the annual effective dose due to thoron inhalation was reported to be 5.1–17.7 mSv.

Future authors should discuss these results and how they can be interpreted from the perspective of previous studies and working hypotheses. The findings and their implications should be discussed in the broadest context possible. Future research directions may also be highlighted.

6. Conclusions

As thoron is a very short half-lived radionuclide, though it is an isotope of radon, it is not easy to measure its activity in air and consequently to assess the resulting dose in the same manner as for radon. Nationwide indoor radon surveys have been conducted in many countries. The annual effective dose for the public is calculated using the indoor radon concentration and an equilibrium factor for radon. The equilibrium factor of radon is typically 0.4 but such an approach is not applicable or meaningful in the case of thoron. The spatial distribution of thoron is so unique that a single value of thoron concentration cannot be given even in a room, due to the short half-life of less than 1 min. Thus, thoron concentrations should not be used for radiation protection purposes because the thoron concentration varies widely with space. Therefore, a direct measurement of thoron progeny concentration will be more effective and useful whereas several assumptions are required in the measurement techniques presented in this paper. As another approach, the surface exhalation rate of thoron may be an index for thoron dose assessment. Although thoron was underestimated in the past, recent findings have revealed that reassessment of risks due to radon exposure may need to take the presence of thoron into account.

Funding: This research was funded by JSPS KAKENHI, grant number JP18KK0261 and JP20H00556.

Conflicts of Interest: The authors declare no conflict of interest.

References

1. United Nations Scientific Committee on the Effects of Atomic Radiation. Volume I: Annex B Exposures from natural radiation sources. In *UNSCEAR 2000 Report, Sources and Effects of Ionizing Radiation*; UNSCEAR: New York, NY, USA, 2000.
2. United Nations Scientific Committee on the Effects of Atomic Radiation. Volume I: Annex B Exposures of the Public and Workers from Various Sources of Radiation. In *UNSCEAR 2008 Report, Sources and Effects of Ionizing Radiation*; UNSCEAR: New York, NY, USA, 2010.
3. World Health Organization. *WHO Handbook on Indoor Radon: A Public Health Perspective*; WHO: Geneva, Switzerland, 2009.
4. International Commission on Radiological Protection. Lung Cancer Risk from radon and Progeny and Statement on Radon. In *Annals of the ICRP*; International Commission on Radiological Protection: New York, NY, USA, 2010.

5. International Commission on Radiological Protection. Radiological Protection against Radon Exposure. In *Annals of the ICRP*; International Commission on Radiological Protection: New York, NY, USA, 2014.
6. International Atomic Energy Agency. *Radiation Protection and Safety of Radiation Sources: International Basic Safety Standards. General Safety Requirements Part 3*; IAEA: Vienna, Austria, 2014.
7. International Atomic Energy Agency. *Protection of the Public against Exposure Indoors due to Radon and Other Natural Sources of Radiation: IAEA Safety Standards for Protecting People and the Environment*; IAEA: Vienna, Austria, 2015.
8. International Commission on Radiological Protection. Protection Against Radon-222 at Home and at Work. In *Annals of the ICRP*; International Commission on Radiological Protection: New York, NY, USA, 1993.
9. Bureau International des Poids et Mesures, Monographie BIPM-5—Table of Radionuclides, Volume 4. Available online: https://www.bipm.org/utils/common/pdf/monographieRI/Monographie_BIPM-5_Tables_Vol4.pdf (accessed on 4 September 2020).
10. Katase, A.; Matsumoto, Y.; Sakae, T.; Ishibashi, K. Indoor concentrations of ^{220}Rn and its decay products. *Health Phys.* **1988**, *54*, 283–286. [CrossRef] [PubMed]
11. Hosoda, M.; Kudo, H.; Iwaoka, K.; Yamada, R.; Suzukia, T.; Tamakuma, Y.; Tokonami, S. Characteristic of thoron (^{220}Rn) in environment. *Appl. Radiat. Isot.* **2017**, *120*, 7–10. [CrossRef] [PubMed]
12. Zhuo, W.; Tokonami, S. *Convenient Methods for Evaluation of Indoor Thoron Progeny Concentrations. High Levels of Natural Radiation and Radon Areas: Radiation Dose and Health Effects*; International Congress Series 1276; Elsevier: Amsterdam, The Netherlands, 2005; pp. 219–220.
13. Stevanovic, N.; Markovic, V.M.; Nikezic, D. Deposition rates of unattached and attached radon progeny in room with turbulent airflow and ventilation. *J. Environ. Radioact.* **2009**, *100*, 585–589. [CrossRef] [PubMed]
14. De With, G.; Smetsers, R.C.G.M.; Slaper, H.; de Jong, P. Thoron exposure in Dutch dwellings—An overview. *J. Environ. Radioact.* **2018**, *183*, 73–81. [CrossRef]
15. Tokonami, S.; Yang, M.; Yonehara, H.; Yamada, Y. Simple, discriminative measurement technique for radon and thoron concentrations with a single scintillation cell. *Rev. Sci. Instrum.* **2002**, *73*, 69–72. [CrossRef]
16. Zhang, L.; Zhuo, W.; Guo, Q.; Guo, L.; Shang, B. Measurement of thoron gas in the environment using a Lucas scintillation cell. *J. Radiol. Prot.* **2010**, *30*, 597–606. [CrossRef]
17. Tokonami, S.; Sun, Q.; Yonehara, H.; Yamada, Y. A simple measurement technique of the equilibrium equivalent thoron concentration with a CR-39 detector. *Jpn. J. Health Phys.* **2002**, *37*, 59–63. [CrossRef]
18. Falk, R.; More, H.; Nyblom, L. Measurements of ^{220}Rn in air using a flow-through Lucas cell and multiple time analysis of recorded pulse events. *Radiat. Prot. Dosim.* **1992**, *45*, 111–113. [CrossRef]
19. Bigu, J.; Elliot, J. An instrument for continuous measurement of ^{220}Rn (and ^{222}Rn) using delayed coincidences between ^{220}Rn and ^{216}Po. *Nucl. Instrum. Methods Phys. Res. A* **1994**, *344*, 415–425. [CrossRef]
20. Takeuchi, Y.; Okumura, K.; Kajita, T.; Tasaka, S.; Hori, H.; Nemoto, M.; Okazawa, H. Development of high sensitivity radon detectors. *Nucl. Instrum. Methods Phys. Res. A* **1999**, *421*, 334–341. [CrossRef]
21. Tokonami, S.; Ichiji, T.; Iimoto, T.; Kurosawa, R. Calculation procedure of potential alpha energy concentration with continuous air sampling. *Health Phys.* **1996**, *71*, 937–943. [CrossRef] [PubMed]
22. Eappen, K.P.; Mayya, Y.S. Calibration factors for LR-115 (type-II) based radon thoron discriminating dosimeter. *Radiat. Meas.* **2004**, *38*, 5–17. [CrossRef]
23. Sahoo, B.K.; Sapra, B.K.; Kanse, S.D.; Gaware, J.J.; Mayya, Y.S. A new pin-hole discriminated ^{222}Rn/^{220}Rn passive measurement device with single entry face. *Radiat. Meas.* **2013**, *58*, 52–60. [CrossRef]
24. Doi, M.; Kobayashi, S. The passive radon-thoron discriminative dosimeter for practical use. *Jpn. J. Health Phys.* **1994**, *29*, 155–166. [CrossRef]
25. Sciocchetti, G.; Sciocchetti, A.; Giovannoli, P.; DeFelice, P.; Cardellini, F.; Cotellessa, G.; Pagliari, M. A new passive radon-thoron discriminative measurement system. *Radiat. Prot. Dosim.* **2010**, *141*, 462–467. [CrossRef]
26. Tokonami, S.; Takahashi, H.; Kobayashi, Y.; Zhuo, W. Up-to-date radon and thoron discriminative detector for a large-scale survey. *Rev. Sci. Instrum.* **2005**, *76*, 113505. [CrossRef]
27. Omori, Y.; Prasad, G.; Sorimachi, A.; Sahoo, S.K.; Ishikawa, T.; Sagar, D.V.; Ramola, R.C.; Tokonami, S. Long-term measurements of residential radon, thoron, and thoron progeny concentrations around the Chhatrapur placer deposit, a high background radiation area in Odisha, India. *J. Environ. Radioact.* **2016**, *162*, 371–378. [CrossRef]
28. Kleinschmidt, R.; Watson, D.; Janik, M.; Gillmore, G. The presence and dosimetry of radon and thoron in a historical, underground metalliferous mine. *J. Sustain. Min.* **2018**, *17*, 120–130. [CrossRef]

29. Autsavapromporn, N.; Klunklin, P.; Threeratana, C.; Tuntiwechapikul, W.; Hosoda, M.; Tokonami, S. Short telomere length as a biomarker risk of lung cancer development induced by high radon levels: A pilot study. *Int. J. Environ. Res. Public Health* **2018**, *15*, 2152. [CrossRef]
30. Adelikhah, M.; Shahrokhi, A.; Chalupnik, S.; Toth-Bordrogi, E.; Kovacs, T. High level of natural ionizing radiation at a thermal bath in Dehloran, Iran. *Heliyon* **2020**, *6*, e04297. [CrossRef]
31. Pornnumpa, C.; Oyama, Y.; Iwaoka, K.; Hosoda, M.; Tokonami, S. Development of radon and thoron exposure systems at Hirosaki University. *Radiat. Environ. Med.* **2018**, *7*, 13–20.
32. International Organization for Standardization. *Measurement of Radioactivity in the Environment—Air—Radon 220: Integrated Measurement Methods for the Determination of the Average Activity Concentration Using Passive Solid-State Nuclear Track Detectors ISO16641*; ISO: Geneva, Switzerland, 2014.
33. International Organization for Standardization. *Determination of the Characteristics Limits (Decision Threshold, Detection Limit and Limits of the Confidential Interval) for Measurements of Ionizing Radiation—Fundamentals and Application—Part 1: Elementary Applications ISO11929*; ISO: Geneva, Switzerland, 2019.
34. Ramola, R.C.; Prasad, M.; Rawat, M.; Dangwal, A.; Gusain, G.S.; Mishra, R.; Sahoo, S.K.; Tokonami, S. Comparative study of various techniques for environmental radon, thoron and progeny measurements. *Radiat. Prot. Dosim.* **2015**, *167*, 22–28. [CrossRef] [PubMed]
35. Zhuo, W.; Iida, T. Estimation of thoron progeny concentrations in dwellings with their deposition rate measurements. *Jpn. J. Health Phys.* **2000**, *35*, 365–370. [CrossRef]
36. Tokonami, S. Why is ^{220}Rn (thoron) measurement important? *Radiat. Prot. Dosim.* **2010**, *141*, 335–339. [CrossRef] [PubMed]
37. Mishra, R.; Mayya, Y.S. Study of a deposition-based direct thoron progeny sensor (DTPS) technique for estimating equilibrium equivalent thoron concentration (EETC) in indoor environment. *Radiat. Meas.* **2008**, *43*, 1408–1416. [CrossRef]
38. Mishra, R.; Mayya, Y.S.; Kushwaha, H.S. Measurement of ^{220}Rn/^{222}Rn progeny deposition velocities on surfaces and their comparison with theoretical models. *J. Aerosol Sci.* **2009**, *40*, 1–15. [CrossRef]
39. Gulan, L.; Milic, G.; Bossew, P.; Omori, Y.; Ishikawa, T.; Mishra, R.; Mayya, Y.S.; Stojanovska, Z.; Nikezic, D.; Vuckovic, B.; et al. Field experience on indoor radon, thoron, their progenies with solid-state detectors in a survey of Kosovo and Metohija (Balkan region). *Radiat. Prot. Dosim.* **2012**, *152*, 189–197. [CrossRef]
40. Stojanovska, Z.; Zunic, Z.S.; Bossew, P.; Bochicchio, F.; Carpentieri, C.; Venso, G.; Mishra, R.; Rout, R.P.; Sapra, B.K.; Burghele, B.D.; et al. Results from time integrated measurements of indoor radon, thoron and their decay product concentrations in schools in the Republic of Macedonia. *Radiat. Prot. Dosim.* **2014**, *162*, 152–156. [CrossRef]
41. Curguz, Z.; Stojanovska, Z.; Zunic, Z.S.; Kolaz, P.; Ishikawa, T.; Omori, Y.; Mishra, R.; Sapra, B.K.; Vaupotic, J.; Ujic, P.; et al. Lon-term measurements of radon, thoron and their airborne progeny in 25 schools in Republic of Srpska. *J. Environ. Radioact.* **2015**, *148*, 163–169. [CrossRef]
42. Zunic, Z.S.; Stojanovska, Z.; Veselinovic, N.; Mishra, R.; Yarmoshenko, V.; Sapra, B.K.; Ishikawa, T.; Omori, Y.; Curguz, Z.; Bossew, P.; et al. Indoor radon, thoron and their progeny concentrations in high thoron rural Serbia environments. *Radiat. Prot. Dosim.* **2017**, *177*, 36–39. [CrossRef]
43. Zunic, Z.S.; Mishra, R.; Celikovic, I.; Stojanovska, Z.; Yarmoshenko, I.V.; Malinovsky, G.; Milic, G.; Kovacs, T.; Sapra, B.K.; Kavasi, N.; et al. Effective doses estimated from the results of direct radon and thoron progeny sensors (DRPS/DTPS), exposed in selected regions of Balkans. *Radiat. Prot. Dosim.* **2019**, *185*, 387–390.
44. Mayya, Y.S.; Mishra, R.; Prajith, R.; Sapra, B.K.; Kushwaha, H.S. Wire-mesh capped deposition sensors: Novel passive tool for coarse fraction flux estimation of radon thoron progeny in indoor environments. *Sci. Total Environ.* **2010**, *409*, 378–383. [CrossRef] [PubMed]
45. Marsh, J.W.; Birchall, A. Letter to the editor—The thoron issue: Monitoring activities, measuring techniques and dose conversion factors. *Radiat. Prot. Dosim.* **1999**, *81*, 311–312. [CrossRef]
46. Marsh, J.W.; Birchall, A. Determination of lung-to-blood absorption rates for lead and bismuth which are appropriate for radon progeny. *Radiat. Prot. Dosim.* **1999**, *83*, 331–337. [CrossRef]
47. Porstendoefer, J. Physical parameters and dose factors of the radon and thoron decay products. *Radiat. Prot. Dosim.* **2001**, *94*, 365–373. [CrossRef] [PubMed]
48. Ishikawa, T.; Tokonami, S.; Nemeth, C. Calculation of dose conversion factors for thoron decay products. *J. Radiol. Prot.* **2007**, *27*, 447–456. [CrossRef] [PubMed]

49. Kendall, G.M.; Phipps, A.W. Effective and organ doses from thoron decay products at different ages. *J. Radiol. Prot.* **2007**, *27*, 427–435. [CrossRef]
50. Hofmann, W.; Winkler-Heil, R.; Truta, L.A.; Tschiersch, J. Application of a monte carlo lung dosimetry code to the inhalation of thoron progeny. *Radiat. Prot. Dosim.* **2014**, *160*, 96–99. [CrossRef]
51. International Commission on Radiological Protection. Occupational Intakes of Radionuclides: Part 3. In *Annals of the ICRP*; International Commission on Radiological Protection: New York, NY, USA, 2017.
52. Bineng, G.S.; Saïdou, S.T.; Hosoda, M.; Siaka, Y.F.; Issa, H.; Suzuki, T.; Kudo, H.; Bouba, O. The importance of direct progeny measurements for correct estimation of effective dose due to radon and thoron. *Front. Public Health* **2020**, *8*, 17. [CrossRef]
53. Chen, J.; Moir, D.; Sorimachi, A.; Janik, M.; Tokonami, S. Determination of thoron equilibrium factor from simultaneous long-term thoron and its progeny measurements. *Radiat. Prot. Dosim.* **2012**, *149*, 155–158. [CrossRef]
54. Chen, J.; Bergman, L.; Falcomer, R.; Whyte, J. Results of simultaneous radon and thoron measurements in 33 metropolitan areas of Canada. *Radiat. Prot. Dosim.* **2015**, *163*, 210–216. [CrossRef] [PubMed]
55. Kudo, H.; Tokonami, S.; Omori, Y.; Ishikawa, T.; Iwaoka, K.; Sahoo, S.K.; Akata, N.; Hosoda, M.; Pornnumpa, C.; Sun, Q.; et al. Comparative dosimetry for radon and thoron in high background radiation areas in China. *Radiat. Prot. Dosim.* **2015**, *167*, 155–159. [CrossRef] [PubMed]
56. Shang, B.; Tschiersch, J.; Cui, H.; Xia, Y. Radon survey in dwellings of Gansu, China: The influence of thoron and an attempt for correction. *Radiat. Environ. Biophys.* **2008**, *47*, 367–373. [CrossRef] [PubMed]
57. Tokonami, S.; Sun, Q.; Akiba, S.; Zhuo, W.; Furukawa, M.; Ishikawa, T.; Hou, C.; Zhang, S.; Narazaki, Y.; Ohji, B.; et al. Radon and Thoron Exposures for cave residents in Shanxi and Shaanxi Provinces. *Radiat. Res.* **2004**, *162*, 390–396. [CrossRef]
58. Kovacs, T. Thoron measurements in Hungary. *Radiat. Prot. Dosim.* **2010**, *141*, 328–334. [CrossRef]
59. Omori, Y.; Tokonami, S.; Sahoo, S.K.; Ishikawa, T.; Sorimachi, A.; Hosoda, M.; Kudo, H.; Pornnumpa, C.; Nair, R.R.K.; Jayalekshmi, P.A.; et al. Radiation dose due to radon and thoron progeny inhalation in high-level natural radiation areas of Kerala, India. *J. Radiol. Prot.* **2017**, *37*, 111–126. [CrossRef]
60. Mc Laughlin, J.P.; Murray, M.; Currivan, L.; Pollard, D.; Smith, V.; Tokonami, S.; Sorimachi, A.; Janik, M. Thoron and its airborne progeny in Irish dwellings. In Proceedings of the Third European IRPA Congress, Helsinki, Finland, 14–18 June 2010; pp. 2607–2612.
61. Nyambura, C.; Tokonami, S.; Hashim, N.O.; Chege, M.W.; Suzuki, T.; Hosoda, M. Annual effective dose assessment due to radon and thoron progenies in dwellings of Kilimanbogo, Kenya. *Radiat. Prot. Dosim.* **2019**, *184*, 430–434. [CrossRef]
62. Kim, C.K.; Kim, Y.J.; Lee, H.Y.; Chang, B.U.; Tokonami, S. ^{220}Rn and its progeny in dwellings of Korea. *Radiat. Meas.* **2007**, *42*, 1409–1414. [CrossRef]
63. Stojanovska, Z.; Bossew, P.; Tokonami, S.; Zunic, Z.; Bochicchio, F.; Boev, B.; Ristova, M.; Januseski, J. National survey of indoor thoron concentration in FYR of Macedonia (continental Europe–Balkan region). *Radiat. Meas.* **2013**, *49*, 57–66. [CrossRef]
64. Martinez, T.; Navarrete, M.; Gonzalez, P.; Ramirez, A. Variation in indoor thoron levels in Mexico City dwellings. *Radiat. Prot. Dosim.* **2004**, *111*, 111–113. [CrossRef]
65. Smetsers, R.C.G.M.; Blaauboer, R.O.; Dekkers, F.; Slaper, H. Radon and thoron progeny in Dutch dwellings. *Radiat. Prot. Dosim.* **2018**, *181*, 11–14. [CrossRef] [PubMed]
66. Vaupotic, J.; Kavasi, N. Preliminary study of thoron and radon levels in various indoor environments in Slovenia. *Radiat. Prot. Dosim.* **2010**, *141*, 383–385. [CrossRef] [PubMed]
67. Saputra, M.A.; Nugraha, E.D.; Purwanti, T.; Arifianto, R.; Laksmana, R.I.; Hutabarat, R.P.; Hosoda, M.; Tokonami, S. Exposures from radon, thoron, and thoron progeny in high background radiation area in Takandeang, Mamuju, Indonesia. *Nukleonika* **2020**, *65*, 89–94. [CrossRef]
68. Wang, Z.; Lubin, J.; Wang, L.; Zhang, S.; Boice, J.; Cui, H.; Zhang, S.; Conrath, S.; Xia, Y.; Shang, B.; et al. Residential radon and lung cancer risk in a high-exposure area of Gansu Province, China. *Am. J. Epidemiol.* **2002**, *155*, 554–564. [CrossRef]
69. Darby, S.; Hill, D.; Auvinen, A.; Barros-Dios, J.M.; Baysson, H.; Bochicchio, F.; Deo, H.; Falk, R.; Forastiere, F.; Hakama, M.; et al. Radon in homes and risk of lung cancer: Collaborative analysis of individual data from 13 European case-control studies. *Br. Med. J.* **2005**, *330*, 223. [CrossRef]

70. Darby, S.; Hill, D.; Deo, H.; Auvinen, A.; Barros-Dios, J.M.; Baysson, H.; Bochicchio, F.; Falk, R.; Farchi, S.; Figueuras, A.; et al. Residential radon and lung cancer—detailed results of a collaborative analysis of individual data on 7148 persons with lung cancer and 14208 persons without lung cancer from 13 epidemiologic studies in Europe. *Scand. J. Work Environ. Health* **2006**, *32*, 1–84.
71. Krewski, D.; Lubin, J.H.; Zielinski, J.M.; Alavanja, M.; Catalan, V.S.; Field, R.W.; Klotz, J.B.; Letourneau, E.G.; Lynch, C.F.; Lyon, J.I.; et al. Residential radon and risk of lung cancer: A combined analysis of 7 North American case-control studies. *Epidemiology* **2005**, *16*, 137–145. [CrossRef]
72. Krewski, D.; Lubin, J.H.; Zielinski, J.M.; Alavanja, M.; Catalan, V.S.; Field, R.W.; Klotz, J.B.; Letourneau, E.G.; Lynch, C.F.; Lyon, J.I.; et al. A combined analysis of North American case-control studies of residential radon and lung cancer. *J. Toxicol. Environ. Health A* **2006**, *69*, 533–598. [CrossRef]
73. Lubin, J.H.; Wang, Z.Y.; Boice, J.D., Jr.; Xu, Z.Y.; Blot, W.J.; Wang, L.D.; Kleinerman, R.A. Risk of lung cancer and residential radon in China: Pooled results of two studies. *Int. J. Cancer* **2004**, *109*, 132–137. [CrossRef]
74. Tokonami, S.; Yang, M.; Sanada, T. Contribution from thoron on the response of passive radon detectors. *Health Phys.* **2001**, *80*, 612–615. [CrossRef]
75. Yamada, Y.; Sun, Q.; Tokonami, S.; Akiba, S.; Zhuo, W.; Hou, C.; Zhang, S.; Ishikawa, T.; Furukawa, M.; Fukutsu, K.; et al. Radon-thoron discriminative measurements in Gansu Province, China, and their implication for dose estimates. *J. Toxic. Environ. Health* **2006**, *69*, 723–734. [CrossRef] [PubMed]
76. Syaeful, H.; Sukadana, I.G.; Sumaryato, A. Radiometric mapping for naturally occurring radioactive materials (NORM) assessment in Mamuju, West Sulawesi. *Atom Indones.* **2014**, *40*, 33–39. [CrossRef]

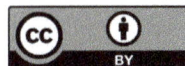

© 2020 by the author. Licensee MDPI, Basel, Switzerland. This article is an open access article distributed under the terms and conditions of the Creative Commons Attribution (CC BY) license (http://creativecommons.org/licenses/by/4.0/).

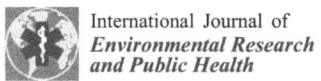

Article

Transition of Radioactive Cesium Deposition in Reproductive Organs of Free-Roaming Cats in Namie Town, Fukushima

Yohei Fujishima [1], Yasushi Kino [2], Takumi Ono [2], Valerie Swee Ting Goh [3], Akifumi Nakata [4], Kentaro Ariyoshi [5], Kosuke Kasai [3], Tadashi Toyoda [6], Toru Akama [7], Hirofumi Tazoe [8], Masatoshi Yamada [9], Mitsuaki A. Yoshida [10] and Tomisato Miura [11]

1. Department of Radiation Biology, Tohoku University School of Medicine, 2-1 Seiryo-machi, Aoba-ku, Sendai, Miyagi 980-8575, Japan; yohei.fujishima@med.tohoku.ac.jp
2. Department of Chemistry, Tohoku University Graduate School of Science, 6-3 Aramaki Aza-Aoba, Aoba-ku, Sendai, Miyagi 980-8578, Japan; yasushi.kino.e5@tohoku.ac.jp (Y.K.); takumi.ono.s4@dc.tohoku.ac.jp (T.O.)
3. Department of Bioscience and Laboratory Medicine, Hirosaki University Graduate School of Health Sciences, 66-1 Hon-cho, Hirosaki, Aomori 036-8564, Japan; h19gg801@hirosaki-u.ac.jp (V.S.T.G.); kokasai@hirosaki-u.ac.jp (K.K.)
4. Department of Pharmacy, Faculty of Pharmaceutical Science, Hokkaido University of Science, Sapporo, 7-Jo 15-4-1 Maeda, Teine, Sapporo, Hokkaido 006-8590, Japan; nakata_a@hus.ac.jp
5. Integrated Center for Science and Humanities, Fukushima Medical University, 1 Hikariga-oka, Fukushima 960-1295, Japan; ariyoshi@fmu.ac.jp
6. Toyoda Animal Hospital, 402-7 Kanairo, Nihonmatsu, Fukushima 964-0915, Japan; tadashit@violin.ocn.ne.jp
7. Akama Industry Co., Ltd., 259-3 Babauchi, Kakura, Namie, Fukushima 979-1536, Japan; kra9791536@yahoo.co.jp
8. Department of International Cooperation and Collaborative Research, Institute of Radiation Emergency Medicine, Hirosaki University, 66-1 Hon-cho, Hirosaki 036-8564, Japan; tazoe@hirosaki-u.ac.jp
9. Central Laboratory, Marine Ecology Research Institute, 300 Iwawada, Onjuku, Isumi, Chiba 299-5105, Japan; m-yamada@kaiseiken.or.jp
10. Institute of Chromosome Life Science, 11-5-409, Fukuokachuo 2-Chome, Fujimino-shi, Saitama 356-0031, Japan; mtak_yoshidad1955@axel.ocn.ne.jp
11. Department of Risk Analysis and Biodosimetry, Institute of Radiation Emergency Medicine, Hirosaki University, 66-1 Hon-cho, Hirosaki, Aomori 036-8564, Japan
* Correspondence: tomisato@hirosaki-u.ac.jp; Tel./Fax: +81-172-39-5966

Abstract: We investigated the internal contamination by radioactive cesium associated with the FDNPP accident, in the testes or uterus and ovaries of free-roaming cats (*Felis silvestris catus*), which were protected by volunteers in the Namie Town, Fukushima. A total of 253 samples (145 testes and 108 uterus and ovaries) obtained from adult cats and 15 fetuses from 3 pregnant female cats were measured. Free-roaming cats in Namie Town had a higher level of radioactive contamination in comparison to the control group in Tokyo, as the ^{134}Cs + ^{137}Cs activity concentration ranged from not detectable to 37,882 Bq kg^{-1} in adult cats. Furthermore, the radioactivity in the fetuses was almost comparable to those in their mother's uterus and ovaries. The radioactivity was also different between several cats protected in the same location, and there was no significant correlation with ambient dose-rates and activity concentrations in soil. Moreover, radioactive cesium levels in cats decreased with each year. Therefore, it is likely that decontamination work in Namie Town and its surroundings could affect radioactive cesium accumulation, and thus possibly reduce the internal radiation exposure of wildlife living in contaminated areas. It is hence necessary to continue radioactivity monitoring efforts for the residents living in Namie Town.

Keywords: Fukushima; free-roaming cat; radioactive cesium; reproductive organ; internal contamination

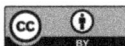

1. Introduction

After the accident in the TEPCO Fukushima Daiichi Nuclear Power Plant (FDNPP), the surrounding areas were contaminated by large amounts of released radionuclides [1,2]. A 20-km radius around the FDNPP was initially established as a restricted zone to avoid unnecessary radiation exposure to residents. As the evacuation order was issued with no advanced warning, all residents living within the 20-km radius had to evacuate immediately without packing and were not allowed to bring along their companion animals during evacuation. Emergency animal shelters were launched in Iino Town, Fukushima Prefecture in April 2011 and in Miharu Town, Fukushima Prefecture in October 2011, to rescue companion animals left behind at the time of evacuation. Large-scale trap and rescue operations for cats were also performed several times by the Ministry of Environment, local government, and local veterinary medical association. Despite multiple efforts to rescue abandoned companion animals, cats (*Felis silvestris catus*) in particular have been reproducing in the restricted zones and Namie Town [3]. Since September 2013, volunteers in Namie Town are managing abandoned (now free-roaming) cats from uncontrolled reproduction and possible disruption to the area's ecosystem, using the "Trap-Neuter-Vaccinate-Return (TNVR) [4]" program.

With regards to radiation, although the ambient dose-rates are gradually decreasing, prolonged effects of chronic low-dose exposure on animals are expected to be seen in the coming years. Therefore, by assessing biological effects from radioactive substances, we are able to understand any possible health effects caused by radiation. To date, several species of animals were evaluated (livestock bulls [5], wild boars [6–8], wild Japanese monkeys [9–11], wild rodents [12–14] and freshwater fish [15–17]) around the evacuation zone of the FDNPP. Furthermore, some studies [18] suggested that some negative biological effects seen in wild animals were likely caused by the release of radionuclides from the FDNPP accident.

Decontamination efforts gradually started from October 2013 to remove radioactive substances released by the FDNPP accident, such that the impact of environmental pollution and radiation exposure on human health and the surrounding environment could be reduced. For example, decontamination work in urban areas involves the removal of contaminated topsoil (0–5 cm) and replacing the surface with non-contaminated soil. As a result, evacuation orders in some parts of Namie Town were able to be lifted on 31 March 2017, due to low ambient dose-rates after decontamination. However, there are fewer reports focusing on the biological effects before and after decontamination work. Moreover, in existing research, the deposition of the radioactive substances in wild animals was not studied in urban areas. Although radioactive substances were heterogeneously distributed, detailed surveys of privately owned land would be difficult in urban areas when evacuated residents return in the future.

Radioactive substances released by the FDNPP accident includes radioisotopes of iodine (^{131}I, ^{132}I and ^{133}I), cesium (^{134}Cs, ^{136}Cs and ^{137}Cs), tellurium (^{132}Te), and inert gases (such as ^{133}Xe) [19,20]. These radionuclides can contribute to ambient dose-rates and be potential health risks immediately after the accident. Among these radionuclides, radioactive cesium has longer half-lives (^{134}Cs, $t_{1/2}$ = 2.06 years; ^{137}Cs, $t_{1/2}$ = 30.1 years), and are most likely the major contributors to radioactive contamination from 2013 to 2016. Hence, in this study, we monitored radioactive cesium (^{134}Cs and ^{137}Cs) derived from the FDNPP accident, in free-roaming cats caught in urban areas. We also measured the ambient dose-rates and soil cesium levels to verify the effectiveness of decontamination work and to evaluate how decontamination work changes the deposition of radioactive cesium in animals. In addition, we also evaluated feline leukemia virus (FeLV) and feline immunodeficiency virus (FIV) infections in free-roaming cats, as they are among the most common infectious diseases in domestic cats and are known to cause immunosuppression.

2. Materials and Methods

2.1. Animal Collection

Free-roaming cats in Namie Town were caught in humane live traps from September 2013 for TNVR [4]. Through surgical castration or ovariohysterectomy, reproductive organs, such as testes or uterus and ovaries, were extracted. In this study, we analyzed 253 samples (145 testes and 108 uterus and ovaries) from free-roaming cats rescued in October 2013 to December 2016 from 18 areas in Namie Town (Figure 1, Table 1). As a control, 10 samples (5 testes and 5 uterus and ovaries) from spayed and neutered free-roaming cats in Tama-area, Tokyo were also analyzed (Figure 1, Table 1). Samples were stored at −20 °C, until radioactivity measurements were performed.

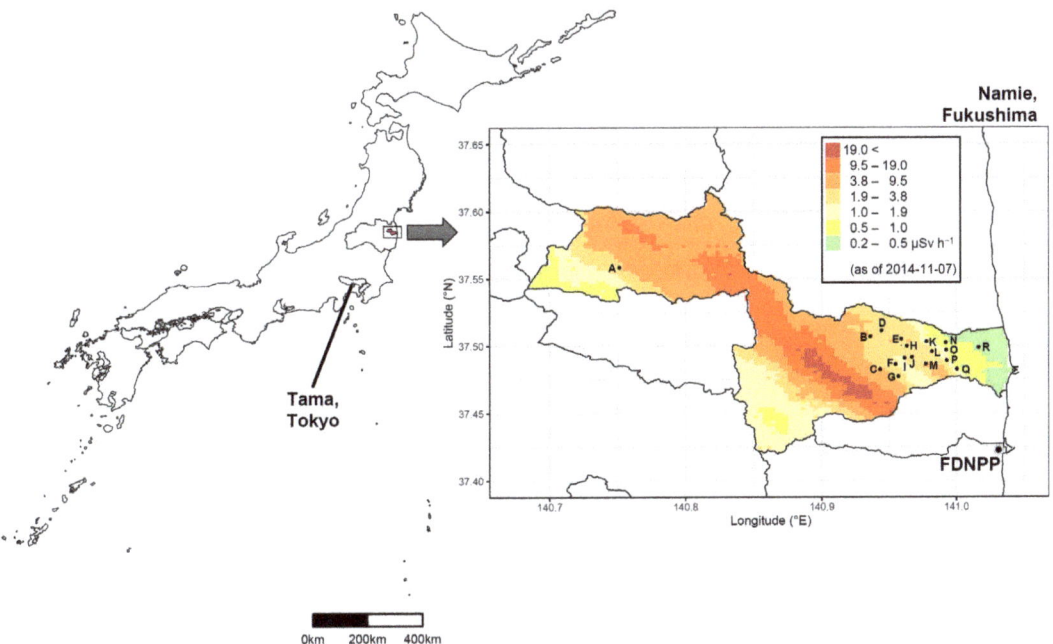

Figure 1. Sampling areas of free-roaming cats protected in Namie Town, Fukushima, and Tama area, Tokyo. The magnified map shows Namie Town and the sampling areas [(A) Tsushima, (B) Murohara, (C) Suenomori, (D) Tatsuno, (E) Karino, (F) Tajiri, (G) Obori, (H) Kakura, (I) Midorigaoka, (J) Uenohara, (K) Sakata, (L) Kawazoe, (M) Ushiwata, (N) Nishidai, (O) Gongendo, (P) Hiwatashi, (Q) Takase and (R) Kiyohashi], as well as the TEPCO Fukushima Daiichi Nuclear Power Plant (FDNPP). The maps were modified shapefiles from the National Land Numerical Information download service (data was retrieved from http://nlftp.mlit.go.jp/ksj/index.html on 5 February 2016). The heat map shows the ambient dose-rates on 7 November 2014 provided by the Nuclear Regulation Authority 9th airborne monitoring survey (data were retrieved from http://radioactivity.nsr.go.jp/ja/list/362/list-1.html on 5 February 2016).

Table 1. Locations and decontamination status of sampling areas.

Sampling Areas		GPS Location Longitude (°)	GPS Location Latitude (°)	Distance from F1-NPP (km)	Decontamination Status [†]
Namie, Fukushima	(A) Tsushima	37°33′30.8″ N	140°45′04.4″ E	29.1	Non-decontaminated
	(B) Murohara	37°30′24.4″ N	140°56′11.0″ E	12.6	Decontaminated
	(C) Suenomori	37°28′56.9″ N	140°56′37.0″ E	10.3	Non-decontaminated
	(D) Tatsuno	37°30′40.3″ N	140°56′40.6″ E	12.5	Non-decontaminated
	(E) Karino	37°30′18.1″ N	140°57′32.9″ E	11.2	Decontaminated
	(F) Tajiri	37°29′10.0″ N	140°57′18.0″ E	9.8	Decontaminated
	(G) Obori	37°28′38.0″ N	140°57′25.3″ E	9.0	Non-decontaminated
	(H) Kakura	37°29′59.4″ N	140°57′47.7″ E	10.5	Decontaminated
	(I) Midorigaoka	37°29′26.7″ N	140°57′41.5″ E	9.8	Decontaminated
	(J) Uenohara	37°29′29.0″ N	140°58′00.8″ E	9.6	Decontaminated
	(K) Sakata	37°30′10.5″ N	140°58′39.1″ E	10.1	Decontaminated
	(L) Kawazoe	37°29′44.1″ N	140°58′53.7″ E	9.3	Decontaminated
	(M) Ushiwata	37°29′11.3″ N	140°58′37.4″ E	8.6	Non-decontaminated
	(N) Nishidai	37°30′08.1″ N	140°59′31.3″ E	9.5	Decontaminated
	(O) Gongendo	37°29′48.2″ N	140°59′32.4″ E	8.9	Decontaminated
	(P) Hiwatashi	37°29′20.5″ N	140°59′34.0″ E	8.1	Decontaminated
	(Q) Takase	37°28′57.3″ N	141°00′01.8″ E	7.2	Decontaminated
	(R) Kiyohashi	37°29′54.9″ N	141°00′59.5″ E	8.5	Decontaminated
Tama area, Tokyo	Chofu Airport *	35°39′58.0″ N	139°31′54.0″ E	236.8	–

* The nearest monitoring post from the sampling point (data was retrieved from https://radioactivity.nsr.go.jp/map/ja/download.html on 15 March 2017). [†] This column represents the decontamination status of each sampling point as of 10–11 September 2016.

2.2. Tests for FeLV and FIV

To evaluate FeLV and FIV, blood from the cephalic antebrachial vein was used. Viral infections were detected with commercial immunochromatography kits of Checkman FeLV (Kyoritsu Seiyaku Corporation/Adtec, Tokyo, Japan) and Checkman FIV (Kyoritsu Seiyaku Corporation/Adtec, Tokyo, Japan).

2.3. Ambient Dose-Rate Measurements

Ambient dose-rates were measured at 4–5 points in a 20 m^2 area centered around the location, where the feline trap was installed on 30–31 July 2014, 22–23 July 2015, and 10–11 September 2016, using a NaI(Tl) scintillation survey meter (TCS-171B, Hitachi Aloka Medical, Ltd., Tokyo, Japan). The measurements were expressed as micro-grays per hour at 1 m above the ground with the time constant of the survey meter set to 10 s. Measurements were recorded after a minimum wait of 30 s for the readings to be stabilized. The ambient dose-rate in Tama area was referenced from the nearest monitoring post data provided by Nuclear Regulation Authority, Japan (data was retrieved from https://radioactivity.nsr.go.jp/map/ja/download.html on 15 March 2017).

2.4. Measurements of Activity Concentrations in Reproductive Organ and Soil Samples

For reproductive organs, samples were homogenized in separate plastic containers (U-8 container, SANPLATEC Co., Ltd., Osaka, Japan) after thawing. As for the soil samples, five surface soil samples of 5 cm depth were collected at each sampling point. The soil samples were completely dried at 120 °C, for 20 h before measurement. Each sample was transferred into separate U-8 plastic containers. The weight and height of the samples in the U-8 container was measured in order to calculate the sample density.

2.5. Gamma-Spectrometry

The activity concentration for the collected samples was determined by gamma-ray spectrometry, using a hyperpure germanium (HPGe) detector (ORTEC GEM-40190, SEIKO-EG&G Co., Ltd., Tokyo, Japan), as previously shown by Fukuda et al. [21]. ^{134}Cs and ^{137}Cs were detected using 604.6 and 795.8 keV gamma-ray energies, respectively, to satisfy measurement uncertainty from counting statistics to below 5% of the corresponding activity concentration. Activity was decay-corrected to the sampling date, and activity concentration was calculated as per kilogram of dry weight of the soil samples.

2.6. Statistics

Correlation analysis was carried out by calculating the Pearson's product-moment correlation coefficient or Spearman's rank correlation coefficient, based on Shapiro-Wilk normality tests. Wilcoxon rank sum test was applied to assess differences between two groups. The results were considered statistically significant if *p*-values below 0.05 were obtained. All statistical analyses were performed using the R version 4.0.3 (R Development Core Team, Austria) [22].

3. Results

3.1. Ambient Dose-Rates and Radioactive Cesium Activity Concentrations in Soil at Namie Town

Ambient dose-rates and radioactive cesium (^{134}Cs + ^{137}Cs) activity concentrations in soil of specimen collection sites were represented in Figure 2A (2014 vs. 2015), Figure 2B (2015 vs. 2016), Figure 2C (2014 vs. 2015), Figure 2D (2015 vs. 2016), respectively. In particular, decontamination work was performed only in 2015 and 2016. The ambient dose-rates in Namie Town in July 2015 decreased by approximately 39%, as compared to July 2014 (Figure 2A). Comparing July 2015 and September 2016, the ambient dose-rates decreased sharply in the decontaminated areas, with an average decrease of 62%. On the other hand, even in the areas where decontamination was not performed, the ambient dose-rates decreased moderately to an average of 38% (Figure 2B). A similar tendency was observed for ^{134}Cs + ^{137}Cs activity concentration in soil, but its distribution was extremely heterogeneous. ^{134}Cs + ^{137}Cs activity concentration in soil at July 2015 decreased by approximately 40%, as compared to July 2014 (Figure 2C). In the decontaminated areas, ^{134}Cs + ^{137}Cs activity concentration in soil significantly reduced by 90% in September 2016 as compared to July 2015. However, in areas where decontamination was not carried out, the average decrease was 44%, and if the points where low ^{134}Cs + ^{137}Cs activity concentration was omitted, the average rate of decrease was only 5% (Figure 2D). In addition, a strong correlation was observed between ambient dose-rate and ^{134}Cs + ^{137}Cs activity concentration in soil (2014: $r = 0.67$, $p < 0.01$; 2015: $r = 0.68$, $p < 0.01$; 2016: $r = 0.60$, $p < 0.01$).

3.2. Infection of FIV/FeLV

Immunochromatography tests for FIV and FeLV were performed on 211 cats. Fifteen cats (7.1%) were positive for FIV antigen and 16 cats (7.6%) were positive for FeLV antibody. Only 2 cats were positive for both FIV and FeLV antigens.

3.3. Radioactive Cesium Activity Concentration in Testes/Uterus and Ovaries

There was no macroscopic abnormality in the testes/uterus and ovaries. Gamma spectrometry was performed in uterus and ovaries (108 samples) and testes (145 samples) of free-roaming cats captured in both non-decontaminated and decontaminated areas in Namie Town. ^{134}Cs + ^{137}Cs activity concentration accumulated in each organ ranged from not detectable to the maximum of 37,882 Bq kg^{-1} (Figure 3A). Cats from Hiwatashi, Kiyohashi, Nishidai, Sakata, and Ushiwata areas showed low ^{134}Cs + ^{137}Cs activity concentrations of 1500 Bq kg^{-1} or less, while cats with high ^{134}Cs + ^{137}Cs activity concentrations were seen in Gongendo, Uehara, Kawazoe, Midorigaoka, and especially, in Tsushima areas (Figure 3B). Moreover, ^{134}Cs + ^{137}Cs activity concentrations differed greatly even in cats caught in the same collection area. As ^{134}Cs + ^{137}Cs activity concentrations were monitored in cats from October 2013 to December 2016, the half-life was approximated to 310 days (Figure 3). On the other hand, all 10 cats from Tama area of Tokyo, which served as the control area, showed radioactive cesium activity concentrations below the detection limit (16.6 Bq kg^{-1}, maximum 35.7 Bq kg^{-1}, minimum 10.6 Bq kg^{-1}), and were significantly lower than cats in Namie Town, Fukushima ($p < 0.01$).

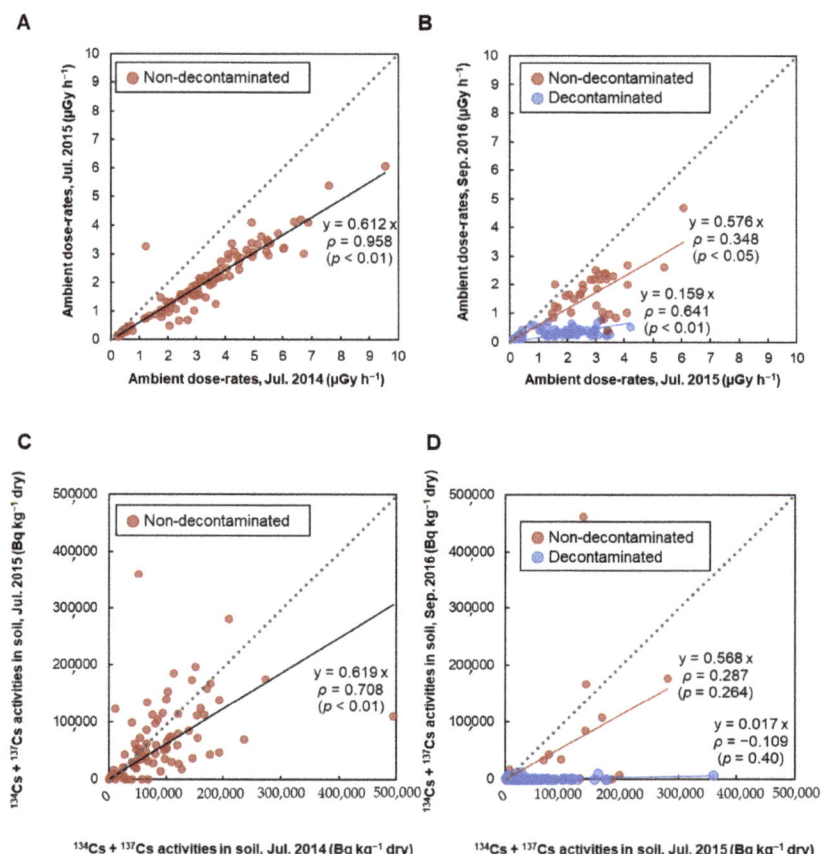

Figure 2. Ambient dose-rates and ^{134}Cs + ^{137}Cs activity concentrations in soil. Comparison of ambient dose-rates measured in (**A**) 2014 vs. 2015, (**B**) 2015 vs. 2016, and of ^{134}Cs + ^{137}Cs activity concentrations in soil measured in (**C**) 2014 vs. 2015, (**D**) 2015 vs. 2016. Red and blue circles represent areas that are non-decontaminated and decontaminated, respectively. Decontamination work in our research location in Namie Town started from September 2015.

There was also no clear correlation between the areas of where the cat was captured (ambient dose-rates and ^{134}Cs + ^{137}Cs activity concentration in soil) and ^{134}Cs + ^{137}Cs activity concentration in the reproductive organs of cats (Figure 4).

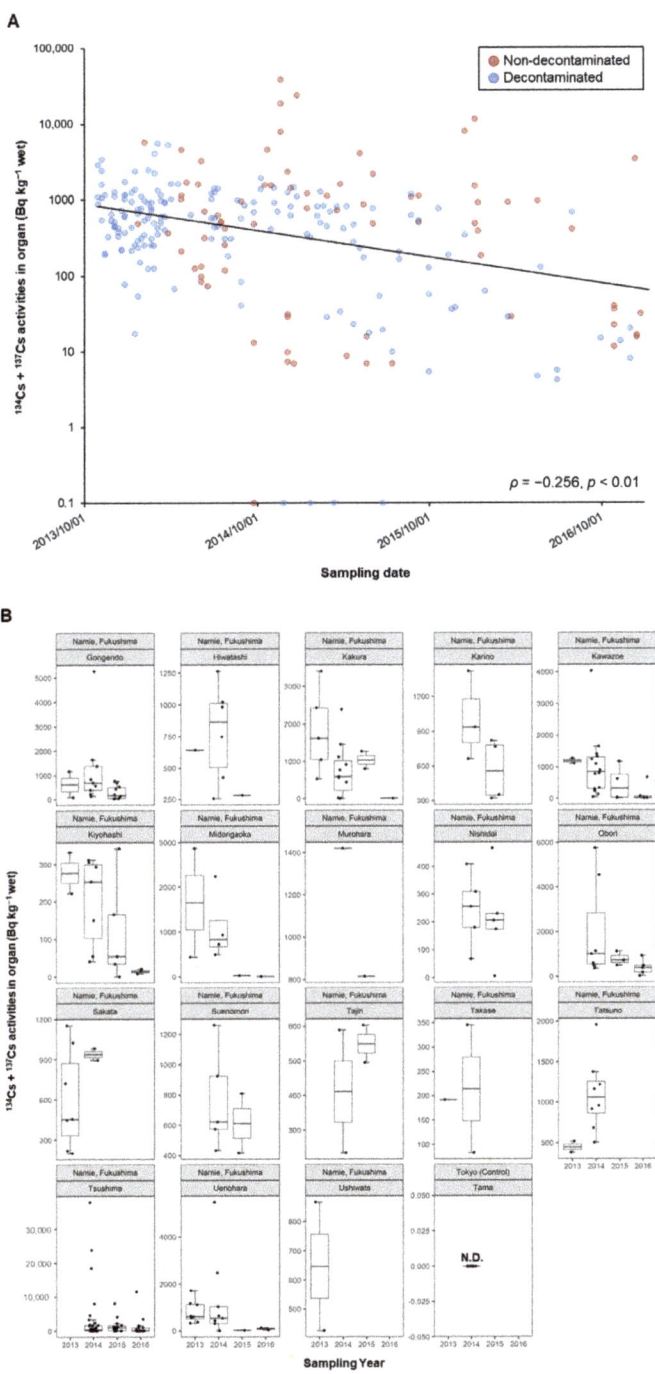

Figure 3. Change in ^{134}Cs + ^{137}Cs activity concentrations in reproductive organs of cats, with respect to (**A**) date caught and (**B**) area caught. In panel (**B**), each boxplot represents its distribution and black dots shows individual ^{134}Cs + ^{137}Cs activity concentrations in reproductive organs. N.D.; not detected.

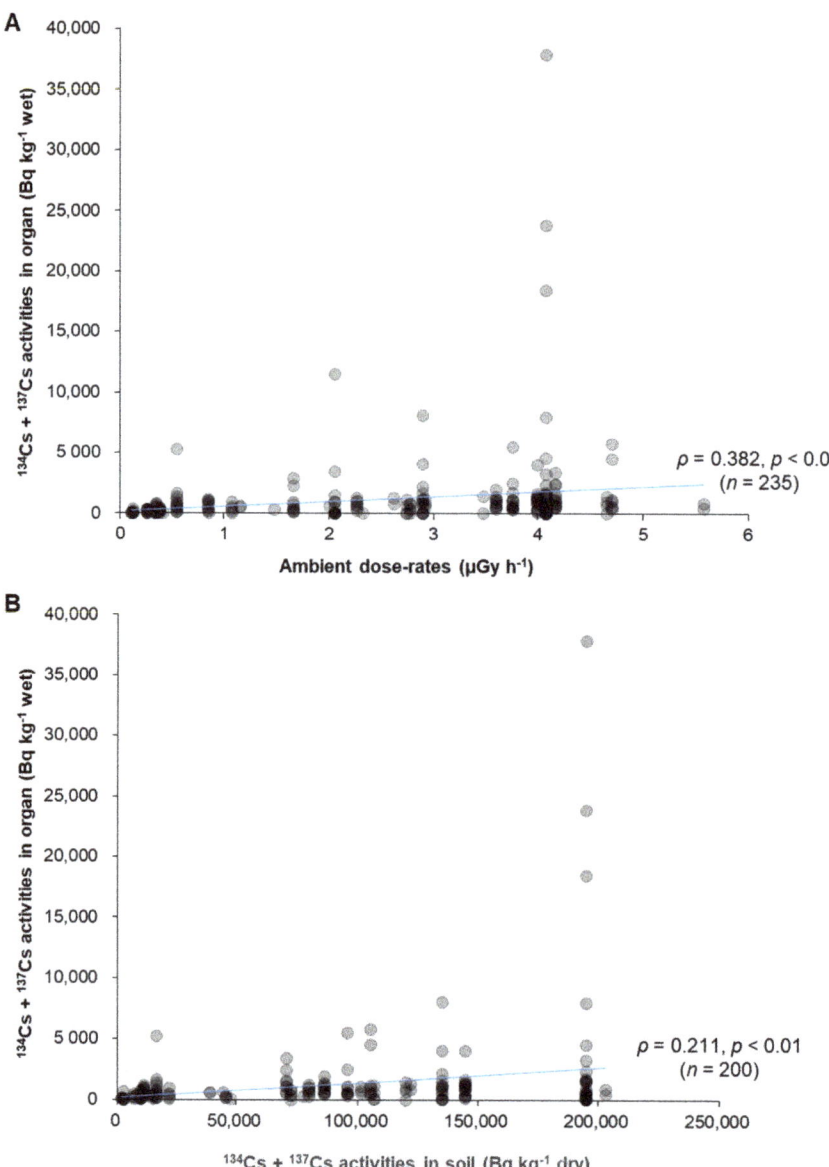

Figure 4. ^{134}Cs + ^{137}Cs activity concentrations in reproductive organs of cats compared with (**A**) ambient dose-rates and (**B**) ^{134}Cs + ^{137}Cs activity concentrations in soil. Grey dots represent individual ^{134}Cs + ^{137}Cs activity concentrations in reproductive organs.

When ^{134}Cs + ^{137}Cs activity concentration in testes and uterus and ovaries were compared, ^{134}Cs + ^{137}Cs activity concentration was higher in male than female cats ($p < 0.01$, Figure 5A). In addition, some age-dependency was observed as younger male cats tended to have a higher accumulation of radioactive cesium in their testes (Figure 5B).

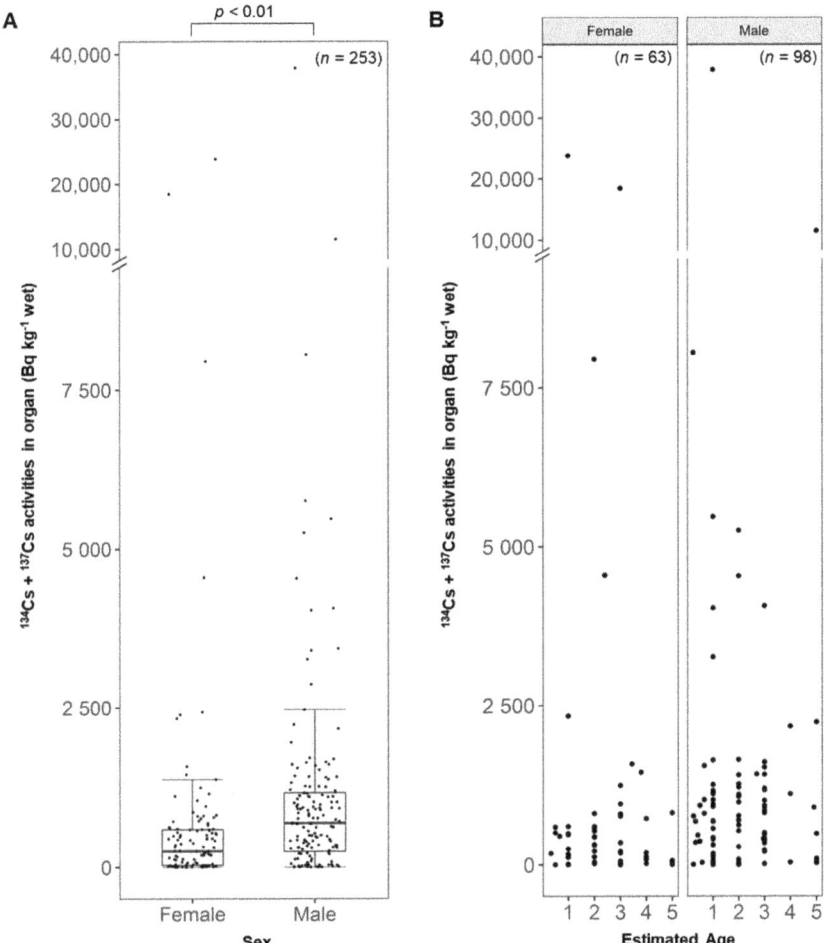

Figure 5. (**A**) An overall comparison and (**B**) a comparison with available estimated age of ^{134}Cs + ^{137}Cs activity concentrations in reproductive organs between male and female cats. Boxplot represents its distribution and black dots shows individual ^{134}Cs + ^{137}Cs activity concentrations in reproductive organs.

3.4. Radioactive Cesium Activity Concentrations Compared between Mother and Fetuses

In this study, we were also able to compare ^{134}Cs + ^{137}Cs activity concentrations in mother's uterus and fetus, as three female cats (caught in February 2014) were discovered to be pregnant while spaying. Only Case 3 (caught in Gongendo area) showed a significantly higher ^{134}Cs + ^{137}Cs activity concentration in the fetus than the maternal uterus. In the other two cases (caught in Kawazoe and Midorigaoka areas), there was no difference in ^{134}Cs + ^{137}Cs activity concentration between the fetus and maternal uterus (Figure 6). There was also no association seen between the areas of where the cats were caught (ambient dose-rate and ^{134}Cs + ^{137}Cs activity concentrations in the soil) and accumulated ^{134}Cs + ^{137}Cs activity concentrations in the fetus and maternal uterus.

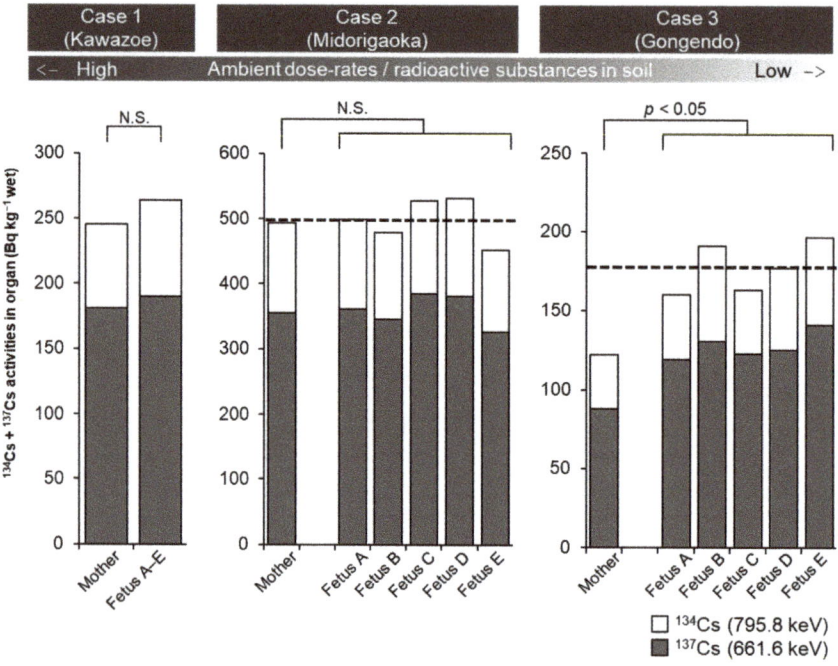

Figure 6. Comparison of ^{134}Cs + ^{137}Cs activity concentrations in the cat maternal uterus and fetuses. Dashed line in Case 2 and 3 represents mean activity concentrations of fetuses.

4. Discussion

Due to the sudden evacuation orders issued to Namie Town residents after the FDNPP accident, the evacuees had to leave their companion animals behind. Companion animals including cats left behind at the time of the evacuation were rescued and neutered by various organizations [3]. However, many free-roaming cats are still found in Namie Town and its surroundings. As evacuation orders are slowly lifting and more residents are returning, population control of free-roaming cats is thus necessary. As proper management of cat population control is required, a volunteer group in Namie Town is now continuing the initial efforts previously carried out by the local government, as recommended by the Ministry of the Environment's Guidelines [23].

No notable deformities such as malformations or growth retardations in reproductive organs of cats were seen with macroscopic observations. In addition, FeLV and FIV infections, which are common infectious diseases in domestic cats, were 7.1% and 7.6% respectively. In comparison to previous reports (FeLV: 0–8.1%; FIV: 0–12.8% [24–29]), FeLV and FIV infection rates in Namie Town were very similar to other non-contaminated areas. In Minamisoma City, dogs were reported to be aggressive and to bite humans. Their aggressiveness could be attributed to intermittent aftershocks and mental stress caused by owner abandonment as a result of immediate evacuation [30]. In contrast, cats rescued in Namie Town were not wary of us based on personal observations. Moreover, as the infection rates of FeLV and FIV were comparable to other general populations of domestic cats, the health of free-roaming cats was well controlled in Namie Town.

From our results, we showed that radioactive cesium activity concentrations in reproductive organs of cats was higher than that of the control area. With regards to the dynamics of radioactive cesium in the body, a model was proposed where radioactive cesium absorbed in the body through the digestive tract was transferred to visceral tissues via blood and finally excreted as urine [31]. Even though reproductive organs were only analyzed in this study, we could also expect radioactive cesium accumulation in other unanalyzed organs. According to a report in radioactive cesium distribution in cattle after the FDPP accident [5], activity concentrations were higher in skeletal muscle, kidney, and liver, as compared to blood, despite individual variations. In addition, as the testis showed the same activity concentration as the kidney and liver [5], it was thus highly likely that high radioactive cesium would be present in the skeletal muscle of free-roaming cats. Furthermore, the activity concentration of the feline testes was higher than that of the uterus and ovaries. Some studies also showed the same tendency in pigs and wild boars [32,33], but the underlying reason why ^{134}Cs + ^{137}Cs activity concentrations between males and females differed so markedly remains unclear. Furthermore, age effect was not observed on the cesium concentration in cats, although some young cats showed high radioactive cesium concentrations in both testes and uterus and ovaries. Wada et al. reported that the biological half-life of the ^{137}Cs in cats was 30.8 days [34]. In this study, the youngest cat analyzed was 3-months old (3 biological half-lives elapsed). Therefore, we speculated that a high amount of radioactive cesium in young cats was likely not dependent on mother–fetus transition.

A slight correlation was seen when ambient dose-rates was compared with ^{134}Cs + ^{137}Cs activity concentrations in reproductive organs, but no correlation was seen with ^{134}Cs + ^{137}Cs activity concentrations in the soil. The weak correlation could be due to (1) heterogeneous contamination by radioactive substances in different habitats, (2) wide home range and movement between habitats (including movement between decontaminated and non-decontaminated areas), and (3) uncontaminated cat food fed to rescued cats. According to previous reports, the home range of cats could range from several hundred meters to several kilometers [35–38], suggesting that extreme outliers of highly contaminated cats caught in some areas (e.g., Uenohara and Gogendo areas in 2014) could be due to cat movement. Furthermore, as decontamination work was carried out in each administrative district, radioactive cesium accumulation in the body could also be affected when a cat moves between non-decontaminated and decontaminated areas.

Moreover, the transfer of radionuclides from mother to fetus was one of the major concerns of exposure to internal radiation. As radioactive cesium was also detected in the fetus, this finding suggests that cesium was able to transfer freely from mother to fetus.

5. Conclusions

Since October 2013, we have been continuously monitoring radioactive cesium activity concentrations in reproductive organs of free-roaming cats in Namie Town. We showed that radioactive cesium levels decreased with each year. Therefore, it is likely that decontamination work in Namie Town and its surroundings could affect radioactive cesium accumulation, and thus possibly reduce the internal radiation exposure of wildlife living in contaminated areas. These findings suggest that analyzing radioactive substance deposition in animals and soil is useful to evaluate the effectiveness of decontamination work and to monitor the environment of urban areas.

Author Contributions: Y.F., T.T., and T.M. designed the study; T.A. and T.T. protected free-roaming cats; T.T. performed tests for FeLV and FIV; Y.F., V.S.T.G., A.N., K.A., K.K., and T.M. measured the ambient dose rate, and collected the soil samples; Y.F., Y.K., T.O., H.T., and M.Y. conducted the gamma spectrometry; Y.F., V.S.T.G., and T.M. processed the data; Y.F., V.S.T.G., M.A.Y., and T.M. wrote the manuscript; M.A.Y. and T.M supervised the study. All authors reviewed and approved the final manuscript.

Funding: This work was supported in part by the Environmental Radioactivity Research Network Center (F-19-31).

Institutional Review Board Statement: Ethical review and approval were waived for this study, as this study was approved by Namie Town local government and conducted by veterinarians and a volunteer group as part of a large-scale trap and rescue operations for cats.

Informed Consent Statement: Not applicable.

Data Availability Statement: The data presented in this study are available on request from the corresponding author.

Acknowledgments: The authors express our deep appreciation to the local government in Namie Town, Fukushima Prefecture, Japan. We are also grateful to Sanae Akama for her continuous care and protection of free-roaming cats in Namie Town. We also thank Ikue Asari, Naomi Sasaki, Yuki Sato, and other members of the laboratory staff for their technical and secretarial support.

Conflicts of Interest: The authors have no conflict of interest to disclose.

References

1. Kinoshita, N.; Sueki, K.; Sasa, K.; Kitagawa, J.; Ikarashi, S.; Nishimura, T.; Wong, Y.-S.; Satou, Y.; Handa, K.; Takahashi, T.; et al. Assessment of Individual Radionuclide Distributions from the Fukushima Nuclear Accident Covering Central-East Japan. *Proc. Natl. Acad. Sci. USA* **2011**, *108*, 19526–19529. [CrossRef] [PubMed]
2. Hosoda, M.; Tokonami, S.; Sorimachi, A.; Monzen, S.; Osanai, M.; Yamada, M.; Kashiwakura, I.; Akiba, S. The Time Variation of Dose Rate Artificially Increased by the Fukushima Nuclear Crisis. *Sci. Rep.* **2011**, *1*, 2–6. [CrossRef] [PubMed]
3. Ministry of the Environment (Japan) (MOE). *The Situation of Companion Animals Affected by the Great East Japan Earthquake*; MOE: Tokyo, Japan, 2019; p. 257. Available online: https://www.env.go.jp/nature/dobutsu/aigo/2_data/pamph/h2508c/cover.pdf (accessed on 15 July 2020). (In Japanese)
4. Schaffner, J.E.; Wandesforde-smith, G.; Wolf, P.J.; Levy, J.; Riley, S.; Farnworth, M.J. *Sustaining Innovation in Compassionate Free-Roaming Cat Management Across the Globe: A Decadal Reappraisal of the Practice and Promise of TNVR*; Schaffner, J.E., Wandesforde-Smith, G., Wolf, P.J., Levy, J., Riley, S., Farnworth, M.J., Eds.; Frontiers Research Topics; Frontiers Media SA: Lausanne, Switzerland, 2019; p. 142, ISBN 978-2-88963-271-8.
5. Yamashiro, H.; Abe, Y.; Fukuda, T.; Kino, Y.; Kawaguchi, I.; Kuwahara, Y.; Fukumoto, M.; Takahashi, S.; Suzuki, M.; Kobayashi, J.; et al. Effects of Radioactive Caesium on Bull Testes after the Fukushima Nuclear Plant Accident. *Sci. Rep.* **2013**, *3*, 1–6. [CrossRef]
6. Steinhauser, G.; Saey, P.R.J. ^{137}Cs in the Meat of Wild Boars: A Comparison of the Impacts of Chernobyl and Fukushima. *J. Radioanal. Nucl. Chem.* **2016**, *307*, 1801–1806. [CrossRef]
7. Tomoko, M.; Nakanishi, K.T. *Agricultural Implications of the Fukushima Nuclear Accident—The First Three Years*; Nakanishi, T.M., Tanoi, K., Eds.; Springer Open; Springer: Tokyo, Japan, 2016; ISBN 978-4-431-55826-2.
8. Anderson, D.; Okuda, K.; Hess, A.; Nanba, K.; Johnson, T.; Takase, T.; Hinton, T. A Comparison of Methods to Derive Aggregated Transfer Factors Using Wild Boar Data from the Fukushima Prefecture. *J. Environ. Radioact.* **2019**, *197*, 101–108. [CrossRef]
9. Hayama, S.; Nakiri, S.; Nakanishi, S.; Ishii, N.; Uno, T.; Kato, T.; Konno, F.; Kawamoto, Y.; Tsuchida, S.; Ochiai, K.; et al. Concentration of Radiocesium in the Wild Japanese Monkey (*Macaca Fuscata*) over the First 15 Months after the Fukushima Daiichi Nuclear Disaster. *PLoS ONE* **2013**, *8*, 1–8. [CrossRef]
10. Ochiai, K.; Hayama, S.-I.; Nakiri, S.; Nakanishi, S.; Ishii, N.; Uno, T.; Kato, T.; Konno, F.; Kawamoto, Y.; Tsuchida, S.; et al. Low Blood Cell Counts in Wild Japanese Monkeys after the Fukushima Daiichi Nuclear Disaster. *Sci. Rep.* **2014**, *4*. [CrossRef]
11. Urushihara, Y.; Suzuki, T.; Shimizu, Y.; Ohtaki, M.; Kuwahara, Y.; Suzuki, M.; Uno, T.; Fujita, S.; Saito, A.; Yamashiro, H.; et al. Haematological Analysis of Japanese Macaques (*Macaca Fuscata*) in the Area Affected by the Fukushima Daiichi Nuclear Power Plant Accident. *Sci. Rep.* **2018**, *8*, 1–10. [CrossRef]
12. Kubota, Y.; Tsuji, H.; Kawagoshi, T.; Shiomi, N.; Takahashi, H.; Watanabe, Y.; Fuma, S.; Doi, K.; Kawaguchi, I.; Aoki, M.; et al. Chromosomal Aberrations in Wild Mice Captured in Areas Differentially Contaminated by the Fukushima Dai-Ichi Nuclear Power Plant Accident. *Environ. Sci. Technol.* **2015**, *49*, 10074–10083. [CrossRef] [PubMed]
13. Kawagoshi, T.; Shiomi, N.; Takahashi, H.; Watanabe, Y.; Fuma, S.; Doi, K.; Kawaguchi, I.; Aoki, M.; Kubota, M.; Furuhata, Y.; et al. Chromosomal Aberrations in Large Japanese Field Mice (*Apodemus Speciosus*) Captured near Fukushima Dai-Ichi Nuclear Power Plant. *Environ. Sci. Technol.* **2017**, *51*, 4632–4641. [CrossRef] [PubMed]
14. Fujishima, Y.; Nakata, A.; Ujiie, R.; Kasai, K.; Ariyoshi, K.; Goh, V.S.T.; Suzuki, K.; Tazoe, H.; Yamada, M.; Yoshida, M.A.; et al. Assessment of Chromosome Aberrations in Large Japanese Field Mice (*Apodemus Speciosus*) in Namie Town, Fukushima. *Int. J. Radiat. Biol.* **2020**, 1–27. [CrossRef] [PubMed]
15. Mizuno, T.; Kubo, H. Overview of Active Cesium Contamination of Freshwater Fish in Fukushima and Eastern Japan. *Sci. Rep.* **2013**, *3*, 7–10. [CrossRef] [PubMed]
16. Wada, T.; Tomiya, A.; Enomoto, M.; Sato, T.; Morishita, D.; Izumi, S.; Niizeki, K.; Suzuki, S.; Morita, T.; Kawata, G. Radiological Impact of the Nuclear Power Plant Accident on Freshwater Fish in Fukushima: An Overview of Monitoring Results. *J. Environ. Radioact.* **2016**, *151*, 144–155. [CrossRef] [PubMed]
17. Fuma, S.; Ihara, S.; Takahashi, H.; Inaba, O.; Sato, Y.; Kubota, Y.; Watanabe, Y.; Kawaguchi, I.; Aono, T.; Soeda, H.; et al. Radiocaesium Contamination and Dose Rate Estimation of Terrestrial and Freshwater Wildlife in the Exclusion Zone of the Fukushima Dai-Ichi Nuclear Power Plant Accident. *J. Environ. Radioact.* **2017**, *171*, 176–188. [CrossRef] [PubMed]

18. Møller, A.P.; Hagiwara, A.; Matsui, S.; Kasahara, S.; Kawatsu, K.; Nishiumi, I.; Suzuki, H.; Ueda, K.; Mousseau, T.A. Abundance of Birds in Fukushima as Judged from Chernobyl. *Environ. Pollut.* **2012**, *164*, 36–39. [CrossRef]
19. González, A.J.; Akashi, M.; Boice Jr, J.D.; Chino, M.; Homma, T.; Ishigure, N.; Kai, M.; Kusumi, S.; Lee, J.-K.; Menzel, H.-G.; et al. Radiological Protection Issues Arising during and after the Fukushima Nuclear Reactor Accident. *J. Radiol. Prot.* **2013**, *33*, 497–571. [CrossRef]
20. Steinhauser, G.; Brandl, A.; Johnson, T.E. Comparison of the Chernobyl and Fukushima Nuclear Accidents: A Review of the Environmental Impacts. *Sci. Total Environ.* **2014**, *470–471*, 800–817. [CrossRef]
21. Fukuda, T.; Kino, Y.; Abe, Y.; Yamashiro, H.; Kuwahara, Y.; Nihei, H.; Sano, Y.; Irisawa, A.; Shimura, T.; Fukumoto, M.; et al. Distribution of Artificial Radionuclides in Abandoned Cattle in the Evacuation Zone of the Evacuation Zone of the Fukushima Daiichi Nuclear Power Plant. *PLoS ONE* **2013**, *8*, 1–7. [CrossRef] [PubMed]
22. R Core Team. *R: A Language and Environment for Statistical Computing*; R Foundation for Statistical Computing: Vienna, Austria, 2020.
23. Ministry of the Environment (Japan) (MOE). *Guidelines for Proper Breeding of Dogs and Cats in Densely Built-up Area*; MOE: Tokyo, Japan, 2010; p. 22. Available online: https://www.env.go.jp/nature/dobutsu/aigo/2_data/pamph/h2202.pdf (accessed on 15 July 2020). (In Japanese)
24. Ishida, T.; Kawai, S.; Fujiwara, K. Detection of Feline Leukemia Virus Infection in Tokyo Area by Enzyme-Linked Immunosorbent Assay (ELISA). *Jpn. J. Vet. Sci.* **1981**, *43*, 871–874. [CrossRef]
25. Furuya, T.; Kawaguchi, Y.; Miyazawa, T.; Fujikawa, Y.; Tohya, Y.; Azetaka, M.; Takahashi, E.; Mikami, T. Existence of Feline Immunodeficiency Virus Infection in Japanese Cat Population since 1968. *Jpn. J. Vet. Sci.* **1990**, *52*, 891–893. [CrossRef] [PubMed]
26. Ishida, T.; Taniguchi, A.; Kanai, T.; Kataoka, Y.; Aimi, K.; Kariya, K.; Washizu, T.; Tomoda, I. Retrospective Serosurvey for Feline Immunodeficiency Virus Infection in Japanese Cats. *Jpn. J. Vet. Sci.* **1990**, *52*, 453–454. [CrossRef]
27. Maruyama, S.; Kabeya, H.; Nakao, R.; Tanaka, S.; Sakai, T.; Xuan, X.; Katsube, Y.; Mikami, T. Seroprevalence of *Bartonella Henselae*, *Toxoplasma Gondii*, FIV and FeLV Infections in Domestic Cats in Japan. *Microbiol. Immunol.* **2003**, *47*, 147–153. [CrossRef] [PubMed]
28. Lee, I.T.; Levy, J.K.; Gorman, S.P.; Crawford, P.C.; Slater, M.R. Prevalence of Feline Leukemia Virus Infection and Serum Antibodies against Feline Immunodeficiency Virus in Unowned Free-Roaming Cats. *J. Am. Vet. Med. Assoc.* **2006**, *220*, 620–622. [CrossRef]
29. Uetake, K.; Yamada, S.; Kaneko, K.; Fujimori, W.; Sato, R.; Tanaka, T. Blood Characteristics and Reproductive Status of Stray Cats (*Felis Silvestris Catus*) in an Urban Residential Area of Japan. *Anim. Behav. Manag.* **2014**, *50*, 1–5. [CrossRef]
30. Mori, J.; Tsubokura, M.; Sugimoto, A.; Tanimoto, T.; Kami, M.; Oikawa, T.; Kanazawa, Y. Increased Incidence of Dog-Bite Injuries after the Fukushima Nuclear Accident. *Prev. Med.* **2013**, *57*, 363–365. [CrossRef] [PubMed]
31. Leggett, R.W.; Williams, L.R.; Melo, D.R.; Lipsztein, J.L. A Physiologically Based Biokinetic Model for Cesium in the Human Body. *Sci. Total Environ.* **2003**, *317*, 235–255. [CrossRef]
32. Green, R.M.; McNeill, K.G.; Robinson, G.A. The Distribution of Potassium and Caesium-137 in the Calf and the Pig. *Can. J. Biochem. Physiol.* **1961**, *39*, 1021–1026. [CrossRef]
33. Tanoi, K.; Uchida, K.; Doi, C.; Nihei, N.; Hirose, A.; Kobayashi, N.I.; Sugita, R.; Nobori, T.; Nakanishi, T.M.; Kanno, M.; et al. Investigation of Radiocesium Distribution in Organs of Wild Boar Grown in Iitate, Fukushima after the Fukushima Daiichi Nuclear Power Plant Accident. *J. Radioanal. Nucl. Chem.* **2016**, *307*, 741–746. [CrossRef]
34. Wada, S.; Ito, N.; Watanabe, M.; Kakizaki, T.; Natsuhori, M.; Kawamata, J.; Urayama, Y. Whole-Body Counter Evaluation of Internal Radioactive Cesium in Dogs and Cats Exposed to the Fukushima Nuclear Disaster. *PLoS ONE* **2017**, *12*, 1–15. [CrossRef]
35. Sakagami, S.F.; Takahashi, H.; Niida, N. A Small Census on the Home Range of Domestic Cats. *Jpn. J. Ecol.* **1957**, *6*, 137–140.
36. Fitzgerald, B.M.; Karl, B.J. Home Range of Feral House Cats (*Felis Catus* L.) in Forest of the Orongorongo Valley, Wellington, New Zealand. *N. Z. J. Ecol.* **1986**, *9*, 71–81. [CrossRef]
37. Horn, J.A.; Mateus-Pinilla, N.; Warner, R.E.; Heske, E.J. Home Range, Habitat Use, and Activity Patterns of Free-Roaming Domestic Cats. *J. Wildl. Manag.* **2011**, *75*, 1177–1185. [CrossRef]
38. Loyd, K.A.T.; Hernandez, S.M.; Carroll, J.P.; Abernathy, K.J.; Marshall, G.J. Quantifying Free-Roaming Domestic Cat Predation Using Animal-Borne Video Cameras. *Biol. Conserv.* **2013**, *160*, 183–189. [CrossRef]

Article

Long-Term Measurements of Radon and Thoron Exhalation Rates from the Ground Using the Vertical Distributions of Their Activity Concentrations

Oumar Bobbo Modibo [1,2], Yuki Tamakuma [1,3], Takahito Suzuki [1], Ryohei Yamada [1], Weihai Zhuo [4], Chutima Kranrod [3], Kazuki Iwaoka [5], Naofumi Akata [3], Masahiro Hosoda [1,3] and Shinji Tokonami [3,*]

1. Department of Radiation Science, Graduate School of Health Sciences, Hirosaki University, 66-1 Honcho, Hirosaki, Aomori 036-8564, Japan; h19gg701@hirosaki-u.ac.jp (O.B.M.); tamakuma@hirosaki-u.ac.jp (Y.T.); suzuki-takahito@fujielectric.com (T.S.); yamada.ryohei@jaea.go.jp (R.Y.); m_hosoda@hirosaki-u.ac.jp (M.H.)
2. Nuclear Technology Section, Institute of Geological and Mining Research, P.O. Box 4110, Yaoundé, Cameroon
3. Institute of Radiation Emergency Medicine, Hirosaki University, 66-1 Honcho, Hirosaki, Aomori 036-8564, Japan; kranrodc@hirosaki-u.ac.jp (C.K.); akata@hirosaki-u.ac.jp (N.A.)
4. Institute of Radiation Medicine, Fudan University, 2094 Xietu Road, Shanghai 200032, China; whzhuo@fudan.edu.cn
5. National Institutes for Quantum and Radiological Science and Technology, 4-9-1 Anagawa, Inage, Chiba 263-0024, Japan; iwaoka.kazuki@qst.go.jp
* Correspondence: tokonami@hirosaki-u.ac.jp; Tel.: +81-172-39-5404

Abstract: A long-term measurement technique of radon exhalation rate was previously developed using a passive type radon and thoron discriminative monitor and a ventilated type accumulation chamber. In the present study, this technique was applied to evaluate the thoron exhalation rate as well, and long-term measurements of radon and thoron exhalation rates were conducted for four years in Gifu Prefecture. The ventilated type accumulation chamber ($0.8 \times 0.8 \times 1.0$ m^3) with an open bottom was embedded 15 cm into the ground. The vertical distributions of radon and thoron activity concentrations from the ground were obtained using passive type radon-thoron discriminative monitors (RADUETs). The RADUETs were placed at 1, 3, 10, 30, and 80 cm above the ground inside the accumulation chamber. The measurements were conducted from autumn 2014 to autumn 2018. These long-term results were found to be in good agreement with the values obtained by another methodology. The radon exhalation rates from the ground showed a clearly seasonal variation. Similar to findings of previous studies, radon exhalation rates from summer to autumn were relatively higher than those from winter to spring. In contrast, thoron exhalation rates were not found to show seasonal variation.

Keywords: exhalation rate; radon; thoron; long-term measurement; seasonal variation

1. Introduction

Radon (^{222}Rn) and thoron (^{220}Rn) are naturally occurring radioactive gases generated from the ^{238}U- and ^{232}Th-series. It is well known that radon and thoron are the biggest contributors to human radiation exposure from natural sources [1]. The World Health Organization (WHO) has recognized them as the second largest cause of lung cancer after smoking [2]. Indoor and outdoor radon and thoron concentrations vary widely from place to place depending on geological features and meteorological condition of an area (see, e.g., [3]). In general, indoor radon concentration is continuously supplied by a portion of outdoor radon, an infiltration rate of 10 Bq m^{-3} h^{-1} was reported [1]. In addition to the health effect assessment due to its inhalation, outdoor radon monitoring is useful in several scientific disciplines as a radioactive tracer. Its half-life of $T_{1/2}$ = 3.82 days is comparable to the air masses' transit time across the major continents. Outdoor radon monitoring serves also on earthquake forecasting, geological faults identifications or ore exploration, and environmental reprocessing in mining [4–7]. Some researchers have reported a positive correlation between outdoor radon concentration and radon exhalation rate from the ground [8–10]. Therefore, the exhalation rates of radon and thoron, which are often called flux or flux density, are useful parameters to understand human health risk due to radon and thoron inhalation, and many researchers have reported data obtained by field and experimental studies [11–14]. Generally, a common technique for exhalation rate measurement is based on placing an accumulation chamber on the ground surface to accumulate radon gas exhaling from the ground and using radon monitor to measure radon concentration and deduce radon exhalation rate, the technique has been applied for short- and long-term radon exhalation rate measurements [15]. However, it is difficult to evaluate both radon and thoron exhalation rates simultaneously using this method due to short half-life of thoron ($T_{1/2}$ = 55.6 s). Alternatively, Zhuo et al. [10] reported on the long-term measurement technique of radon exhalation rate using a passive type radon and thoron discriminative monitor and a ventilated type accumulation chamber. However, their report did not evaluate thoron exhalation rate. It was reported that thoron activity concentrations from a source such as the materials of building walls and the ground have a unique distribution [16–19]. In the present study, long-term radon and thoron exhalation rates from the ground were simultaneously measured for a period of four years by applying the previously reported technique of ventilated type accumulation chamber [9]. From the results obtained, the seasonal variations of radon and thoron exhalation rates from the ground were discussed.

2. Materials and Methods

2.1. Ventilated-Type Accumulation Chamber System for Measuring Radon-Thoron Exhalation Rates from the Ground

A naturally ventilated accumulation chamber (0.8 × 0.8 × 1.0 m^3) which is a stainless-steel box with an open bottom was embedded 15 cm into the ground on the campus of the National Institute of Fusion Science (NIFS) located in Gifu Prefecture, Japan (N35.325°, E137.168°), as shown in Figure 1. Two rectangle openings (20 × 10 cm^2) were perforated at the upper right and lower left walls of the stainless-steel box to get air ventilation, and each opening was covered on the inside side by a fiber filter (Whatman® No. 41) and the outside side by a rain/wind shelter. Thus, the change of particles (dust) outside cannot interfere with the inside environment of the stainless-steel box as the two openings are covered with filters. According to the report by Zhuo et al. [10], wind speed inside and outside of the ventilated accumulation chamber was monitored, and it was found that the inside wind speed could hardly be affected by the change of outside winds. Additionally, the air and soil conditions (pressure, temperature, relative humidity, and water potential) monitored simultaneously inside and outside of the stainless-steel box showed that except for the air humidity both the soil and air conditions inside and outside were nearly the same throughout the year, and it showed that the passive radon-thoron monitor used here is not affected by air humidity [10]. The vertical distributions of radon and thoron concentrations inside the accumulation chamber were obtained using a passive type radon-thoron discriminative monitor (RADUET, Radosys Ltd., Budapest, Hungary) [20]. The Raduets are composed of two different diffusion chambers of the same inner volume of about 30 cm^3. The chambers are made of electroconductive plastic with a cylindrical form. The radon–thoron discrimination principle is based on the diffusion characteristics of each chamber. Radon in the air with its longer diffusion length is able to diffuse through an invisible air gap of one of the chambers located between its lid and bottom. Thoron can scarcely diffuse into that chamber with such a small pathway due to its very short half-life and lower diffusion length compared to that of radon. The second chamber has 6 holes of 6 mm of diameter opened at the side of the chamber which allow the diffusion of thoron as well as radon, the 6 holes are recovered by an electroconductive sponge to block the passage of charges particulate in the diffusion chamber [20]. The detection limits for the typical measurement period (3 months) were estimated to be 3 and 14 Bq m^{-3} for radon and thoron, respectively [21]. The RADUETs were placed at heights of 1, 3,

10, 30, and 80 cm from the ground surface inside the accumulation chamber. For laboratory analysis, the RADUETs were exchanged every three months: spring, March–May; summer, June–August; autumn, September–November; winter, December–February. The solid-state track detectors (CR-39; BARYOTRAK, Nagase Landauer, Ltd., Tsukuba, Japan), which were installed in the RADUETs, were taken out and chemically etched for 24 h in a 6M NaOH solution at 60 °C [21]. The number of alpha tracks was counted using an optical microscope and image analysis software (ImageJ, National Institutes of Health, Bethesda, Maryland, USA). Radon and thoron concentrations were calculated according to the International Organization for Standardization (ISO) 16641 [22]. The conversion factors from track densities of CR-39s to radon and thoron concentrations had been already evaluated using the radon-thoron calibration chamber in Hirosaki University [23]. Environmental parameters of temperature, relative humidity and atmospheric pressure inside the accumulation chamber were measured continuously using a portable type meteorological monitor (TR-73U, T&D Corp., Matsumoto, Japan).

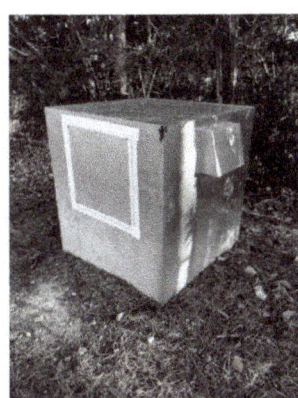
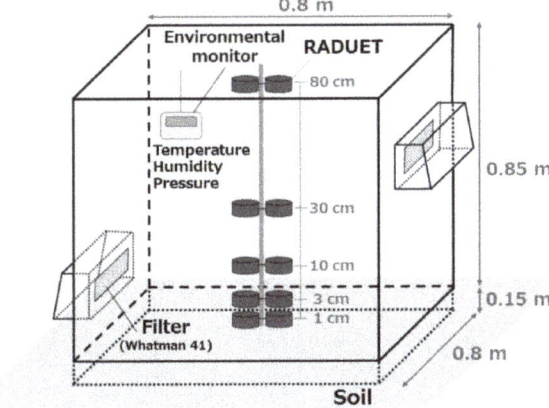

Figure 1. Photo and schematic drawing of the ventilation-type accumulation chamber system for measuring radon and thoron exhalation rates from the ground.

2.2. Evaluation of Radon and Thoron Exhalation Rates Using the Ventilated Type Accumulation Chamber

According to Zhuo et al. [10], the radon exhalation rate E_{Rn} (mBq m^{-2} s^{-1}) obtained using the ventilated type accumulation chamber can be calculated by Equation (1).

$$E_{Rn} = 1000 \times C_{Rn} \times Z_{max} \times \frac{Q + \lambda_{Rn}}{3600} \quad (1)$$

Here, C_{Rn} is the average radon concentration at each height (Bq m^{-3}), Z_{max} is the height of the chamber from the ground surface (=0.85 m), Q is air exchange rate in the accumulation chamber, and λ_{Rn} is the decay constant of radon (7.6 × 10^{-3} h^{-1}). Air exchange rate in the chamber was evaluated using carbon dioxide (CO_2) gas and a CO_2 monitor (TR-76Ui, T&D Corporation). Generally, the air exchange rate is much larger than the decay constant of radon. Therefore, the decay constant of radon can be neglected ($Q \gg \lambda_{Rn}$, $Q + \lambda_{Rn} \approx Q$).

According to the one-dimensional diffusion equation reported by Katase et al. [24], the thoron concentration $C_{Tn}(z)$ at a height z (m) above the ground is given by Equation (2).

$$C_{Tn}(Z) = \frac{E_{Tn}}{\sqrt{(Q + \lambda_{Tn})D_e}} \cdot \exp\left(-\sqrt{\frac{Q + \lambda_{Tn}}{D_e}} z\right) \quad (2)$$

Here, E_{Tn} is the thoron exhalation rate from the ground (Bq m^{-2} s^{-1}), λ_{Tn} is the decay constant of thoron (44.9 h^{-1}), and D_e is the effective diffusion coefficient in free air (1.2 × 10^{-5} m^2 s^{-1}) [25]. In this study, the following exponential regression formula was applied to the vertical distribution of thoron concentration in each season for the simplified estimation of thoron concentration at 0 m.

$$C_{Tn}(Z) = a \cdot \exp(-bz) \tag{3}$$

Thoron concentration at the ground surface ($z = 0$ m) was estimated by Equation (3). Then, thoron exhalation rate E_{Tn} (mBq m^{-2} s^{-1}) was evaluated by Equation (4) obtained by substituting $z = 0$ into Equation (2).

$$E_{Tn} = 1000 \times C_{Tn,0} \times \sqrt{D \cdot \frac{(Q + \lambda_{Tn})}{3600}} \tag{4}$$

Here, $C_{Tn,0}$ is the thoron activity concentration at 0 m (Bq m^{-3}).

2.3. Soil Parameters and Its Activity Concentrations of ^{226}Ra and ^{228}Ra

Five soil core samples from the ground surface to 5 cm depth were collected using a stainless-steel soil sampler, which had a volume of 100 mL [26]. Dry bulk density, soil particle density, porosity, and soil textures were evaluated after drying samples for 24 h at 110 °C. The dry bulk density ρ_b was calculated as the mass of the dried soil divided by the soil volume. The soil particle density ρ_s was evaluated using a specific gravity bottle according to the test procedure of Japan Industrial Standards (JIS) A1202 [27]. The porosity ε was calculated by $\varepsilon = 1 - \rho_b/\rho_s$. Soil particle size distribution was evaluated using a standard stainless-steel sieve for 0.075–2.0 mm particle size range and the sedimentation analysis for particles below 0.075 mm was made according to the test procedure of JIS A1204 [28] to determine the soil textures of the samples. The percentages of sand, silt, and clay for each soil sample were evaluated using the sample particle size distribution curves.

The activity concentrations of ^{226}Ra and ^{228}Ra were evaluated using a high-purity germanium semiconductor detector (GEM-100210, ORTEC, USA) with a relative efficiency of 30%, 1.85 keV energy resolution (FWHM) at 1.33 MeV of ^{60}Co. The efficiency calibration of the detector was made using the standard volumetric sources which are contained ^{109}Cd, ^{57}Co, ^{139}Ce, ^{51}Cr, ^{85}Sr, ^{137}Cs, ^{54}Mn, ^{88}Y, and ^{60}Co supplied by Japan Radioisotope Association. The detector was enclosed in a shielding made out of compacted lead of 10 cm of thickness. Each soil sample was enclosed in a cylindrical polypropylene container (U8 type container, 100 cm^3) after drying for 24 h at 110 °C. The prepared soil sample was then enclosed in an air-tight container for 40 days to allow radioactive equilibrium between ^{226}Ra and ^{222}Rn to be reached. The measurement time was set as 80,000 s. In this study, the weighted average concentration of ^{214}Pb and ^{214}Bi were used as the ^{226}Ra concentration in the soil samples by counting photons in the photoelectric peak channels of 352 keV for ^{214}Pb and 609 keV for ^{214}Bi. ^{228}Ra was measured by counting photons in the photoelectric peak channel of 911 keV for ^{228}Ac. The uncertainty for the activity concentration was evaluated taking into account the uncertainties of the counts for the sample and background. Coincidence summing, self-attenuation and decay corrections were applied using software (Gamma Studio, SEIKO EG&G, Tokyo, Japan).

2.4. Comparison of the Exhalation Rates with the Other Methods

2.4.1. Accumulation Chamber with Scintillation Cell

The stainless-steel accumulation chamber was set on the ground surface. Radon gas exhaled from the ground was accumulated for 1.5 to 3 h. Then, the radon gas inside the accumulation chamber was collected into a scintillation cell (Pylon 300A, Pylon Electrics, Inc., Toronto, Ontario Canada) at a sampling flow rate of 0.5 L min^{-1} and a sampling time of 5 min. After 3.5 h, the alpha counts from radon gas in the scintillation cell were measured using a portable radiation monitor (AB-5, Pylon Electrics, Inc., Toronto, Ontario Canada) [29]. The radon exhalation rate by grab sampling can be calculated by applying Equation (5).

$$E_{Rn} = \frac{(N - N_b) \cdot CF \cdot V \cdot \lambda_{Rn}}{S \cdot [1 - \exp(-\lambda_{Rn} \cdot t)]} \quad (5)$$

Here, N and N_b are the count rates of the sample and background (cpm), CF is the conversion factor from count rate to radon concentration (27.0 Bq m^{-3} cpm^{-1}) [30], V is the volume of the accumulation chamber (1.4 × 10^{-2} m^3), λ_{Rn} is the decay constant of radon (2.1 × 10^{-6} s^{-1}), S is the area under the accumulation chamber (9.9 × 10^{-2} m^2), and T is the accumulation time (s).

2.4.2. In Situ Radon and Thoron Exhalation Rate Monitor

Radon and thoron exhalation rates from the ground was also measured with an *in-situ* radon and thoron exhalation rate monitor (MSZ). The details of the method have been described by Saegusa et al. [31]. The monitor was composed of an accumulation chamber (volume, 13 L), a ZnS(Ag) scintillation detector with an aluminized mylar sheet, a light guide, a photomultiplier tube, a pulse counting part and scaler, and a timer. The area of an acrylic board coated with ZnS(Ag) scintillator was 0.12 m^2. Count rates were recorded over consecutive 30-s intervals during a total recording period of 30 min after the monitor was set up on the ground. The conversion factors from count rates of 10 min and 30 min to exhalation rates of radon and thoron were 0.521 ± 0.040 mBq m^{-2} s^{-1} cpm^{-1} and 18.1 ± 3.2 mBq m^{-2} s^{-1} cpm^{-1}, respectively. The measurement uncertainties for radon and thoron exhalation rates using the MSZ have been reported as ~20% and ~6%, respectively [11].

3. Results and Discussion

3.1. Physical Parameters of Soil and ^{226}Ra and ^{228}Ra Activity Concentrations at the Study Site

The percentages of sand, silt and clay for each soil sample collected at the study site were evaluated as 63 ± 4%, 16 ± 2%, and 21 ± 3%, respectively. As a result, the textural class of all soil samples was decided as sandy clay loam (SCL) based on a soil texture triangle. In general, the characteristics of SCL are reported to be high water retention and low air permeability [32]. Dry bulk density, soil particle density and porosity were evaluated as 1340 ± 19 kg m^{-3}, 2657 ± 27 kg m^{-3}, and 0.50 ± 0.07, respectively. These obtained values were not significantly different from the typical values of 1300–1350 kg m^{-3} for dry bulk density, 2600–2700 kg m^{-3} for soil particle density, and 0.3–0.6 for porosity [33]. Activity concentrations of ^{226}Ra and ^{228}Ra were evaluated to be 24.1 ± 0.4 Bq kg^{-1} and 34.0 ± 0.9 Bq kg^{-1}, respectively. According to the UNSCEAR [1], the Japanese mean activity concentrations of ^{226}Ra and ^{228}Ra (assuming radioactive equilibrium with ^{232}Th) are reported as 33 Bq kg^{-1} and 28 Bq kg^{-1}, respectively. Thus, radium activity concentrations in soil at the study site were found to be slightly lower than those of the national mean.

3.2. Radon and Thoron Concentration in the Ventilated-Type Accumulation Chamber

An example of the vertical distribution of thoron concentration inside the ventilated type accumulation chamber is shown in Figure 2. Thoron concentration decreased exponentially with the height above the ground surface. On the other hand, radon concentrations inside the accumulation chamber did not depend on the height above the ground. These observations were similar to the previously reported findings [16,17,19]. The results obtained at the 10 cm and above height from the ground were not considered in the calculation of thoron exhalation rate because the thoron concentrations at these heights were below the lower limit of detection. Additionally, the air exchange rate of the accumulation chamber was evaluated as 0.30 h^{-1} which was similar to the literature [9].

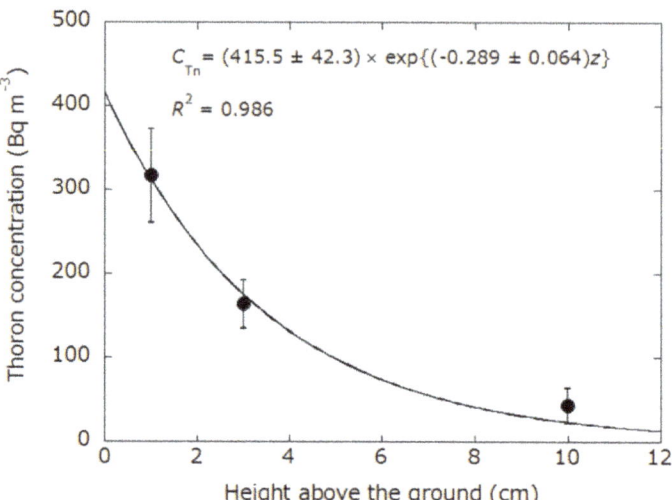

Figure 2. Example of the vertical distribution of thoron concentration inside the ventilated type accumulation chamber. The thoron concentration at ground level ($z = 0$ cm) was determined to be 416 ± 42 Bq m^{-3}.

3.3. Comparison of Radon and Thoron Exhalation Rates Obtained by the Present System to Those Obtained by the Other Methods

Comparison of radon and thoron exhalation rates obtained by the ventilated-type accumulation chamber, accumulation chamber with scintillation cell and in situ monitor are shown in Table 1. Radon exhalation rates obtained by the passive method were in relatively good agreement with the results measured by the accumulation chamber with scintillation cell and in situ monitor (MSZ) taking into account the measurement uncertainty. Statistical analyses were conducted using the "EZR software" (Easy R) [34]. The difference was considered significant for $p < 0.05$. A one-way ANOVA test was performed for the comparison of radon exhalation rates obtained by each technique. Consequently, the radon exhalation rate measured by the present system and those obtained by the other methods are not significantly different ($p = 0.128$). Furthermore, the thoron exhalation rate obtained by the ventilated-type accumulation chamber in the first measurements was also in agreement with the result obtained by the in situ monitor ($p = 0.156$). However, in the second measurements, thoron exhalation rate obtained by the ventilated-type accumulation chamber was approximately half that of the value obtained by the in situ monitor. Theoretically, the diffusion length of thoron is reported as a few centimeters which is much shorter than that of radon due to the short half-life of thoron. Therefore, thoron exhalation rate is considered to be more strongly affected by the soil surface condition compared with the radon exhalation rate. Thus, it is necessary to make intercomparison experiments repeatedly to ensure the quality of the data obtained by the present ventilated-type accumulation chamber. However, the present method can offer an easy and low-cost system for the measurements of both radon and thoron exhalation rates, as no electric power supply is needed and operation and maintenance are easy.

Table 1. Comparison of radon and thoron exhalation rates obtained by the ventilated-type accumulation chamber, accumulation chamber with scintillation cell, and in situ monitor (MSZ) method.

Intercomparison	Methods	Radon Exhalation Rate (mBq m^{-2} s^{-1})	Thoron Exhalation Rate (mBq m^{-2} s^{-1})
1st measurement	Ventilated-type accumulation chamber	3.6 ± 0.5	797 ± 336
	Accumulation chamber with scintillation cell	4.6 ± 2.9	-
	In situ monitor (MSZ) method	1.1 ± 0.1	584 ± 103
2nd measurement	Ventilated type accumulation chamber	4.3 ± 0.5	1120 ± 321
	Accumulation chamber with scintillation cell	8.8 ± 5.3	-
	In situ monitor (MSZ) method	5.1 ± 1.8	474 ± 177

3.4. Seasonal Variations of the Radon and Thoron Exhalation Rates

Seasonal variations of radon and thoron exhalation rates are shown in Figure 3. The median values (range) of radon exhalation rate in spring, summer, autumn and winter were estimated to be 3.5 ± 0.5 (2.4−5.8), 5.4 ± 1.1 (4.0−6.4), 5.6 ± 0.3 (4.0−7.1), and 3.5 ± 0.3 (2.1−4.8) mBq m^{-2} s^{-1}, respectively. The median values (range) of thoron exhalation rates were evaluated as 614 ± 126 (159−848), 555 ± 110 (295−1110), 563 ± 395 (61−1524), and 593 ± 138 (318−797) mBq m^{-2} s^{-1} for spring, summer, autumn and winter, respectively. Annual means of the radon and thoron exhalation rates were evaluated to be 4.5 ± 0.3 mBq m^{-2} s^{-1} and 581 ± 113 mBq m^{-2} s^{-1}, respectively. According to the results of a large-scale survey in Japan [12,35], average radon and thoron exhalation rates from the ground were 8.6 mBq m^{-2} s^{-1} (N = 111) and 790 mBq m^{-2} s^{-1} (N = 405), respectively. Therefore, radon and thoron exhalation rates at the present measurement site were 52% and 74% of the Japanese averages. Furthermore, average radon exhalation rates in summer and autumn were higher than the annual mean. The ratio of the radon exhalation rate in summer to the radon exhalation rate in winter (or spring) is 1.5 and the ratio of the radon exhalation rate in autumn to the radon exhalation rate in winter (or spring) is 1.6. A one-way ANOVA was performed to determine whether there are any statistically significant differences between the means of each season. Consequently, it showed no statistically significant difference in the average radon exhalation rate between the seasons in this study (p = 0.103). However, the median values of radon exhalation rate tend to be higher from summer to autumn and lower from winter to spring (Figure 3a). Zhuo et al. [36] reported a similar seasonal variation of radon exhalation rate from the ground in China. Zhuo et al. [9] have also reported a negative correlation between radon exhalation rate and precipitation. On the other hand, Hosoda et al. [12] reported that when the variation of moisture saturation was small, the soil temperature appeared to induce a strong effect on the exhalation rate. However, when the variation of moisture saturation was large, the influence of moisture saturation appears to be larger than the soil surface temperature [12]. Furthermore, it has been also reported that an increase in the soil temperature markedly decreased the amount of adsorption of gases which contributed to the increase of emanation and diffusion coefficients [37,38]. Precipitation data from a location near the monitoring site were reported by the Japan Meteorological Agency [39], and cumulative precipitations in spring, summer, autumn, and winter during the measurement period were 424, 586, 441, and 177 mm, respectively. Additionally, their respective mean temperatures were 14.1, 25.2, 17.9, and 4.2 °C. Therefore, the radon exhalation rate in winter at the measurement site might be affected by low precipitation and temperature. On the other hand, in summer the high temperature might affect the radon exhalation rate.

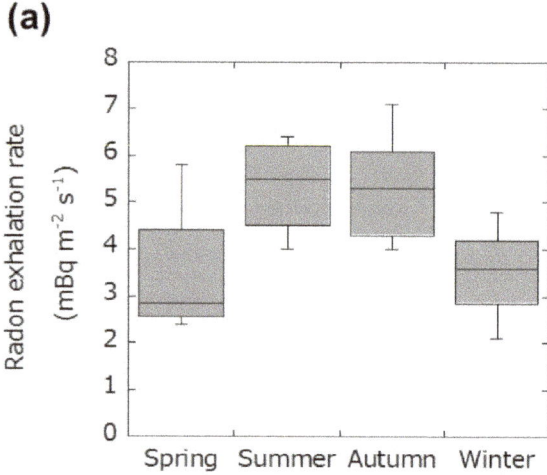

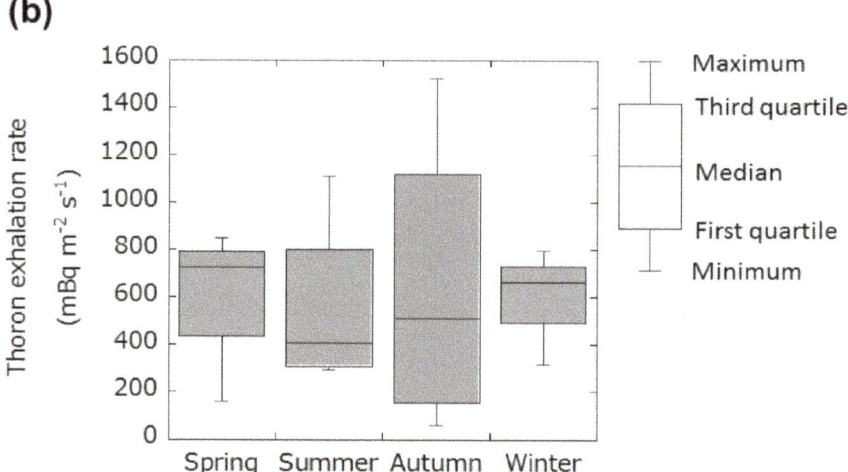

Figure 3. Seasonal variations of radon (**a**) and thoron (**b**) exhalation rates. The lines from top to bottom of the box-plot from top to bottom are defined as maximum, third quartile (75th percentile), median (50th percentile), first quartile (25th percentile), and minimum values.

The statistical analysis using the one-way ANOVA test showed that there was no significant difference between the averages of thoron exhalation rate for the different seasons (p = 0.982) (Figure 3b). According to the report by Prasad et al. [40], radon and thoron exhalation rates in summer and autumn were higher than those in spring and winter. However, the reported diffusion length of radon and thoron were a few meters and a few centimeters, respectively [11,26]. That is, thoron exhalation rate from the ground would be affected by such environmental parameters as moisture saturation and temperature around the surface soil. Therefore, the soil temperature and moisture saturation were measured continuously for three months in summer at 10 cm depth from the surface inside and outside of the accumulation chamber. The average surface soil temperature inside and outside the accumulation chamber were 22.3 ± 3.5 (RSD: 18%) and 22.2 ± 3.9 °C (RSD: 16%), respectively. The results suggested that the accumulation chamber setup was not affected by the surface soil temperature as same with the previous report [10]. On the other hand, the average moisture saturation (convert from volumetric water content using porosity) inside and outside the accumulation chamber were evaluated to be 0.364 ± 0.172 (RSD: 47%) and 0.114 ± 0.028 (RSD: 24%), respectively. As we mentioned above, Zhuo et al. reported that the water potential inside and outside of the stainless-steel box shown nearly the same throughout the year [10]. It is well known that the water potential is related parameter to volumetric water content which is influential parameter of exhalation rate. However, both the average moisture saturation and its variation inside the accumulation chamber were smaller than those outside the chamber. Additionally, the accumulation chamber was embedded 15 cm into the soil. That is, it is considered that this measurement condition was not easy for water due to rainfall to move from outside the chamber to under the chamber by passing through pore spaces in the surface soil. However, the thoron exhalation rates obtained in this study may be considered as baseline level at the measurement site. Thus, we will develop the correction method of thoron exhalation rates with the variation of the environmental factors. Additionally, it might be possible to evaluate the seasonal variations of thoron exhalation rate if a passive type radon and thoron discriminative monitor was set in a small size accumulation chamber.

4. Conclusions

In this study, radon and thoron exhalation rates from the ground were simultaneously evaluated for four years by applying the naturally ventilated accumulation chamber of a previous report. The results were compared to the data obtained by the accumulation chamber with scintillation cell and in situ radon and thoron exhalation rate monitor. The results of the present method had relatively good agreement with results of the other methods. Relationships between radon exhalation rates with environmental parameters were also observed and their variations with seasons were determined. The baseline level of thoron exhalation rate at the measurement site was evaluated. However, thoron exhalation rates did not show clear seasonal variations, most likely due to limitations of the present methodology. Therefore, the methodology will be modified based on the present results to allow the season variation of thoron exhalation rate from the ground to be obtained.

Author Contributions: Conceptualization, M.H. and S.T.; methodology, W.Z., N.A., M.H., and S.T.; validation, C.K., K.I., N.A., and M.H.; formal analysis, Y.T., T.S., and R.Y.; investigation, Y.T., T.S., R.Y., K.I., N.A., M.H., and S.T.; resources, N.A., M.H., and S.T.; data curation, T.S. and M.H.; writing—original draft preparation, O.B.M.; writing—review and editing, Y.T., T.S., R.Y., W.Z., C.K., K.I., N.A., M.H., and S.T.; visualization, T.S. and M.H.; supervision, C.K., N.A., M.H., and S.T.; project administration, N.A., M.H., and S.T.; funding acquisition, M.H. and S.T. All authors have read and agreed to the published version of the manuscript.

Funding: This work has been partially supported by the Research Foundation for the Electrotechnology of Chubu, the NIFS Collaboration Research Program (NIFS17KLEA034), the Radiation Effects Association, the JSPS KAKENHI (Grant Number 16H02667, 16K15358, and 18K10023), and the Hirosaki University Institutional Research Grant.

Institutional Review Board Statement: Not applicable.

Informed Consent Statement: Not applicable.

Data Availability Statement: Not applicable.

Conflicts of Interest: The authors declare no conflict of interest.

References

1. United Nations Scientific Committee on the Effects of Atomic Radiation. *UNSCEAR 2008 Report, Effects of Ionizing Radiation. Volume I: Annex B Exposures of the Public and Workers from Various Sources of Radiation*; UNSCEAR: New York, NY, USA, 2010.
2. World Health Organization. *WHO Handbook on Indoor Radon: A Public Health Perspective*; WHO: Geneva, Switzerland, 2009.
3. Sanada, T.; Fujimoto, K.; Miyano, K.; Doi, M.; Tokonami, S.; Uesugi, M.; Takata, Y. Measurement of nationwide indoor Rn concentrations in Japan. *J. Environ. Radioact.* **1999**, *45*, 129–137. [CrossRef]

4. Chambers, S.D.; Preunkert, S.; Weller, R.; Hong, S.B.; Humphries, R.S.; Tositti, L.; Angot, H.; Legrand, M.; Williams, A.G.; Griffiths, A.D.; et al. Characterizing Atmospheric Transport Pathways to Antarctica and the Remote Southern Ocean Using Radon-222. *Front. Earth Sci.* **2018**, *6*, 1–28. [CrossRef]
5. Hwa, O.Y.; Kim, G. A radon-thoron isotope pair as a reliable earthquake precursor. *Sci. Rep.* **2015**, *5*, 1–6. [CrossRef] [PubMed]
6. Igarashi, G.; Saeki, S.; Takahata, N.; Sumikawa, K.; Tasaka, S.; Sasaki, Y.; Takahashi, M.; Sano, Y. Ground-Water Radon Anomaly Before the Kobe Earthquake in Japan. *Science* **1995**, *269*, 60–61. [CrossRef] [PubMed]
7. Lawrence, C.E.; Akber, R.A.; Bollhöfer, A.; Martin, P. Radon-222 exhalation from open ground on and around a uranium mine in the wet-dry tropics. *J. Environ. Radioac.* **2009**, *100*, 1–8. [CrossRef]
8. Ikebe, Y.; Yamanishi, H.; Tojo, K.; Iida, T. Relationship between radon exhalation rate from ground and atmospheric radon concentration. *Nippon Genshiryoku Gakkai-Shi* **1993**, *35*, 735–738. (In Japanese)
9. Zhuo, W.; Furukawa, M.; Qiuju, G.; Yoon, S.K. Soil radon flux and outdoor radon concentration in East Asia. *Int. Congr. Ser.* **2005**, *1276*, 285–286. [CrossRef]
10. Zhuo, W.; Furukawa, M.; Tokonami, S. A naturally ventilated accumulator for integrating measurements of radon flux from soil. *J. Nucl. Sci. Technol.* **2007**, *44*, 1100–1105. [CrossRef]
11. Hosoda, M.; Shimo, M.; Sugino, M.; Furukawa, M.; Fukushi, M. Effect of soil moisture content on radon and thoron exhalation. *J. Nucl. Sci. Technol.* **2007**, *44*, 664–672. [CrossRef]
12. Hosoda, M.; Tokonami, S.; Sorimachi, A.; Ishikawa, T.; Sahoo, S.K.; Furukawa, M.; Shiroma, Y.; Yasuoka, Y.; Janik, M.; Kavasi, N.; et al. Influence of soil environmental parameters on thoron exhalation rate. *Radiat. Prot. Dosim.* **2010**, *141*, 420–423. [CrossRef]
13. Griffiths, A.D.; Zahorowski, W.; Element, A.; Werczynski, S. A map of radon flux at the Australian land surface. *Atmos. Chem. Phys.* **2010**, *10*, 8969–8982. [CrossRef]
14. Lucchetti, C.; Briganti, A.; Castelluccio, M.; Galli, G.; Santilli, S.; Soligo, M.; Tuccimei, P. Integrating radon and thoron flux data with gamma radiation mapping in radon-prone areas. The case of volcanic outcrops in a highly-urbanized city (Roma, Italy). *J. Environ. Radioact.* **2019**, *202*, 41–50. [CrossRef] [PubMed]
15. International Commission on Radiation Units and Measurements. Report 88: Measurement and reporting of radon exposures. *J. ICRU* **2012**, *12*, 1–19.
16. Doi, M.; Fujimoto, K.; Kobayashi, S.; Yonehara, H. Spatial distribution of thoron and radon concentrations in the indoor air of a traditional Japanese wooden house. *Health Phys.* **1994**, *66*, 43–49. [CrossRef]
17. Tokonami, S. Why is ^{220}Rn (Thoron) measurement important? *Radiat. Prot. Dosim.* **2010**, *141*, 335–339. [CrossRef]
18. Tschiersch, J.; Meisenberg, O. The HMGU thoron experimental house: A new tool for exposure assessment. *Radiat. Prot. Dosim.* **2010**, *141*, 395–399. [CrossRef]
19. Hosoda, M.; Kudo, H.; Iwaoka, K.; Yamada, R.; Suzuki, T.; Tamakuma, Y.; Tokonami, S. Characteristic of thoron (^{220}Rn) in environment. *Appl. Radiat. Isot.* **2017**, *120*, 7–10. [CrossRef]
20. Tokonami, S.; Takahashi, H.; Kobayashi, Y.; Zhuo, W.; Hulber, E. Up-to-date radon-thoron discriminative detector for a large scale survey. *Rev. Sci. Instrum.* **2005**, *76*, 113505. [CrossRef]
21. Kranrod, C.; Tamakuma, Y.; Hosoda, M.; Tokonami, S. Importance of discriminative measurement for radon isotopes and its utilization in the environment and lessons learned from using the RADUET monitor. *Int. J. Environ. Res.Public Health* **2020**, *17*, 4141. [CrossRef]
22. International Organization for Standardization. *Measurement of Radioactivity in the Environment-Air-Radon 220: Integrated Measurement Methods for the Determination of the Average Activity Concentration Using Passive Solid-State Nuclear Track Detectors ISO16641*; ISO: Geneva, Switzerland, 2014.
23. Pornumpa, C.; Oyama, Y.; Iwaoka, K.; Hosoda, M.; Tokonami, S. Development of radon and thoron exposure systems at Hirosaki University. *Radiat. Environ. Med.* **2018**, *7*, 13–20.
24. Katase, A.; Matsumoto, Y.; Sakae, T.; Ishibashi, K. Indoor concentrations of ^{220}Rn and its decay products. *Health Phys.* **1988**, *54*, 283–286. [CrossRef]
25. Hirst, W.; Harrison, G.E. The diffusion of radon gas mixtures. *Proc. R. Soc. A* **1939**, *169*, 573–586.
26. Hosoda, M.; Sorimachi, A.; Yasuoka, Y.; Ishikawa, T.; Sahoo, S.K.; Furukawa, M.; Hassan, N.M.; Tokonami, S.; Uchida, S. Simultaneous measurements of radon and thoron exhalation rates and comparison with values calculated by UNSCEAR equation. *J. Radiat. Res.* **2009**, *50*, 333–343. [CrossRef] [PubMed]
27. Japanese Standards Association. *Test Methods for Particle Size Distribution of Soils JIS A 1204*; JSA: Tokyo, Japan, 2020.
28. Japanese Standards Association. *Test Methods for Density of Soil Particles JIS A 1202*; JSA: Tokyo, Japan, 2020.
29. Hosoda, M.; Nugraha, E.D.; Akata, N.; Yamada, R.; Tamakuma, Y.; Sasaki, M.; Kelleher, K.; Yoshinaga, S.; Suzuki, T.; Pornumpa Tattanapongs, C.; et al. A unique high natural background radiation area—Dose assessment and perspectives. *Sci. Total Environ.* **2021**, *750*, 142364. [CrossRef] [PubMed]
30. Tokonami, S.; Yang, M.; Yonehara, H.; Yamada, Y. Simple, discriminative measurement technique for radon and thoron concentrations with a single scintillation cell. *Rev. Sci. Instrum.* **2002**, *73*, 69–72. [CrossRef]
31. Saegusa, J.; Yamasaki, K.; Tsujimoto, T. Development of an apparatus for measuring ground exhalatin rates of ^{222}Rn and ^{220}Rn. *Environ. Int.* **1996**, *22*, 483–490. [CrossRef]
32. Ministry of Agriculture, Foresty and Fisheries. Available online: https://www.maff.go.jp/j/seisan/kankyo/hozen_type/h_sehi_kizyun/pdf/ntuti4.pdf (accessed on 24 January 2021). (In Japanese).

33. Hillei, D. General physical characteristics of soil. In *Environmental Soil Physics*; Academic Press: London, UK, 2012; pp. 3–17.
34. Kanda, Y. Investigation of the freely-available easy-to-use software "EZR" (Easy R) for medical statistics. *Bone Marrow Transplant.* **2013**, *48*, 452–458. [CrossRef]
35. Hosoda, M.; Shimo, M.; Sugino, M.; Furukawa, M.; Minami, K.; Ejiri, K. Radon and thoron exhalation rate map in Japan. *AIP Conf. Proc.* **2008**, *1034*, 177–180.
36. Zhuo, W.; Guo, Q.; Chen, B.; Chen, G. Estimating amount and distribution of radon flux density from the soil surface in China. *J. Environ. Radioact.* **2008**, *99*, 1143–1148. [CrossRef]
37. Iskander, D.; Yamazawa, H.; Iida, T. Quantification of the dependency of radon emanation power on soil temperature. *Appl. Radiat. Isot.* **2004**, *60*, 971–973. [CrossRef]
38. Zhuo, W.; Iida, T.; Furukawa, M. Modeling radon flux density from the Earth's surface. *J. Nucl. Sci. Technol.* **2006**, *43*, 479–482. [CrossRef]
39. Meteorological Data. Available online: http://www.data.jma.go.jp/obd/stats/etrn/ (accessed on 24 January 2021). (In Japanese).
40. Prasad, G.; Ishikawa, T.; Hosoda, M.; Sorimachi, A.; Sahoo, S.K.; Kavasi, N.; Tokonami, S.; Sugino, M.; Uchida, S. Seasonal and diurnal variations of radon/thoron exhalation rate in Kanto-loam area in Japan. *J. Radioanal. Nucl. Chem.* **2012**, *292*, 1385–1390. [CrossRef]

Article
A New Methodology for Defining Radon Priority Areas in Spain

Alicia Fernández, Carlos Sainz, Santiago Celaya *, Luis Quindós, Daniel Rábago and Ismael Fuente

Environmental Radioactivity Laboratory of the University of Cantabria (LaRUC), University of Cantabria, Santander, 39011 Cantabria, Spain; alicia.fernandezv@unican.es (A.F.); sainzc@unican.es (C.S.); luis.quindos@unican.es (L.Q.); daniel.rabago@unican.es (D.R.); fuentei@unican.es (I.F.)
* Correspondence: santiago.celaya@unican.es

Abstract: One of the requirements of EU-BSS (European Basic Safety Standards) is the design and implementation of a National Radon Action Plan in the member states. This should define, as accurately as possible, areas of risk for the presence of radon gas (^{222}Rn) in homes and workplaces. The concept used by the Spanish Nuclear Safety Council (CSN), the body responsible for nuclear safety and radiation protection in Spain, to identify "radon priority areas" is that of radon potential. This paper establishes a different methodology from that used by the CSN, using the same study variables (indoor radon measurements, gamma radiation exposure data, and geological information) to prepare a radon potential map that improves the definition of the areas potentially exposed to radon in Spain. The main advantage of this methodology is that by using simple data processing the definition of these areas is improved. In addition, the application of this methodology can improve the delimitation of radon priority areas and can be applied within the cartographic system used by the European Commission-Joint Research Center (EC-JRC) in the representation of different environmental parameters.

Keywords: radon potential map; geography information systems; geology; risk

1. Introduction

Numerous studies have shown that there is a clear correlation between indoor radon exposure and the risk of developing lung cancer [1,2]. Radon gas is considered to be the second leading cause of lung cancer after tobacco, and is responsible for between 3 and 14% of deaths caused by this disease in the first world [3,4] and the main source of ionizing radiation for the population [5–8].

The World Health Organization (WHO) recommended a reference level of 100 Bq/m^3 annual average radon concentration to initiate action plans to minimize health hazards due to indoor radon exposure. However, if this level cannot be reached under the country-specific conditions, the chosen reference level should not exceed 300 Bq/m^3, which represents approximately 10 mSv per year [4].

The interest in radon exposure maps is because the concentration of radon in buildings varies according to their geographical location. This variability is due to a large number of factors that affect the presence of radon indoors. These maps will be a useful instrument for applying the requirements of European legislation [5], which must be implemented in member states at all administrative levels: national, regional and local, to the radon problem. An overview of indoor radon mapping in Europe [9,10] showed the heterogeneity of the data: each country used different sampling strategies, measurement techniques, and representations of the data obtained.

In 2013, the EU-BSS (European Basic Safety Standards) required the design and implementation of National Radon Action Plans in the member states to identify areas of risk for the presence of radon gas in homes and workplaces. It establishes that the indoor radon concentration level in homes and workplaces be set at 300 Bq/m^3, and requires the radon priority areas (RPA) to be delimited. The BSS defines the RPA as an area where it is expected that in a significant number of houses the average annual radon concentration exceeds the national reference level [5].

The problem was that different interpretations of RPA were introduced in each country [11–17]. In Europe, both mapping methodologies and the definitions of RPAs are diverse [18–26].

The concept of radon potential, soil radon potential, or geogenic radon potential is used by the different member states to define and delineate the Radon Priority Areas. Projects currently under development, such as the EURAMET MetroRADON [27–29], or the European Atlas of Natural Radiation [30–35], try to homogenize concepts, mapping methodologies that permit a clear definition of these areas.

The Spanish Nuclear Safety Council (CSN) published a radon potential map in 2017 [36,37]. The concept used in Spain, and defined by the CSN to identify "radon priority areas", is that of radon potential. The CSN defines these areas using the 90th percentile to generate a cartography of the radon potential map of Spain. The variables used by CSN are the national ^{222}Rn concentration database measurements in homes, geological information (lithostratigraphies), and exposure rates to terrestrial gamma radiation.

The CSN generated the radon potential map by combining these three variables: Radon measurements in homes were grouped by lithostratigraphic unit and level of exposure to gamma radiation, and units with homogeneous radon levels were obtained from these data groups. For these units, the 90th percentile (P90) of the radon concentration distribution was considered to be a limit with higher than 90% confidence, and the units were represented by rank in 5 categories based on radon levels from the use of the 90th percentile: P90 > 400 Bq/m^3; P90 301–400 Bq/m^3; P90 201–300 Bq/m^3; P90 101–200 Bq/m^3 and P90 < 100 Bq/m^3. A radon concentration value is calculated using the 90th percentile, meaning that 90% of the values in an area are below that value, and 10% are above it. The CSN identified the areas of Spain where there are a significant percentage of homes with radon concentrations with a given probability of exceeding 300 Bq/m^3 [36,37].

This paper sets out a mapping methodology that improves the definition of radon priority areas in Spain using the same variables used by the CSN (^{222}Rn concentration measurements in homes, lithostratigraphies, and gamma radiation exposure data), but with a different approach. In addition, following the steps taken by the European Commission-Joint Research Centre (EC-JRC) in the production of the European Atlas of Natural Radiation and the European Radon Map [30–35], their reference coordinate system (the GISCO-LAEA projection) will be used and the 10 km × 10 km cell system to represent the data obtained. This cell system ensures the confidentiality of the radon samples taken in private homes and harmonizes the maps from the different countries.

2. Materials and Methods

2.1. Input Data

In order to produce a Spanish radon potential map with this new methodology, we used the following data sources:

2.1.1. Concentration of ^{222}Rn in Homes

There were 11,500 data points on radon concentration measurements throughout Spain used in the preparation of this study. These measurements are taken from the national ^{222}Rn concentration database in homes carried out in sampling campaigns between 1991 and 2016 grouped by municipalities [38]. The samples were taken inside houses, on the ground floor, and the measurements were made with track detectors (CR39) exposed for a period of three to six months.

The bulk of these 9500 measurements were collected by the University of Cantabria through different projects sponsored by CSN according to the internal location protocol of the Environmental Radioactivity Laboratory of the University of Cantabria (LaRUC), created using the indications of the CSN Safety Guide 11.01 [39]. The LaRUC Laboratory has been validated by Public Health England (PHE) since 2002 [40] and accredited since 2016 through UNE-EN ISO/IEC 17025, ENAC [41], to carry out this type of radon measurement on air. This will be the dependent variable (variable 0) in this study.

2.1.2. Gamma Radiation Exposure Data

The gamma radiation exposure data were obtained from the Natural Gamma Radiation Map (MARNA) [42]. This map assesses the rate of exposure to terrestrial gamma radiation at a height of 1 meter above the ground. It was produced by taking aerial and terrestrial measurements with a variety of analysis techniques, and these were later correlated through the MARNA project [43].

Terrestrial gamma radiation rates in Spain range from 44 to 287 nGy/h. This information is identified in 22 individualized rates. The information about the 22 terrestrial gamma radiation rates (rates of 44 at 287 nGy/h) in Spain was extracted after downloading the map image in high quality (.tiff) offered by the CSN website [42]. This will be the first independent variable (variable 1) analyzed.

2.1.3. Lithostratigraphies

The Lithostratigraphic, Permeability and Hydrogeological Map of Spain at a scale of 1:200,000 [44] produced by the Geological and Mining Institute of Spain (IGME) was used, and 329 lithostratigraphic units were analyzed. This map includes the permeability of the lithological units, homogeneously representing the lithostratigraphies and grouping them by similar permeability values. This cartography is used because numerous studies show the importance of soil permeability in determining the radon potential inside buildings [45,46]. The digital cartography was downloaded in a compatible format (.shp) with the use of Geographic Information System (GIS) programs. This will be the second independent variable (variable 2) analyzed.

2.1.4. Radon Potential

Information about radon potential in Spain was obtained after downloading the map image from the CSN website [11,36]. The 5 units shown were analyzed with homogeneous radon levels based on radon levels from the use of the 90th percentile: Unit 1 (>400 Bq/m^3), Unit 2 (301–400 Bq/m^3), Unit 3 (201–300 Bq/m^3), Unit 4 (101–200 Bq/m^3), and Unit 5 (<100 Bq/m^3). This will be the variable (variable 3) used to perform the comparison of the data obtained in this work.

2.2. General Procedure

2.2.1. Framework

A Geographical Information System program (ESRI ArcGis v. 10.0, Environmental Systems Research Institute: Redlands, CA, USA) [47] was used to produce the cartography for this paper. The KaleidaGraph v. 4.1 (Synergy Software: PA, USA) [48] program was used to analyze the data obtained and to make graphs.

To follow a similar scheme to other EU member countries, we began working with a continental level projection system (GISCO-LAEA), and defined the European working area with a 10 km × 10 km grid with established limits (coordinates) as suggested by the Joint Research Centre of the European Commission EC-JRC [30,33]. To define the Spanish working area, we used the administrative boundaries provided by the National Geographic Institute [49], generating a total of 5478 cells of 10 km × 10 km. For each cell, an identifying code was created and its centroid in meters ("x" and "y" coordinates) was calculated.

2.2.2. Harmonization of Input Data

The formats in which the source information for these variables appears are different, and so it was necessary to harmonize this information to later process the data:

Concentration of ^{222}Rn in Homes

The radon concentration variable was analyzed using the 11,500 data points obtained in the various measurement campaigns mentioned above. This information was stored in the GIS database and transferred to the 10 km × 10 km cell system: the transposition of the values into the cell system was performed by calculating the arithmetic mean of the radon concentration points data (in Bq/m^3) contained in each 10 km × 10 km cell. This variable therefore contains information on 5478 fields in its attribute table, corresponding to the average radon concentration (in Bq/m^3) for each of the 5478 Spanish cells. The decision to use the arithmetic mean was taken because the EC-JRC suggested it in the European Radon Atlas [30–35] as the most appropriate parameter in the representation of this variable, due to the great variability of the concentrations obtained per 10 km × 10 km cell and because it is used in most epidemiological studies.

Exposure Rate to Terrestrial Gamma Radiation, Lithostratigraphy and Radon Potential

The information about the Spanish lithostratigraphic units was downloaded in a shape format, and so we worked with geological data of the 329 polygons and the attribute table of lithostratigraphic units provided by IGME. The data for the rates of exposure to terrestrial gamma radiation and radon potential in Spain were downloaded in a high-quality image format. These images were georeferenced to the Spanish administrative boundaries, and its polygons were later digitized in as much detail as possible (at an approximate scale of between 1:3000 and 1:5000): the 5 units with homogeneous radon level were digitized as 5 polygons, assigning them their value in Bq/m^3. There were 22 terrestrial gamma radiation rates digitized as 22 polygons, assigning them their value in nGy/h. A noteworthy fact is that there are no data on exposure to terrestrial gamma radiation for the Balearic Islands or the Canary Islands, so this variable could not be taken into account when conducting the study in these areas.

As mentioned above, each of these variables in shape format contains the graphical unit/polygon (field) information stored in its attribute table, with each field being a record with information about the typology of the element or surface coverage to be analyzed (it is a homogeneous category of information). For the subsequent data analysis, it was necessary to calculate, for each variable, which was the unit or field (polygon) with the largest surface area contained in each 10 km × 10 km cell. To do this, the cell system was intersected with the variables gamma radiation, lithostratigraphies and radon potential, and the surface of the majority field was calculated in each one. In this way, each 10 km × 10 km cell was assigned the value of the field with the highest probability of occurrence in those 100 km^2.

2.2.3. Data Processing

The data processing was different for the input data depending on the origin of the source information: for the dependent variable (concentration of ^{222}Rn in homes) the arithmetic mean data of the radon concentration points (in Bq/m^3) contained in each 10 km × 10 km cell was transferred to the cell system. The data for the independent variables (exposure rate to terrestrial gamma radiation and lithostratigraphy), and the data for performing the comparison of the data and validating the study results (CSN radon potential) were transferred to the cell system by the generation of density maps.

The methodology of the density map creation process is shown in Figure 1 and is as follows:

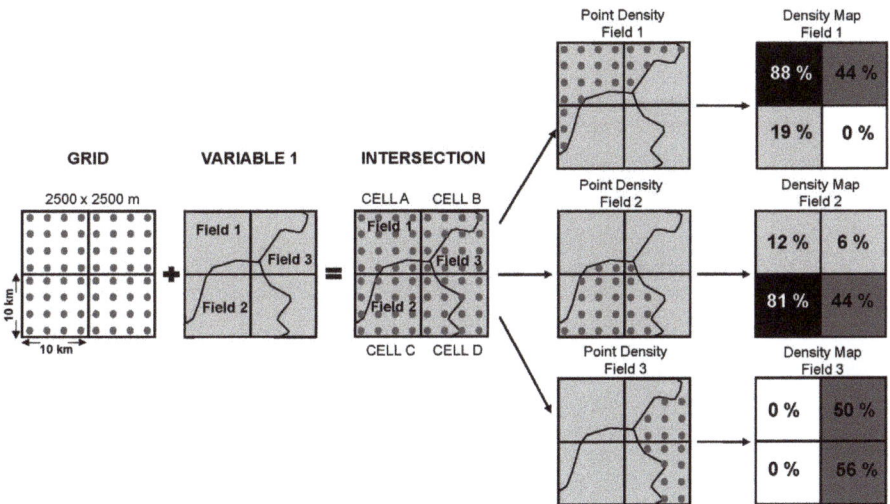

Figure 1. Diagram of the methodology for creating the density maps.

The first step was to create a 2500 m × 2500 m dot mesh on each side, fitted to the limits of the 10 km × 10 km cells in Spain. This meant that each cell was covered homogeneously by a total of 16 points. This dot mesh allowed the extraction, for each 10 km × 10 km cell, of the points contained in each field of the study variables. The process was carried out by intersecting the dot mesh with each of the previously selected fields; in this way a series of layers were created that indicated the density of points per 10 km × 10 km cell: the minimum value (0) corresponded to the absence of that field in that cell, and the maximum value (16) was related to the total presence of that field in that cell. Thus, 22-point layers related to variable 1 (exposure rate to terrestrial gamma radiation), 329-point layers were associated with variable 2 (lithostratigraphies), and 5-point layers were created for variable 3 (CSN radon potential). Density maps were generated with each of these point layers, and fitted the limits of the 10 km × 10 km cells from the point density tool [50].

Once the density maps of each variable were generated, the relationship between the dependent variable (concentration of ^{222}Rn in homes) and the independent variables (exposure rate to terrestrial gamma radiation and lithostratigraphy) was analyzed. In previous steps, the centroid ("x" and "y" coordinates) of the 5478 cells 10 km × 10 km had been calculated, and an identification code added to each of them. Using the extract-by-points tool, the radon concentration value transferred to the cell system (dependent variable) was extracted. In the same way, with this tool, the value of the gamma rate information was extracted for each of the cells of the 22 density maps related to the fields of variable 1. The same procedure was carried out with the 329 fields of variable 2, extracting the information from the lithostratigraphic typology.

Using the data extracted, a simple linear correlation analysis was performed to check the positive or negative relationship between the two parameters for each cell. For example, in a cell with code 1 the Pearson correlation coefficient (R) of the average radon concentration is calculated, and so is the exposure rate to terrestrial gamma radiation with the field 44 nGy/h, for that same cell, the field 88 nGy/h and so on for each field of each variable. The degree of adjustment was quantified through the Pearson correlation coefficient (R), giving for each of the correlations, a value between −1 and +1. The data of these correlations were normalized into 9 categories: value 1 R > +0.75, value 2 (R +0.74 to +0.5), value 3 (R +0.49 to +0.25), value 4 (R +0.24 to +0.1), value 5 (R = 0), value 6 (R −0.1 to −0.24), value 7 (R −0.25 to −0.49), value 8 (R −0.50 to −0.74), and value 9 (R < −0.75). This grouping into ranges of values facilitated the process of representing the correlations obtained between the radon concentration with respect to exposure to gamma radiation and lithostratigraphy.

2.3. Development of the Relationship Maps between Independent Variables and the ^{222}Rn Concentration in Homes and the New Radon Potential Map

For the variable terrestrial gamma radiation exposure rate, the data were represented graphically using the cell system, which gathers the 22 fields into 5 categories, defined by their radon concentrations: 44 nGy/h correspond to 100 Bq/m^3 and 89 nGy/h with 300 Bq/m^3 [51]. The correlations obtained between the radon concentrations with respect to exposure to gamma radiation were represented graphically in 9 categories according to the ranges mentioned above. Similarly, the lithostratigraphy variable was represented graphically in the cell system, bringing together the 329 lithostratigraphic fields of the Iberian Peninsula, the Balearic Islands, and the Canary Islands. The correlations obtained between the radon concentrations with respect to the lithostratigraphies were also represented graphically in 9 categories.

From these two correlation maps, a new radon potential map (Radon Potential Map Calculated) was generated. The sum of the categories of both maps was represented on this calculated map, and so the numerical range of each cell was between 1 and 18: Values from 13 to 18 indicate a positive linear relationship with radon and therefore a high probability of finding high concentrations. Values from 8 to 12 indicate the absence of a relationship and therefore an average probability of finding high concentrations. Values from 1 to 7 indicate a negative linear relationship with radon and therefore a low probability of finding high concentrations.

To facilitate the interpretation of the results, and to represent the data according to their possible radon concentration range, the values were reclassified into 5 categories: Category 1 (>400 Bq/m^3), Category 2 (301–400 Bq/m^3), Category 3 (201–300 Bq/m^3), Category 4 (101–200 Bq/m^3), and Category 5 (<100 Bq/m^3). The equivalences applied to the entire process are shown in Table 1 below:

Table 1. Equivalences and data grouping by ranges of values.

^{222}Rn Concentration (Bq/m^3)	Calculated Potential Radon Map (Value)	Pearson's Correlation Coefficient (R)	Lithostratigraphies and Terrestrial Gamma Radiation Rates Intersections Value (Value)
>400	18 to 14	>+0.75	9
301–400	13 to 10	+0.74 to +0.26	7 to 8
201–300	9 to 7	+0.25 to −0.25	6 to 4
101–200	6 to 4	−0.26 to −0.74	3 to 2
<100	3 to 1	<−0.75	1

The methodology used to evaluate the results was as follows: the success or failure capacity per 10 km × 10 km cell was compared for each of the variables analyzed (^{222}Rn concentration measurements in homes, exposure rate to terrestrial gamma radiation and lithostratigraphies), from both the CSN P90 Radon Potential Map and the Radon Potential Calculated Map. It was considered a success if a cell was in the same concentration or range of values (see Table 1 equivalences) and it was considered a failure if the cell was not a match.

3. Results

3.1. Analysis of Variables

3.1.1. Concentration of ^{222}Rn in Homes

Regarding the concentration of ^{222}Rn in homes, the 11,500 data points on the concentration of ^{222}Rn in air were analyzed using as a starting point the central trend measures and dispersion, and according to the shape of the distribution sample. Table 2 offers the updated data regarding previous publications [52,53] showing the main parameters obtained:

Table 2. Statistics on radon concentration data for Spain.

	Number of Measurements	Arithmetic Mean (Bq/m^3)	Arithmetic Standard Deviation	Geometric Mean (Bq/m^3)	Geometric Standard Deviation	1-st Quartile (Bq/m^3)	Median (Bq/m^3)	3-rd Quartile (Bq/m^3)	Range (Bq/m^3)	Skewness	Kurtosis
Spain	11,500	101	260.6	58	2.6	30	56	110	10–15,400	31.5	1497

The central trend measures show that the data do not follow a normal distribution, since the arithmetic mean (101 Bq/m^3) is far from the median (56 Bq/m^3). Furthermore, the standard deviation of the arithmetic mean is 260.6 Bq/m^3, which shows a high dispersion of the data.

Analysis of the shape of the sample distribution shows a high coefficient of kutorsis (K = 1497), indicating a leptokurtic distribution, whereas the asymmetry coefficient (CS = 31.5) indicates a positive asymmetry: The distribution of measurements is log-normal. The distribution of measurements is log-normal, as shown in the histogram (Figure 2). This distribution is usual for radon concentration measurements since most of the measurements obtained are in low concentrations, whereas only a few measurements appear in the high concentration range.

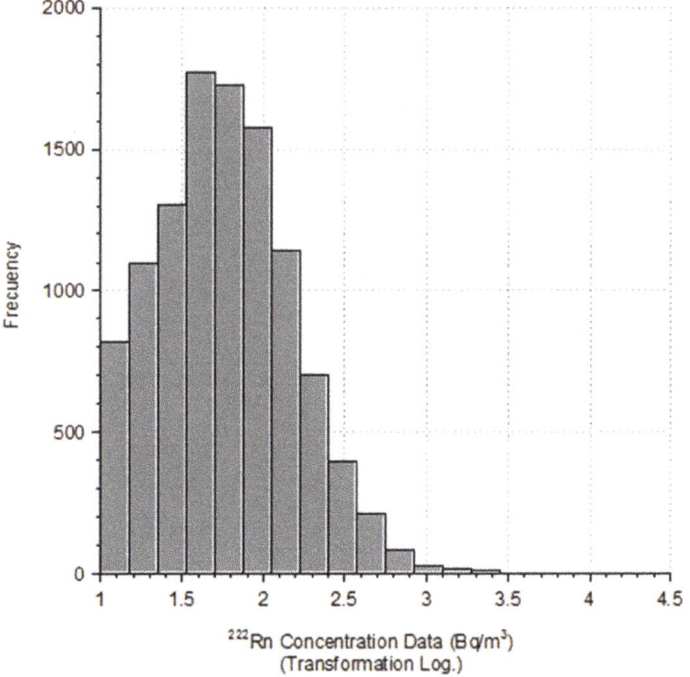

Figure 2. Histogram of the radon concentration data.

Analyzing these 11,500 data points, it is seen that 27% of the samples exceed the level of 100 Bq/m^3 to initiate action plans (5% of the measurements exceed 300 Bq/m^3 and 22% are in the range of between 100 and 300 Bq/m^3).

On transposing these data to the cell system, it is seen (Table 3) that the majority (76%) are in the range of low concentrations (<100 Bq/m^3), 22% between 100–300 Bq/m^3, and that the percentage of cells in high concentrations (>300 Bq/m^3) is reduced to 2%.

Table 3. Mean concentration of ^{222}Rn and number of measurements per 10 × 10 cell.

^{222}Rn Concentration Arithmetic Mean (A.M) (Bq/m^3)	No of 10 km × 10 km Cells (%)	No of Measurements per Cell (Average)	1 Measurements (%)	2 to 6 Measurements (%)	>6 Measurements (%)
>400	1	3.9	32	52	16
301–400	1	4.2	34	45	21
201–300	4	5.2	37	40	23
101–200	18	4.9	37	42	21
<100	76	2.8	50	41	9

It is also clear that the sampling in Spain is not heterogeneous, since there are areas where the measurement density is much higher than others; this is because the sampling in Spain was defined based on a series of criteria that concentrated the number of measurements in areas with potentially high radon concentrations. The decision of how many measurements to be carried out in each 10 km × 10 km cell was made by the CSN, taking into account the general objectives established by the EC-JRC in the creation of the European Radon Map, considering superficial, population and lithostratigraphic criteria, and according to the rate of exposure to terrestrial gamma radiation [51,52].

Despite efforts to try to cover the entire country with at least one measurement per 10 km × 10 km cell, it can be seen that a large part of its surface does not have any measurements (40%). Of the cells for which measurements are available, it is representative that a large percentage of Spain is covered with only one measurement (47%) or with two measurements (19%), whereas cells with more than 6 measurements represent 15% of the total.

Analyzing cell percentage according to concentration category and measurements, it is seen that 68% of cells with concentrations greater than 400 Bq/m^3 have more than two measurements (in 52% of cases from 2 to 6 measurements, and in 16% more than 6 measurements), and that in the concentration range between 301 and 400 Bq/m^3 this percentage of cells is also high (66%). The percentage is slightly lower for the intermediate concentrations (101–300 Bq/m^3) where 63% of cells have more than 2 measurements. Low concentrations (<100 Bq/m^3), despite being the most numerous category, is the one with the fewest measurements. Half of its cells have a single measurement, reducing the number of cells with more than 6 measurements to 9%.

It is clear that as the number of measurements per cell increases, the concentration ranges are better defined.

3.1.2. Exposure Rate to Terrestrial Gamma Radiation

From the analysis of the rates of exposure to terrestrial gamma radiation (Figure 3a), 95% of the peninsula is found to have medium and low rates: 2% of the country is below 44 nGy/h, and 93% between 45 and 122 nGy/h. The areas with rates higher than 122 nGy/h are few (5%), and are mainly in the northwest area of the peninsula and in the Central System. In these areas, there is a clear correspondence between the presence of high radon concentrations and high rates of gamma exposure [43,54].

Analyzing the data of this variable with respect to radon concentrations (Figure 3b), a positive linear relationship is observed between the two parameters starting at 78 nGy/h, the relationship becoming clearer in the case of the identified areas of high rates. These areas correspond once again to those previously mentioned, along with areas of the Catalan Coastal Cordillera and the Pyrenees, corroborating the correspondence of high radon concentrations and high rates of gamma exposure.

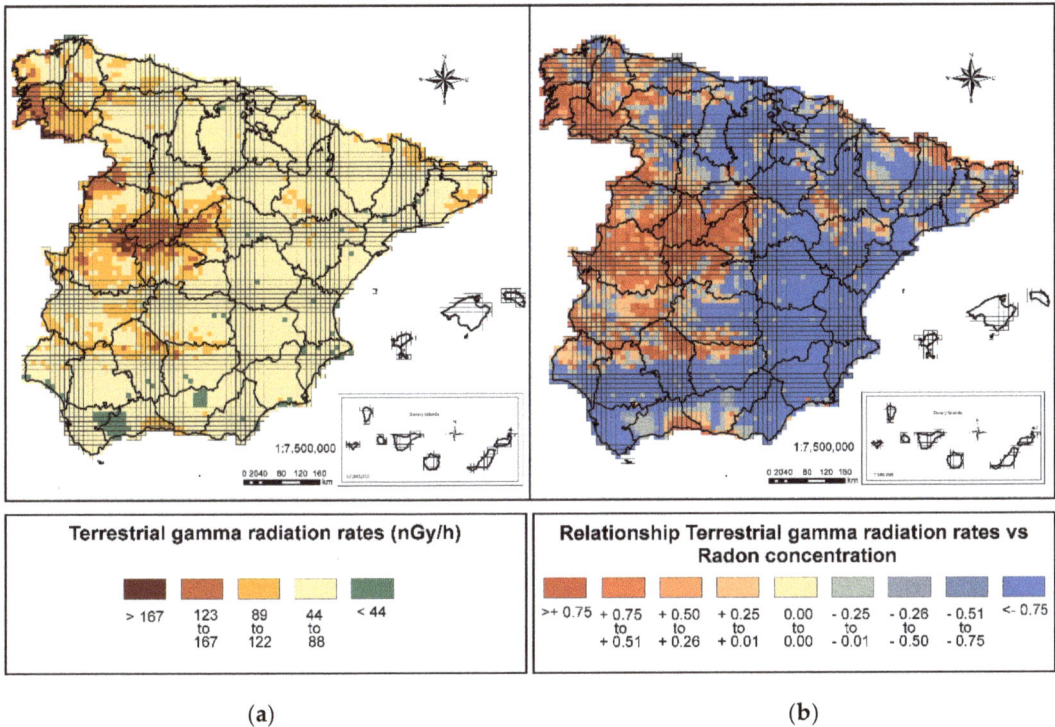

Figure 3. (a) Figure Terrestrial gamma radiation rates (nGy/h) and (b) Relationship between terrestrial gamma radiation rates and radon concentration.

3.1.3. Lithostratigraphies

Regarding the lithostratigraphy variable, it is known that the main indicator in determining a higher or lower probability of high concentrations of radon in an area is the presence of uranium in soils and rocks, for which reason the lithological formations with a high proportion of uranium will generate a high proportion of radium and therefore a higher proportion of radon. In general, the highest uranium values (>2.88 ppm) [55], are associated with acidic intrusive plutonic rocks such as granites.

The analysis of lithostratigraphies (Figure 4a) in Spain suggests that the geologies most commonly found in Spain are acidic plutonic rocks such as granites, granodiorites, and quartz diorites (8% of the territory). Due to the large number of lithostratigraphies present in Spain, the legend of this figure only shows the most numerous (more than 2% of the territory), the complete legend is available in the IGME [56]. It is also noteworthy that 4% of the territory is made up of slates and greywacke. Both shales (metamorphic rocks produced by silt-clay sedimentary rocks) and greywacke (detrital sedimentary rocks derived from the dismantling of acidic plutonic rocks) generally also have high uranium content [43].

In the areas where these two formations are present, there may be a high probability of finding high radon concentrations, which was confirmed after performing the correlation analyses of the two variables.

The results of the relation between lithostratigraphies and radon concentrations (Figure 4b) show that 100 lithostratigraphies show a positive relationship. The clearest relation (>+0.75) appears in a single case, in the geologies corresponding to acidic, Hercynian plutonic rocks (granites, granodiorites, quartz diorites). It has been confirmed that this geology is associated with a high presence of radon.

In addition, six other lithostratigraphies show a marked relationship with the presence of high radon concentrations (between +0.51 and +0.75), representing another 8% of the peninsular surface. They mainly correspond to metamorphic rocks such as shales, gneiss, schists, or quartzites (these are rocks with high concentrations of uranium) [43] and detrital sedimentary rocks such as greywacke derived from acidic plutonic rocks.

On analyzing the geographical distribution of these areas, it is seen that they correspond to the northwest area of the peninsula and the area of the Central System. A close relationship is also observed with the geological formations in the west of the peninsula and their extension towards Sierra Morena, specific areas of the Pyrenean Range, and in the area of the Catalan Coastal Cordilleras.

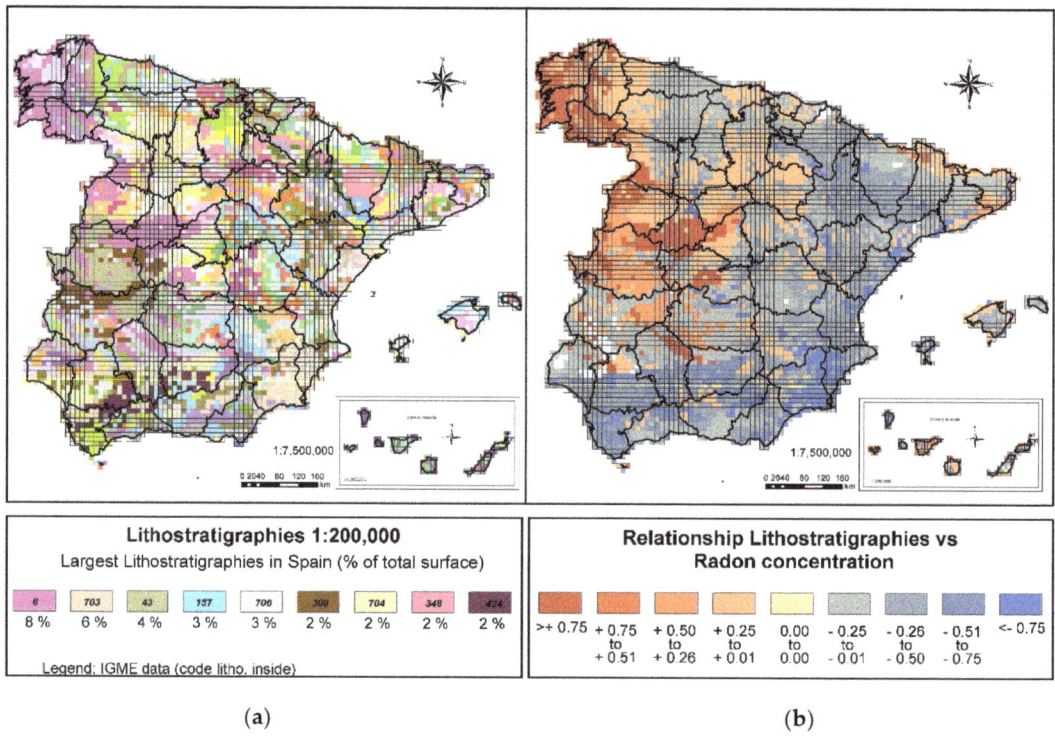

Figure 4. (a) Figure Lithostratigraphies 1:200,000 and (b) Figure Relationship lithostratigraphies and radon concentration.

3.2. Comparison of Radon Potential Maps Generated

As shown in Figure 5, where the P90 Radon Potential Map generated by the CSN (hereafter P90 Potential Map) and the Radon Potential Map Calculated in the present study are compared, both maps show a similar percentage of cells in the range of radon concentrations greater than 400 Bq/m^3 (17% in the case of the Calculated Map and 16% in the P90 Potential Map). In both maps, the areas defined in this range correspond once again to the northwest of the peninsula, the Central System area, the west of the peninsula extending towards Sierra Morena, south of the Pyrenees, and in the area of the Catalan Coastal Cordilleras.

The increase in the weight of the cells with concentrations between 301 Bq/m^3 and 400 Bq/m^3 is significant: it goes from 2% in the P90 Potential Map to 19% in the case of the Calculated Map. As will be seen later, the calculation of this new zoning fits possible radon concentrations more reliably. It is mainly seen in the west of the peninsula surrounding the highest concentrations. The area of Sierra Morena up to the border with Portugal is also clearly defined in this range, and in some areas to the north of the peninsula, areas of the Penibaetic System or areas to the west of the Ebro valley.

Both maps have a similar percentage of cells in the concentration range between 201–300 Bq/m^3 (20% in the case of the Calculated Map and 21% in the P90 Potential Map). However, analyzing Figure 4 shows changes in zoning: in the CSN P90 Potential Map these areas were defined as mainly bordering the areas of greater concentrations in the west of the peninsula and certain areas in the south of the Ebro valley, while with the Calculated Map these areas are mainly found in the south of the Iberian System and the south of the Ebro valley.

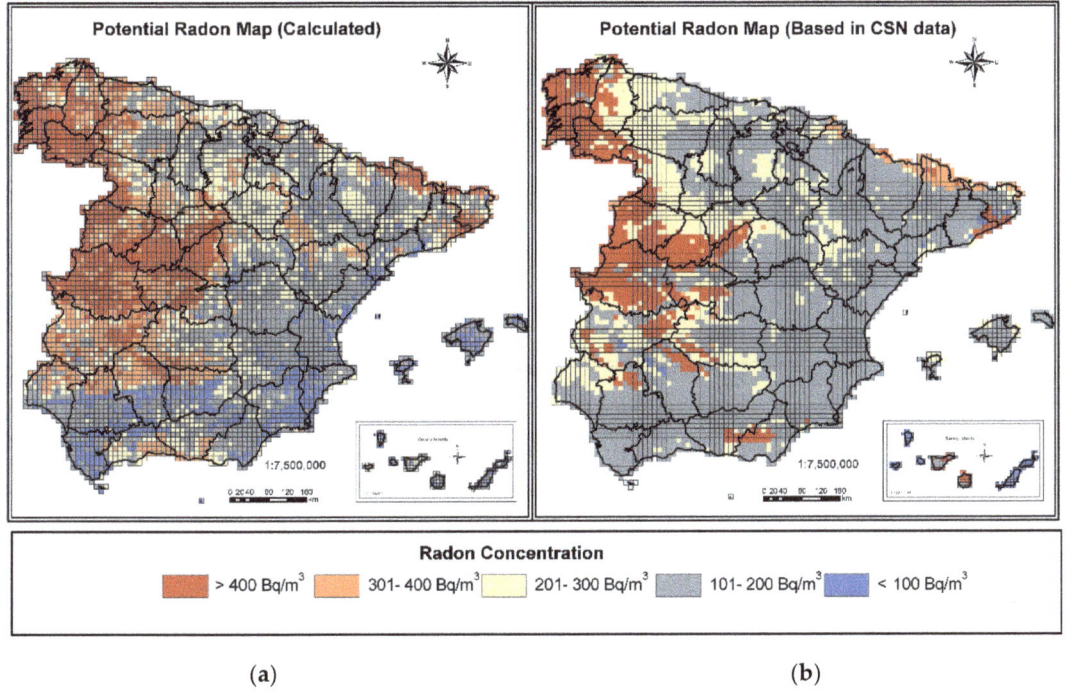

Figure 5. Potential Radon Map. (**a**) Calculated Map and (**b**) Map based on Spanish Nuclear Safety Council (CSN) data.

The most significant change occurs in the cells between 101 and 200 Bq/m^3, where it drops from 59% in the case of the P90 Potential Map to 35% in the Calculated Map. The reduction is this percentage is accompanied by a large group of the cells located in this category switching, on the Calculated Map, to the range between 301–400 Bq/m^3 and cells of less than 100 Bq/m^3.

Regarding the range of cells with concentrations below 100 Bq/m^3, an increase in the number of cells is observed, going from 2% on the P90 Potential Map to 7% on the Calculated Map. This increase in cells is due to a large number of the cells identified in the CSN map as in the range between 101–200 Bq/m^3 having moved to this range of lower concentrations. The area in this category lies mainly in the south of Spain in the Guadalquivir Valley and the Levante.

3.3. Assessment of the Degree of Identification of the Maps

To quantify the degree of identification of the Radon Potential Calculated Map with respect to radon concentrations, the cells are analyzed, identifying for each variable the percentage of failures or successes in each of the ranges. Table 4 reflects the degree of identification of each of the study variables.

Table 4. Degree of identification between the variables of the maps Potential Radon Map Calculated and P90 CSN.

^{222}Rn Concentration A.M (Bq/m^3)	Success (%)	Failure (%)	Gamma Radiation Rate (nGy/h)	Success (%)	Failure (%)	Lithostratigraphies 1:200,000 (Class)	Success (%)	Failure (%)
Radon Potential Calculated Map
>400	68	32	>167	90	10	9	96	4
301–400	20	80	123–167	8	92	8, 7	36	64
201–300	15	85	89–122	3	97	6, 5, 4	27	73
101–200	15	85	45–88	41	59	3, 2	65	35
<100	11	89	<48	0	100	1	80	20
	12	86		32	68		47	53
Radon Potential Map P90 CSN
>400	64	36	>167	53	47	9	89	11
301–400	3	97	123–167	2	98	8, 7	0	100
201–300	30	70	89–122	31	69	6, 5, 4	31	69
101–200	37	63	45–88	72	28	3, 2	91	9
<100	2	98	<48	0	100	1	0	100
	10	90		57	38		47	53

3.3.1. Degree of Identification Regarding Radon Concentrations

Regarding radon concentrations, both maps show a high capacity to identify cells with concentrations greater than 400 Bq/m^3, but the Calculated Potential Map improves the data obtained with respect to the P90 Potential Map: it returns 68% correct identification of these areas compared to 64%.

The increase in the identification capacity of the Calculated Potential Map in areas with concentrations between 301–400 Bq/m^3 is of special interest, from 20% to 3% reported by potential radon map CSN, Directive 2013/59/Euratom sets the first value as a reference level to be considered when devising National Action Plans against radon gas in order to define Radon Priority Areas that, with the proposed method, becomes easier to define.

In the intermediate concentration ranges, the identification capacity of the P90 Potential Map is superior to that of the Calculated Potential Map: In the range 201–300 Bq/m^3 and 101–200 Bq/m^3 it identifies appropriately 30% and 37% of the cells. The Calculated Potential Map correctly identifies 15% of cases.

The greater capacity of identification of the P90 Potential Map in these ranges of mean concentrations is mainly due to the scarcity of measurements made in these areas. As previously shown, a higher sampling density per cell more precisely defines the concentrations, and many of the cells identified as having average concentrations would move to another range of concentrations as the number of measurements in them increases. This greater identification capacity is also due to the fact that the CSN map assigned a high weight to the gamma radiation variable, while when creating the Calculated Potential Map, the weight of the variables was homogenized.

In the lower concentration ranges, the identification capacity of the Calculated Potential Map improves to 12% as against 3% of the P90 Potential Map.

3.3.2. Degree of Identification Regarding the Rates of Exposure to Terrestrial Gamma Radiation

Regarding the rates of exposure to terrestrial gamma radiation, the P90 Potential Map has a greater capacity of identification (57%) as compared to the Calculated Potential Map (32%). However, when analyzing the different ranges in detail, it is found that this reduction in global accuracy is mainly due to low identification in the cells corresponding to the average rates (between 45 nGy/h and 122 nGy/h), because the data on radon concentration in this grid is limited. On the other hand, the increase in the identification of cells with higher rates is notable: in cells with more than 167 nGy/h the level of identification increases to 90%, and in cells between 123 nGy/h and 167 nGy/h it rises to 8%.

3.3.3. Degree of Identification Regarding the Lithostratigraphies

With respect to lithostratigraphies, both maps correctly identify 47% of the cells. The differences emerge when analyzing the different classes associated with concentrations.

In the cells corresponding to lithostratigraphies associated with concentrations of more than 400 Bq/m^3 (Class 9), the Calculated Potential Map increases identification to 96% as against 89% of the P90 Potential Map.

It is of particular interest that the Calculated Potential Map correctly identifies 36% of the cells associated with Classes 7 and 8 (lithostratigraphies linked to radon concentrations between 301 Bq/m^3 and 400 Bq/m^3), since the CSN map does not have the capacity to identify these areas. Again, Directive 2013/59/Euratom sets the value 300 Bq/m^3 as the reference level for producing National Action Plans against radon gas.

The identification of cells associated with concentrations between 201 Bq/m^3 and 300 Bq/m^3 (Classes 4, 5 and 6) is similar in both maps: 27% in the case of the Calculated Potential Map and 31% of the P90 Potential Map.

The identification capacity of the Calculated Potential Map drops to 65% compared to 91% of the P90 Potential Map in Class 2 and 3 cells (lithostratigraphies associated with concentrations between 101 Bq/m^3 and 200 Bq/m^3). This is due to the existence of lithostratigraphies that were previously identified with intermediate concentrations, but now have come to be placed in the category of low concentrations: in Class 1 (lithostratigraphies associated with radon concentrations of less than 100 Bq/m^3) the Calculated Potential Map has an accuracy of 80% as opposed to the null capacity of the P90 Potential Map.

4. Conclusions

In conclusion, it has been shown that:

- The Calculated Potential Map correctly identifies 12% of the cells in terms of the probability of finding a radon concentration in a given area, improving the percentage of the P90 Potential Map (which correctly identifies 10% of the cells).
- Regarding the probability of finding an exposure rate to terrestrial gamma radiation associated with a radon concentration, the P90 Potential Map properly identifies 57% of the cells, while the Calculated Potential Map identifies 32% of the cells. This is because when making the map, the CSN gave great weight to this variable, whereas when making the Calculated Potential Map, the weight of the study variables was homogenized.
- Regarding the probability of finding lithostratigraphies related to the greater or lesser presence of radon, both maps correctly identify 47% of the cells. In general, it is seen that the Calculated Radon Potential Map improves the identification of cells in terms of the probability of finding a radon concentration associated with a type of lithostratigraphy, since it homogenizes the ability to place a type correctly in all concentration ranges. Its identification capacity is markedly better in the ranges of higher concentrations (>300 Bq/m^3) and lower concentrations (<100 Bq/m^3).
- The Calculated Radon Potential Map in this study prepared from joining together the correlation maps shows that in 36% of the country there is a probability of finding radon concentrations higher than 300 Bq/m^3 (17% above 400 Bq/m^3 and 19% between 301 Bq/m^3 and 400 Bq/m^3). With this map, the areas of Spain with probable high radon concentrations (more than 300 Bq/m^3) are precisely defined.

The map also identifies the areas with a probability of finding radon concentrations of between 100 Bq/m^3 and 300 Bq/m^3 more reliably, by homogenizing the weights of the variables. This range of concentrations is also of particular interest, as the WHO designates 100 Bq/m^3 as the recommended reference level to start action plans against radon gas.

Author Contributions: Conceptualization, A.F., C.S., and L.Q.; methodology, A.F., C.S., S.C., L.Q., D.R., and I.F.; software, A.F.; validation, A.F.; formal analysis, A.F., C.S., and L.Q.; investigation, A.F., C.S., S.C., L.Q., D.R., and I.F.; writing—original draft preparation, A.F., C.S., and L.Q.; writing—review and editing, A.F., C.S., and L.Q.; visualization, A.F. All authors have read and agreed to the published version of the manuscript.

Funding: This research received no external funding.

Institutional Review Board Statement: Not applicable.

Informed Consent Statement: Not applicable.

Data Availability Statement: The data presented in this study are available in article.

Conflicts of Interest: The authors declare no conflict of interest.

References

1. Tirmarche, M.; Harrison, J.D.; Laurier, D.; Paquet, F.; Blanchardon, E.J.M.; International Commission on Radiological Protection (ICRP). *Lung Cancer Risk from Radon and Progeny and Statement on Radon*; ICRP Publication 115, Ann. ICRP; Elsevier: Exeter, UK, 2010; Volume 40, ISBN 978-0-7020-4977-4. [CrossRef]
2. Lecomte, J.F.; Solomon, S.; Takala, J.; Jung, T.; Strand, P.; Murith, C.; Kiselev, S.; Zhuo, W.; Shannoun, F.; Janssens, A.; et al. *Radiological Protection against Radon Exposure*; ICRP Publication 126, Ann ICRP; SAGE Publications: London, UK, 2014; Volume 43, pp. 5–73, ISBN 978-14-7-3s91658-6.
3. International Atomic Energy Agency (IAEA). *Radiation Protection and Safety of Radiation Sources: International Basic Safety Standards*; General Safety Requirements Part 3, Interim Edition; International Atomic Energy Agency: Vienna, Austria, 2014; ISBN 978-92-0-120910-8.
4. World Health Organization (WHO). *WHO Handbook on Indoor Radon: A Public Health Perspective*; Zeeb, H., Shannoun, F., Eds.; WHO Library Cataloguing in Publication Data; World Health Organization: Geneva, Switzerland, 2009; ISBN 978-92-4-154767-3.
5. *Council Directive (2013/59/Euratom) on Basic Safety Standards for Protection against the Dangers arising from Exposure to Ionising Radiation of 5 December*; European Commission (EC): Luxembourg, 2013.
6. *Commission Recommendation (90/143/Euratom) on the Protection of the Public against Indoor Exposure to Radon of 21 February 1990*; European Commission (EC): Luxembourg, 1990.
7. Council Directive (96/29/Euratom). *Laying Down Basic Safety Standards for the Protection of Health of Workers and the General Public against the Danger Arising from Ionizing Radiation*; European Commission (EC): Luxembourg, 1996.
8. International Commision on Radiological Protection (ICRP). *Human Respiratory Tract Model for Radiological Protection*; ICRP publication 66, Ann. ICRP; Pergamon: Ottawa, ON, Canada, 1994; Volume 24.
9. Dubois, G. *An Overview of Radon Surveys in Europe*; Report EUR21892; EC, Office for Official Publications of the European Communities: Luxembourg, 2005; ISBN 92-79-01066-2.
10. Pantelić, G.; Čeliković, I.; Živanović, M.; Vukanac, I.; Nikolić, J.K.; Cinelli, G.; Gruber, V. Qualitative overview of indoor radon surveys in Europe. *J. Environ. Radioat.* **2019**, *204*, 163–174. [CrossRef]
11. Spanish Nuclear Safety Council (CSN). Natural Radiation Maps. Viewer: Spanish Radon Potential Map. 2017. Available online: https://www.csn.es/mapa-del-potencial-de-radon-en-espana (accessed on 30 June 2020).
12. Federal Office for Radiation Protection (BfS) Viewer: Radon Potential Mapping. Available online: https://www.bfs.de/EN/topics/ion/environment/radon/maps/soil-air.html (accessed on 9 November 2020).
13. Institute for Radiological Protection and Nuclear Safety (IRSN) Viewer: Radon Potential Mapping. Available online: https://www.irsn.fr/FR/connaissances/Environnement/expertises-radioactivite-naturelle/radon/Pages/5-cartographie-potentiel-radon-commune.aspx#.X6kGZ_NKiM8 (accessed on 9 November 2020).
14. Public Health England (PHE) Viewer: Radon Map. Available online: https://www.ukradon.org/information/ukmaps (accessed on 9 November 2020).
15. Austrian Agency for Health and Food Safety Ltd. (AGES) Viewer: Radon Potential Mapping. Available online: https://geogis.ages.at/GEOGIS_RADON.html (accessed on 9 November 2020).
16. Federal Agency for Nuclear Control (FANC) Viewer: Radon Potential Mapping. Available online: https://fanc.maps.arcgis.com/apps/Viewer/index.html?appid=015b627fde334c15a28e5f71d0e4011e (accessed on 9 November 2020).
17. Environmental Protection Agency of Ireland. (EPA) Viewer: Radon Map. Available online: https://www.epa.ie/radiation/radonmap/ (accessed on 9 November 2020).
18. Talavera, G.M.; Pérez, G.A.; Rey, C.; Ramos, L. Mapping radon-prone areas using radiation dose rate and geological information. *J. Radiol. Prot.* **2013**, *33*, 605–620. [CrossRef]
19. Bossew, P. Radon Priority Areas. Definition, estimation and uncertainty. *Nucl. Techn. Radiat. Prot.* **2018**, *33*, 286–292. [CrossRef]
20. Bossew, P.; Cinelli, G.; Ciotoli, G.; Crowley, Q.G.; de Cort, M.; Medina, J.E.; Gruber, V.; Petermann, E.; Tollefsen, T. Development of a Geogenic Radon Hazard Index. Concept, History, Experiences. *Int. J. Environ. Res. Public Health* **2020**, *17*, 4134. [CrossRef] [PubMed]

21. Ielsch, G.; Cushing, M.E.; Combes, P.; Cuney, M. Mapping of the geogenic radon potential in France to improve radon risk management: Methodology and first applications to region Bourgogne. *J. Environ. Radioact.* **2010**, *101*, 813–820. [CrossRef] [PubMed]
22. Ielsch, G.; Cuney, M.; Buscail, F.; Rossi, F.; Leon, A.; Cushing, M.E. Estimation and mapping of uranium content of geological units in France. *J. Environ. Radioact.* **2017**, *166*, 210–219. [CrossRef] [PubMed]
23. Miles, J.C.H.; Appleton, J.D.; Rees, D.M.; Green, B.M.R.; Adlam, K.A.M.; Myers, A.H. Indicative Atlas of Radon in England and Wales. In *Health Protection Agency and British Geological Survey*; Health Protection Agency: Chilton, UK, 2007; ISBN 978-0-85951-608-2.
24. Bochicchio, F.; Campos-Venuti, G.; Piermattei, S.; Nuccetelli, C.; Risica, S.; Tommasino, L.; Torri, G.; Magnoni, M.; Agnesod, G.; Sgorbati, G.; et al. Annual average and seasonal variations of residential radon concentration for all the Italian Regions. *Radiat. Meas.* **2005**, *40*, 686–694. [CrossRef]
25. Cafaro, C.; Bossew, P.; Giovani, C.; Garavaglia, M. Definition of radon prone areas in Friuli Venezia Giulia region, Italy, using geostatistical tools. *J. Environ. Radioact.* **2014**, *138*, 208–219. [CrossRef] [PubMed]
26. Dowdall, A.; Murphy, P.; Pollard, D.; Fenton, D. Update of Ireland's national average indoor radon concentration. Application of a new survey protocol. *J. Environ. Radioact.* **2016**, *169–170*, 1–8. [CrossRef]
27. Metro RADON—Metrology for Radon Monitoring. Available online: http://metroradon.eu/ (accessed on 20 April 2020).
28. Ciotoli, G.; Procesi, M.; Finoia, M.; Bossew, P.; Cinelli, G.; Tollefsen, T.; Elìo, J.; Gruber, V. Spatial Multicriteria Decision Analysis (SMCDA) for the construction of the European Geogenic Radon Migration map. In Proceedings of the European Geosciences Union (EGU) General Assembly, Online. 4–8 May 2020. EGU2020-7350. [CrossRef]
29. Pantelić, G.; Čeliković, I.; Živanović, M.; Vukanac, I.; Nikolić, J.K.; Cinelli, G.; Gruber, V. *EC-JRC Technical Reports. Literature Review of Indoor Radon Surveys in Europe*; Publications Office of the European Union: Luxembourg, 2018; ISBN 978-92-79-97643-8.
30. Tollefsen, T.; Cinelli, G.; Bossew, P.; Gruber, V.; De Cort, M. From the European indoor radon map towards an atlas of natural radiation. *Radiat. Prot. Dosim.* **2014**, *162*, 129–134. [CrossRef] [PubMed]
31. European Commission-Joint Research Centre (JRC-EC). Nuclear Saferty and Security, REM Project. Indoor Radon Concentration Map. 2018. Available online: https://remon.jrc.ec.europa.eu/About/Atlas-of-Natural-Radiation/Digital-Atlas/Indoor-radon-AM/Indoor-radon-concentration (accessed on 30 June 2020).
32. European Commission-EUROSTAT. The GISCO Database Reference System: GISCO Database Manual. 2004. Available online: https://ec.europa.eu/eurostat/web/gisco (accessed on 30 June 2020).
33. Dubois, G.; Bossew, P.; Tollefsen, T.; De Cort, M. First steps towards a European atlas of natural radiation: Status of the European indoor radon map. *J. Environ. Radioat.* **2010**, *101*, 786–798. [CrossRef] [PubMed]
34. Bossew, P.; Tollefsen, T.; Cinelli, G.; Gruber, V.; De Cort, M. Status of the European Atlas of Natural Radiation. *Radiat. Prot. Dosim.* **2015**, *167*, 29–36. [CrossRef]
35. Cinelli, G.; Tollefsen, T.; Bossew, P.; Gruber, V.; Bogucarsis, K.; De Felice, L.; De Cort, M. Digital version of the European Atlas of natural radiation. *J. Environ. Radioat.* **2019**, *196*, 240–252. [CrossRef] [PubMed]
36. Spanish Nuclear Safety Council (CSN). Natural Radiation Maps. Brochures, Posters and Triptych: FDE-02.17_Cartography of radon Potential in Spain. 2017. Available online: https://www.csn.es/documents/10182/914801/FDE-02.17+Cartograf%C3%ADa+del+potencial+de+rad%C3%B3n+de+Espa%C3%B1a/de116476-df51-49d9-8efb-665d7036d76c (accessed on 30 June 2020).
37. García-Talavera, S.M.M.; Acevedo, F.J.L. *CSN Technical Reports Collection 51.2019. INT-04.41 Cartography of Radon Potential in Spain*; Legal deposit: M-24725-2019; Nuclear Safety Council (CSN): Madrid, Spain, 2019.
38. Spanish Nuclear Safety Council (CSN). 2020. Available online: https://www.csn.es/radon (accessed on 30 June 2020).
39. Spanish Nuclear Safety Council (CSN). *CSN Security Guide Collection 11.01. Guidelines on the Competence of Laboratories and Radon Measurement Services in Air*; Nuclear Safety Council (CSN): Madrid, Spain, 2010.
40. Public Health England (PHE). PHE Validation Scheme for Laboratories. 2018. Available online: https://www.phe-protectionservices.org.uk/cms/assets/gfx/content/resource_3462cs9edda0fd4d.pdf (accessed on 30 June 2020).
41. Spanish National Accreditation Entity (ENAC). Accredited Entities. 2019. Available online: https://www.enac.es/ (accessed on 30 June 2020).
42. Spanish Nuclear Safety Council (CSN). Download: Map of Natural Gamma Radiation in Spain (MARNA) at a Scale of 1: 1,000,000. 2001. Available online: https://www.csn.es/mapa-de-radiacion-gamma-natural-marna-mapa (accessed on 30 June 2020).
43. Mahou, E.S.; Amigot, J.A.F.; Espasa, J.B.; Benito, M.C.M.; Pomar, D.G.; Del Pozo, J.M.; Del Busto, J.L. *CSN Technical Reports Collection 5.2000. INT-04-02. Marna Project. Map of Natural Gamma Radiation*; Legal deposit: M-668-2001; Nuclear Safety Council (CSN): Madrid, Spain, 2000; ISBN 84-95341-12-3.
44. Geological and Mining Institute of Spain (IGME). Download: Lithostratigraphic, Permeability and Hydrogeological Map of Spain at a Scale of 1: 200,000. 2009. Available online: http://info.igme.es/cartografiadigital/portada/default.aspx?Intranet=false&language=es (accessed on 30 June 2020).
45. Kemski, J.; Siehl, A.; Stegemann, R.; Valdivia-Manchego, M. Mapping the geogenic radon potential in Germany. *Sci. Total Environ.* **2001**, *272*, 217–230. [CrossRef]
46. Kemski, J.; Klinger, R.; Siehl, A.; Valdivia-Manchego, M. From radon hazard to risk prediction-based on geological maps, soil gas and indoor measurements in Germany. *Environ. Geol.* **2009**, *56*, 1269–1279. [CrossRef]
47. *ESRI 2011 ArcGIS Desktop: Release 10*; Environmental Systems Research Institute: Redlands, CA, USA, 2011.

48. *Synergy Software*; Kaleida Graph Version 4.1; Synergy Software: Reading, PA, USA, 2016.
49. Spanish National Geographic Institute (IGN)-Spanish National Center of Geographic Information (CNIG). Download: National Atlas of Spain at a Scale of 1:3,000,000. 2019. Available online: http://centrodedescargas.cnig.es/ (accessed on 30 June 2020).
50. Environmental Systems Research Institute (ESRI). ESRI Data & Maps: Point Density. 2019. Available online: http://desktop.arcgis.com/es/arcmap/10.3/tools/spatial-analyst-toolbox/point-density.htm (accessed on 30 June 2020).
51. Miguel, M.G.T.S.; Matarranz, J.L.M.; De Miengo, R.G.; Cadierno, J.P.G.; Mahou, E.S. *CSN Technical Reports Collection 38.2013. INT-04-31. Predictive Map of Radon Exposure in Spain*; Legal deposit: M-1014-2013; Nuclear Safety Council (CSN): Madrid, Spain, 2013.
52. Fernández, C.S.; Villar, A.F.; Merino, I.F.; Gutiérrez-Villanueva, J.L.; Matarranz, J.L.M.; Talavera, M.G.; Poncela, L.S.Q. The Spanish indoor radon mapping strategy. *Radiat. Prot. Dosim.* **2014**, *162*, 58–62. [CrossRef] [PubMed]
53. Fernández, C.S.; Poncela, L.S.Q.; Villar, A.F.; Merino, I.F.; Villanueva, J.L.G.; González, S.C.; Talavera, M.G. Spanish experience on the design of radon surveys based on the use of geogenic information. *J. Environ. Radioat.* **2017**, *166*, 390–397. [CrossRef]
54. Poncela, L.S.Q.; Soto, J.; Fernández, L. Geology and radon levels in Spanish homes. *Rev. Esp. Fis.* **1992**, *6*, 35–37.
55. Salminen, R.; Batista, M.J.; Bidovec, M.; Demetriades, A.; De Vivo, B.; De Vos, W.; Duris, M.; Gilucis, A.; Gregorauskiene, V.; Halamic, J.; et al. *FOREGS-Geochemical Atlas of Europe, Part 1: Background Information, Methodology and Maps*; Geological Survey of Finland: Espoo, Finland, 2005; ISBN 951-690-913-2.
56. Geological and Mining Institute of Spain (IGME). Legend Lithostratigraphic, Permeability and Hydrogeological Map of Spain at a Scale of 1: 200,000. 2009. Available online: http://info.igme.es/cartografiadigital/datos/tematicos/Leyendas/Leyenda_litoestratigrafia_A0.pdf (accessed on 30 June 2020).

Article

Measurement of Indoor Thoron Gas Concentrations Using a Radon-Thoron Discriminative Passive Type Monitor: Nationwide Survey in Japan

Tetsuya Sanada

Department of Radiological Technology, Faculty of Health Sciences, Hokkaido University of Science, Sapporo, Hokkaido 006-8585, Japan; sanada-t@hus.ac.jp

Abstract: As part of a nationwide survey of thoron (^{220}Rn) in Japan, the indoor ^{220}Rn gas concentrations in 940 dwellings were measured throughout one year, from 1993 to 1996, using a passive type ^{222}Rn-^{220}Rn discriminative monitor. The monitor was placed in a bedroom or a living room in each house for four successive three-month periods. The mean annual indoor ^{220}Rn concentration was estimated from the four measurements in each house. The arithmetic mean, the median and the geometric mean for indoor ^{220}Rn concentrations in 899 dwellings were 20.1, 9.6 and 10.0 Bq m^{-3}, respectively. The ^{220}Rn concentrations exhibited a log-normal distribution. It was found that the ^{220}Rn concentrations were dependent on the nature of the materials used for wall construction and also on the distance of measurement from the wall. Significant seasonal variations in the ^{220}Rn concentration were not observed. It would seem that the nature of the wall material contributed to the increased indoor ^{220}Rn concentrations.

Keywords: thoron; radon; indoor; radioactivity; environment; nationwide survey; SSNTD

1. Introduction

Radon (^{222}Rn), thoron (^{220}Rn) and their progeny species are large contributors to the annual exposure of an effective dose to the general population. ^{222}Rn and its progeny species contribute about half of the annual effective dose due to natural radiation based on the world mean dose. According to the United Nations Scientific Committee on the Effects of Atomic Radiation [1], the annual effective dose from natural radiation sources has been calculated to be 2.4 mSv as the worldwide average, whereas ^{222}Rn and ^{220}Rn contribute 1.2 and 0.1 mSv, respectively. ^{222}Rn and ^{220}Rn are products of the decay chains of natural radionuclides, such as the ^{238}U and ^{232}Th series, and have half-lives of 3.825 days and 55 s, respectively. The ^{220}Rn half-life is very short compared with ^{222}Rn. Thus, only a very small amount of ^{220}Rn can enter a room from the outside. It is considered that a ^{220}Rn concentration gradient exists near the mud-based walls and floors in low ventilated houses [2]. Therefore, if a mud mortar wall is present in housing materials which have high concentrations of thorium, ^{220}Rn and its decay products may enter houses and cause potential health problems. In particular, traditional wooden houses with mud mortar walls are a common house type in Japan.

The International Commission on Radiological Protection (ICRP) [3] have issued new dose conversion factors for ^{222}Rn and ^{220}Rn progeny species based on a dosimetric approach in Publication 137. The values specified are 16.8 and 107 nSv (Bq m^{-3} h)$^{-1}$, respectively. This means that even small amounts of ^{220}Rn progeny species will cause higher radiation exposure compared to ^{222}Rn [4]. Therefore, interest in ^{220}Rn exposure is growing among the health sciences communities. Recently, a number of ^{220}Rn surveys have been carried out in local regions and nationwide, and the results have been published enabling an evaluation of exposures from ^{220}Rn [5–21]. Also, the need to adopt reliable ^{220}Rn measurement techniques has been argued in several papers [22].

An indoor ^{222}Rn survey was conducted on 940 houses nationwide in Japan from 1993 to 1996 using ^{222}Rn–^{220}Rn discriminative passive type monitors [23]. The passive monitor, developed by Doi and Kobayashi [2], was placed in either a bedroom or a living room where residents spent most of their time. Indoor ^{222}Rn concentrations were determined at 20 dwellings in each prefecture for four successive three-month periods to cover an entire year. In the survey, to eliminate the influence of ^{220}Rn on ^{222}Rn measurement, the ^{220}Rn concentration was performed at the same time for referencing purposes. The ^{222}Rn and ^{220}Rn calibration experiments were performed in a standard radon chamber at the National Radiological Protection Board (Didcot, UK) and using the ^{222}Rn–^{220}Rn mixed chamber of Waseda University (Tokyo, Japan), respectively. This study is concerned with the results for the indoor ^{220}Rn concentrations using the reference data from the nationwide survey which was conducted to determine the ^{222}Rn concentrations in Japan [23]. Furthermore, the seasonal and regional variations were investigated, and the influence of the type of house structure was examined as mentioned previously. However, this study does not include a dose assessment of ^{220}Rn because the ^{220}Rn concentration varies widely in rooms and it is not easy to measure the activity concentration given the short half-life of the radioisotope [22].

2. Materials and Methods

2.1. ^{220}Rn Monitor and Measurement Periods

The solid-state nuclear track detector (SSNTD) was developed at the National Institute of Radiological Sciences (Chiba, Japan) as a ^{222}Rn and ^{220}Rn discriminative monitor [2]. The monitor consists of two electroconductive hemispheres and there are two polycarbonate films installed in the center of the two hemispheres. To isolate and separate the progeny species of ^{222}Rn and ^{220}Rn, a glass fiber filter is located in the first hemisphere. Therefore, only gaseous ^{222}Rn and ^{220}Rn can pass through the filter and enter the first hemisphere. This monitor has two different diffusion chambers which have relatively large and small ventilation rates. This system has been developed based on the large difference in half-lives of ^{222}Rn and ^{220}Rn. After being exposed, the film was first subjected to chemical etching with a mixed solution of 8 mol L^{-1} KOH and 20% C_2H_5OH at 30 °C for 30 min [23]. Then the films were electrochemically etched at 800 V and 2000 Hz for 2 h. A control film, which was exposed to particles from an ^{241}Am source and which had been etched simultaneously with the sample films, was also prepared to assure the stability of the etching condition. The track density was converted to the average ^{220}Rn concentration by the calibration factor after subtraction of the background track density, i.e., 3.5 ± 1.8 tracks cm^{-2}. In the case of the three month long exposure period, the detection limit (DL) for the concentration of ^{220}Rn was estimated to be 7.4 Bq m^{-3} (k = 1.65), the definition of DL being based on the definition of Currie [24]. Four monitors were used in the survey to determine the mean annual ^{220}Rn concentration. Consequently, the DL for the mean annual ^{220}Rn concentration was estimated to be about 1/2 of DL value specified above. The measurements were carried out for four successive three-month periods to cover a whole year (i.e., January–March, April–June, July–September and October–December) for estimation of the mean annual indoor ^{220}Rn concentration. The survey was carried out for four years (January 1993–June 1996) and conducted in the same manner as reported previously [23].

2.2. ^{220}Rn Calibration Experiments

The ^{222}Rn and ^{220}Rn calibration experiments were performed in a standard radon chamber at the National Radiological Protection Board in the UK and at the ^{222}Rn–^{220}Rn mixed chamber of Waseda University, Tokyo, respectively [25]. ^{220}Rn conversion factor was evaluated to be 0.0098 ± 0.0016 (tracks cm^{-2} per Bq m^{-3} d).

3. Results and Discussion

3.1. Distribution of ^{220}Rn Concentration

The mean annual ^{220}Rn concentrations were obtained for 899 houses, the number of houses monitored being reduced from the original 940 houses as was the case for ^{222}Rn [23]. The annual arithmetic mean, and the median were calculated and values less than the DL (<4 Bq m^{-3}) were included in each quarter value. In addition, if a negative value was obtained due to statistical variation as a result of background subtraction, this value was assigned as a zero. The histogram for the mean annual indoor ^{220}Rn concentrations is presented in Figure 1. The mean annual ^{220}Rn concentration was found to vary from <4 to 383 Bq m^{-3}. The arithmetic mean, the median, the geometric mean and the geometric standard deviation were 20.1 ± 36.8, 9.6, 10.0 Bq m^{-3} and 3.2, respectively. The ^{222}Rn concentrations varied from 3.1 to 208 Bq m^{-3}. The arithmetic mean, the median, the geometric mean and the geometric standard deviation were 15.5 ± 13.5, 11.7, 12.7 Bq m^{-3} and 1.78, respectively [23]. As a comparison, Kim et al. reported that the geometric mean for ^{220}Rn concentrations in Korea was 10.7 Bq m^{-3}. The log-normal cumulative frequency distribution for the indoor ^{220}Rn concentrations is shown in Figure 2. The ^{220}Rn concentration distribution would appear to be close to a log-normal distribution. The distribution of the mean annual indoor ^{220}Rn concentrations was accepted as a log-normal distribution based on the Kolmogorov–Smirnov test at a significance level of 95%.

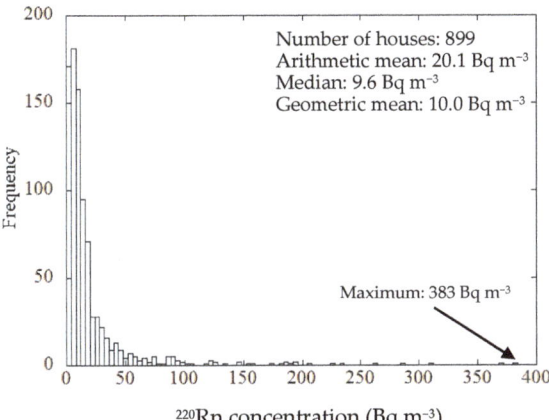

Figure 1. Histogram for indoor ^{220}Rn concentrations.

3.2. Seasonal Variation

The indoor ^{220}Rn concentration data for each season are presented in Table 1. Negative values in this dataset were eliminated for calculation of the geometric mean. A significant seasonal variation in the ^{220}Rn concentrations for the four seasons was not found. According to Kim et al. [15] and Stjanovska et al. [16], a temporal pattern in the ^{220}Rn concentration data was observed with values in the winter and spring seasons being higher than those in the summer and autumn. Martinez et al. [17] found that the highest concentrations for Mexico City were in the autumn season and the lowest concentrations were in summer.

In the present study, slight differences were noted in the ^{220}Rn concentrations depending on the periods of exposure. The lowest ^{220}Rn concentrations for all types of houses were observed in the winter season (October–December). However, a different relationship was noted for the ^{222}Rn concentrations, namely, that the ^{222}Rn concentrations tended to be higher in winter compared to the other seasons [23]. This was probably because the residents used domestic heaters to maintain a comfortable room temperature in winter, and consequently there would have been increased ventilation rates due to the contribution of convection and/or stack effect in the rooms.

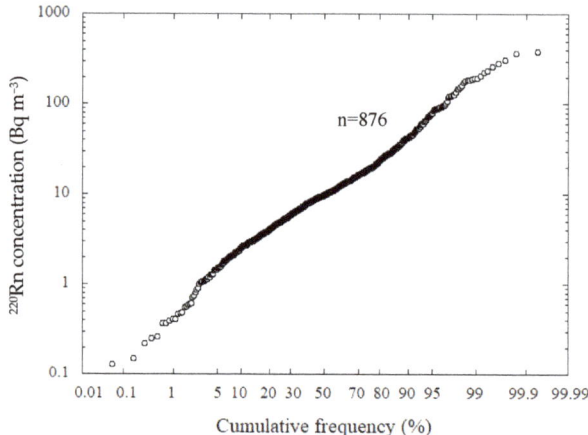

Figure 2. Cumulative frequency distribution for indoor ^{220}Rn concentrations. This figure has been prepared using the mean annual ^{220}Rn concentrations in excess of zero Bq m^{-3}.

Table 1. ^{220}Rn concentrations measured in the different seasons.

Measurement Period	Number of Houses	^{220}Rn (Bq m^{-3})			GSD
		AM	SD	GM (Number of Houses)	
January–March		18.9	40.0	14.6 (576)	3.5
April–June	899	22.8	39.2	14.4 (733)	3.5
July–September		21.9	42.3	14.0 (713)	3.3
October–December		16.6	41.0	13.0 (492)	3.9

AM: Arithmetic mean; SD: Standard deviation; GM: Geometric mean; GSD: Geometric standard deviation (dimensionless).

The variation of the ^{220}Rn concentration in the rooms was slightly different from that of ^{222}Rn, which may reflect the differences in the half-lives and sources of ^{220}Rn, despite the fact that there were large fluctuations in the standard deviations for the seasonal variations of ^{220}Rn concentrations. The reason why the indoor ^{220}Rn concentrations did not display a variation similar to ^{222}Rn is unclear at this time.

3.3. Nature of Housing

Indoor ^{220}Rn concentrations were categorized in terms of the structural features of the housing. The annual mean, the standard deviation, and the geometric mean for the indoor ^{220}Rn concentrations together with number of houses monitored are given in Table 2. The arithmetic and geometric mean concentrations for wooden and concrete-based houses have higher values than those of other structures, although there were large fluctuations in the data. The maximum value was found for a wooden house with a mud wall, the highest ^{220}Rn concentration being 383 Bq m^{-3}. The cause of the high ^{220}Rn concentration of wooden houses is that they have relatively high ratio of the mud wall in comparison to other house structure types. Table 3 lists the ratio of the mud wall in each housing type. Accordingly, the ^{220}Rn concentrations in wooden houses are higher than those for other housing types.

Table 2. The mean annual ^{220}Rn concentration for each type of house.

Structure	Number of Houses	^{220}Rn (Bq m^{-3})		
		AM	SD	GM
Wooden	597	23.1	40.7	10.8
Concrete	182	16.3	32.5	9.6
Steel frame	90	8.6	8.9	6.1
Concrete block	16	21.8	25.6	13.8
Prefabricated	6	3.4	2.6	2.7

AM: Arithmetic mean; SD: Standard deviation; GM: Geometric mean.

Table 3. Ratio of mud wall in each structure type.

Structure Type	Total Number of Houses	Number of Mud Wall Houses	Ratio of Mud Wall in the House (%)
Wooden	597	190	31.8
Concrete	182	3	1.6
Steel frame	90	0	0
Concrete block	16	1	6.3
Prefabricated	6	0	0

With respect to the ^{220}Rn concentrations by region, the overall ratios for wooden houses with mud walls in the Hokkaido—Tohoku, Kanto and Kyushu—Okinawa areas are lower than for those in other areas of Japan. Therefore, the ^{220}Rn concentrations in these former areas also tends to be lower than the values found in the other areas.

3.4. Dependency of ^{220}Rn Concentration on Wall Structure and Distance from Wall

The present survey on ^{220}Rn concentrations considered four categories of material which were used for wall construction in the houses. The mean annual ^{220}Rn concentrations obtained by passive measurement for the different wall materials in the houses are presented in Figure 3. Inspection of the results (Figure 3) reveals that high ^{220}Rn concentrations occurred for houses with mud walls, and the values decreased gradually with distance from the surface of the wall as shown in Figure 4. Yonehara et al. reported similar behavior for ^{220}Rn concentrations at locations near the wall surfaces in Japanese dwellings [26].

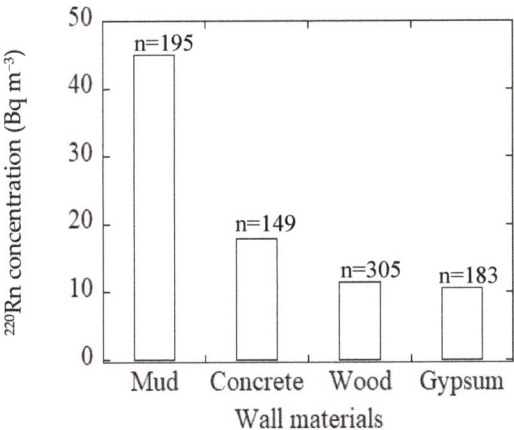

Figure 3. ^{220}Rn concentrations for various wall materials.

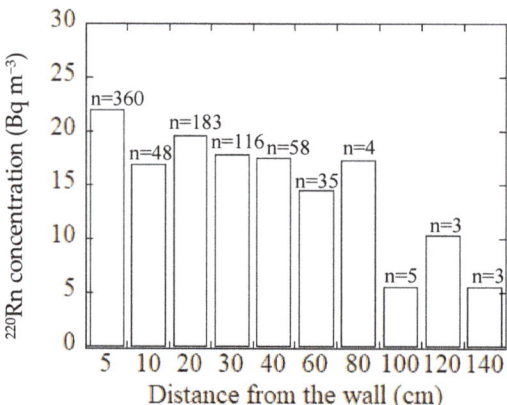

Figure 4. ^{220}Rn concentrations at different distances from the wall surface for all wall materials.

3.5. ^{220}Rn and ^{222}Rn Correlation

The correlation between the indoor ^{220}Rn and ^{222}Rn concentrations was investigated. The relationship between the ^{220}Rn and the ^{222}Rn concentrations is illustrated in Figure 5. The concentration distributions for both radioisotopes follow approximately a log-normal distribution. Consequently, both datasets were calculated after taking the logarithms of the respective data. The linear regression analysis shows a weak positive correlation (R = 0.25). The ratio for the concentrations of ^{220}Rn/^{222}Rn ranged from 0.007 to 40.3 and reveal a log-normal plot. The arithmetic mean for ^{220}Rn/^{222}Rn was 1.64 and geometric mean was 0.78.

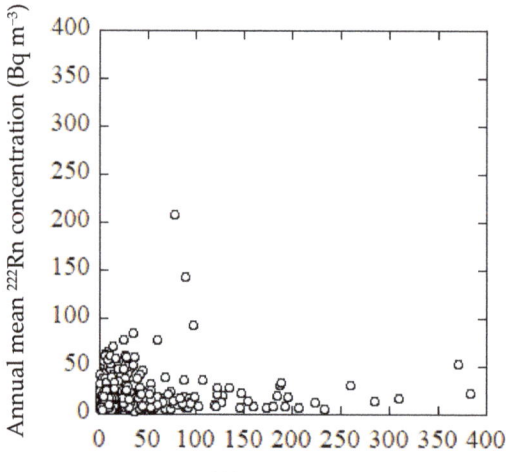

Figure 5. Correlation between the mean annual concentrations of ^{220}Rn and ^{222}Rn.

4. Conclusions

The mean annual indoor ^{220}Rn concentrations were measured in 899 houses using a passive ^{222}Rn–^{220}Rn discriminative monitor. The arithmetic mean, the median and the geometric mean were 20.1, 9.6 and 10.0 Bq m^{-3}, respectively. The ^{220}Rn concentration plot exhibited a log-normal distribution. The maximum ^{220}Rn concentration found in the present survey was 383 Bq m^{-3} for a wooden house with mud walls. The survey data for the indoor ^{220}Rn concentrations in Japan did not exhibit a significant seasonal variation. There was a marked difference in the ^{220}Rn concentration depending on the nature of the house structure. Relatively higher concentrations of ^{220}Rn were found in wooden and concrete block houses compared to other housing types. In general, the ^{220}Rn concentrations in traditional wooden houses with mud walls tended to be higher than those for houses with different wall types. Further, it was demonstrated that the ^{220}Rn concentrations decreased with distance of measurement from the wall.

Funding: This research was carried out in collaboration with 47 prefectural institutes under the auspices of the former Science and Technology Agency of Japan.

Institutional Review Board Statement: Not applicable for studies not involving humans or animals.

Informed Consent Statement: Not applicable for studies not involving humans.

Data Availability Statement: The data presented in this study are available on request from the corresponding author.

Conflicts of Interest: The author declares no conflict of interest.

References

1. United Nations Scientific Committee on the Effects of Atomic Radiation. Volume I: Annex B Exposures of the Public and Workers from Various Sources of Radiation. In *UNSCEAR 2008 Report, Sources and Effects of Ionizing Radiation*; UNSCEAR: New York, NY, USA, 2010.
2. Doi, M.; Kobayashi, S. The passive radon-thoron discriminative dosimeter for practical use. *Hoken Butsuri*. **1994**, *29*, 155–166. [CrossRef]
3. International Commission on Radiological Protection. Occupational intakes of radionuclides: Part 3. In *Annals of the ICRP 46 (3/4)*; ICRP Publication 137: London, UK, 2017.
4. Tokonami, S. Characteristic of Thoron (^{220}Rn) and its progeny in the indoor environment. *Int. J. Environ. Res. Public Health* **2020**, *17*, 8769. [CrossRef]
5. Bineng, G.S.; Saïdou, S.T.; Hosoda, M.; Siaka, Y.F.; Issa, H.; Suzuki, T.; Kudo, H.; Bouba, O. The importance of direct progeny measurements for correct estimation of effective dose due to radon and thoron. *Front. Public Health* **2020**, *8*, 17. [CrossRef] [PubMed]
6. Chen, J.; Moir, D.; Sorimachi, A.; Janik, M.; Tokonami, S. Determination of thoron equilibrium factor from simultaneous long-term thoron and its progeny measurements. *Radiat. Prot. Dosim.* **2012**, *149*, 155–158. [CrossRef]
7. Chen, J.; Bergman, L.; Falcomer, R.; Whyte, J. Results of simultaneous radon and thoron measurements in 33 metropolitan areas of Canada. *Radiat. Prot. Dosim.* **2015**, *163*, 210–216. [CrossRef] [PubMed]
8. Kudo, H.; Tokonami, S.; Omori, Y.; Ishikawa, T.; Iwaoka, K.; Sahoo, S.K.; Akata, N.; Hosoda, M.; Pornnumpa, C.; Sun, Q.; et al. Comparative dosimetry for radon and thoron in high background radiation areas in China. *Radiat. Prot. Dosim.* **2015**, *167*, 155–159. [CrossRef] [PubMed]
9. Shang, B.; Tschiersch, J.; Cui, H.; Xia, Y. Radon survey in dwellings of Gansu, China: The influence of thoron and an attempt for correction. *Radiat. Environ. Biophys.* **2008**, *47*, 367–373. [CrossRef]
10. Tokonami, S.; Sun, Q.; Akiba, S.; Zhuo, W.; Furukawa, M.; Ishikawa, T.; Hou, C.; Zhang, S.; Narazaki, Y.; Ohji, B.; et al. Radon and thoron exposures for cave residents in Shanxi and Shaanxi Provinces. *Radiat. Res.* **2004**, *162*, 390–396. [CrossRef]
11. Kovacs, T. Thoron measurements in Hungary. *Radiat. Prot. Dosim.* **2010**, *141*, 328–334. [CrossRef]
12. Omori, Y.; Tokonami, S.; Sahoo, S.K.; Ishikawa, T.; Sorimachi, A.; Hosoda, M.; Kudo, H.; Pornnumpa, C.; Nair, R.R.K.; Jayalekshmi, P.A.; et al. Radiation dose due to radon and thoron progeny inhalation in high-level natural radiation areas of Kerala, India. *J. Radiol. Prot.* **2017**, *37*, 111–126. [CrossRef]
13. Mc Laughlin, J.P.; Murray, M.; Currivan, L.; Pollard, D.; Smith, V.; Tokonami, S.; Sorimachi, A.; Janik, M. Thoron and its airborne progeny in Irish dwellings. In Proceedings of the Third European IRPA Congress, Helsinki, Finland, 14–18 June 2010; pp. 2607–2612.
14. Nyambura, C.; Tokonami, S.; Hashim, N.O.; Chege, M.W.; Suzuki, T.; Hosoda, M. Annual effective dose assessment due to radon and thoron progenies in dwellings of Kilimanbogo, Kenya. *Radiat. Prot. Dosim.* **2019**, *184*, 430–434. [CrossRef] [PubMed]
15. Kim, C.K.; Kim, Y.J.; Lee, H.Y.; Chang, B.U.; Tokonami, S. ^{220}Rn and its progeny in dwellings of Korea. *Radiat. Meas.* **2007**, *42*, 1409–1414. [CrossRef]
16. Stojanovska, Z.; Bossew, P.; Tokonami, S.; Zunic, Z.; Bochicchio, F.; Boev, B.; Ristova, M.; Januseski, J. National survey of indoor thoron concentration in FYR of Macedonia (continental Europe–Balkan region). *Radiat. Meas.* **2013**, *49*, 57–66. [CrossRef]
17. Martinez, T.; Navarrete, M.; Gonzalez, P.; Ramirez, A. Variation in indoor thoron levels in Mexico City dwellings. *Radiat. Prot. Dosim.* **2004**, *111*, 111–113. [CrossRef]

18. Smetsers, R.C.G.M.; Blaauboer, R.O.; Dekkers, F.; Slaper, H. Radon and thoron progeny in Dutch dwellings. *Radiat. Prot. Dosim.* **2018**, *181*, 11–14. [CrossRef]
19. Vaupotic, J.; Kavasi, N. Preliminary study of thoron and radon levels in various indoor environments in Slovenia. *Radiat. Prot. Dosim.* **2010**, *141*, 383–385. [CrossRef]
20. Saputra, M.A.; Nugraha, E.D.; Purwanti, T.; Arifianto, R.; Laksmana, R.I.; Hutabarat, R.P.; Hosoda, M.; Tokonami, S. Exposures from radon, thoron, and thoron progeny in high background radiation area in Takandeang, Mamuju, Indonesia. *Nukleonika* **2020**, *65*, 89–94. [CrossRef]
21. Wang, Z.; Lubin, J.; Wang, L.; Zhang, S.; Boice, J.; Cui, H.; Zhang, S.; Conrath, S.; Xia, Y.; Shang, B.; et al. Residential radon and lung cancer risk in a high-exposure area of Gansu Province, China. *Am. J. Epidemiol.* **2002**, *155*, 554–564. [CrossRef]
22. Hosoda, M.; Kudo, H.; Iwaoka, K.; Yamada, R.; Suzuki, T.; Tamakuma, Y.; Tokonami, S. Characteristic of thoron (^{220}Rn) in environment. *Appl. Radiat. Isot.* **2017**, *120*, 7–10. [CrossRef]
23. Sanada, T.; Fujimoto, K.; Miyano, K.; Doi, M.; Tokonami, S.; Uesugi, M.; Takata, Y. Measurement of nationwide indoor Rn concentration in Japan. *J. Environ. Radioact.* **1999**, 129–137. [CrossRef]
24. Currie, L.A. Limits for qualitative detection and quantitative determination. *Anal. Chem.* **1968**, *40*, 586–593. [CrossRef]
25. Kurosawa, R.; Tokonami, S.; Kamota, F. On the convenient test chamber for calibration of passive integrating radon-thoron monitor, environmental radon. In Proceedings of the '91 Radon Symposium, Kumatori, Japan, 8–10 August 1992; pp. 464–475.
26. Yonehara, H.; Tokonami, S.; Zhuo, W.; Ishikawa, T.; Fukutsu, K.; Yamada, Y. Thoron in the living environments of Japan. *Int. Congr. Ser.* **2005**, *1276*, 58–61. [CrossRef]

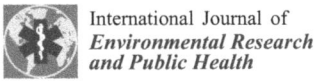

Article

Temporal and Spatial Variation of Radon Concentrations in Environmental Water from Okinawa Island, Southwestern Part of Japan

Shunya Nakasone [1,*], Akinobu Ishimine [2], Shuhei Shiroma [3], Natsumi Masuda [3], Kaori Nakamura [1], Yoshitaka Shiroma [4], Sohei Ooka [5], Masahiro Tanaka [6,7], Akemi Kato [8], Masahiro Hosoda [9], Naofumi Akata [10], Yumi Yasuoka [11] and Masahide Furukawa [1]

1. Graduate School of Engineering and Science, University of the Ryukyus, Nishihara, Okinawa 903–0213, Japan; k198345@eve.u-ryukyu.ac.jp (K.N.); m_furu@sci.u-ryukyu.ac.jp (M.F.)
2. Department of Radioecology, Institute for Environmental Sciences, Rokkasho, Aomori 039–3212, Japan; aki_ishi@ies.or.jp
3. Faculty of Science, University of the Ryukyus, Nishihara, Okinawa 903–0213, Japan; shiromashuhei1101@gmail.com (S.S.); 83ka.ha.ho@gmail.com (N.M.)
4. Faculty of Education, University of the Ryukyus, Nishihara, Okinawa 903–0213, Japan; y_shiro@cs.u-ryukyu.ac.jp
5. Nanto Co., Ltd., Naha, Okinawa 900–0013, Japan; oooka@gyokusendo.co.jp
6. Department of Helical Plasma Research, National Institute for Fusion Science, National Institutes of Natural Sciences, Toki, Gifu 509–5292, Japan; tanaka.masahiro@nifs.ac.jp
7. School of Physical Sciences, The Graduate University for Advanced Studies, SOKENDAI, Toki, Gifu 509–5292, Japan
8. Department of Engineering and Technical Services, National Institute for Fusion Science, National Institutes of Natural Sciences, Toki, Gifu 509–5292, Japan; kakemi@nifs.ac.jp
9. Department of Radiation Science, Hirosaki University Graduate School of Health Sciences, Hirosaki, Aomori 036–8564, Japan; m_hosoda@hirosaki-u.ac.jp
10. Department of Radiation Chemistry, Institute of Radiation Emergency Medicine, Hirosaki University, Hirosaki, Aomori 036–8564, Japan; akata@hirosaki-u.ac.jp
11. Radioisotope Research Center, Kobe Pharmaceutical University, Kobe, Hyogo 658–8558, Japan; yasuoka@kobepharma-u.ac.jp
* Correspondence: k198602@eve.u-ryukyu.ac.jp; Tel.: +81–3998-1029

Abstract: In this study, to get a better understanding in characterizing groundwater and ensure its effective management, the radon concentrations in water samples were measured through Ryukyu limestone in southern Okinawa Island, Japan. Water samples were collected from a limestone cave (Gyokusendo cave, dropping water) and two springs (Ukinju and Komesu, spring water), and the radon concentrations were measured by liquid scintillation counters. The radon concentrations in the samples from the Gyokusendo cave, and Ukinju and Komesu springs were 10 ± 1.3 Bq L^{-1}, 3.2 ± 1.0 Bq L^{-1}, and 3.1 ± 1.1 Bq L^{-1}, respectively. The radon concentrations showed a gradually increasing trend from summer to autumn and decreased during winter. The variation of radon concentrations in the dripping water sample from the Gyokusendo cave showed a lagged response to precipitation changes by approximately 2–3 months. The estimated radon concentrations in the dripping water sample were calculated with the measured radon concentrations from the dripping water obtained during the study period. Based on our results, groundwater in the Gyokusendo cave system was estimated to percolate through the Ryukyu limestone in 7–10 days, and the residence time of groundwater in the soil above Gyokusendo cave was estimated to be approximately 50–80 days. This work makes a valuable contribution to the understanding of groundwater processes in limestone aquifers, which is essential for ensuring groundwater sustainability.

Keywords: radon concentration; groundwater; residence time; limestone aquifer; Okinawa Island

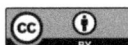

Citation: Nakasone, S.; Ishimine, A.; Shiroma, S.; Masuda, N.; Nakamura, K.; Shiroma, Y.; Ooka, S.; Tanaka, M.; Kato, A.; Hosoda, M.; et al. Temporal and Spatial Variation of Radon Concentrations in Environmental Water from Okinawa Island, Southwestern Part of Japan. *IJERPH* 2021, *18*, 998. https://doi.org/10.3390/ijerph18030998

Academic Editor: Paul B. Tchounwou
Received: 28 December 2020
Accepted: 20 January 2021
Published: 23 January 2021

Publisher's Note: MDPI stays neutral with regard to jurisdictional claims in published maps and institutional affiliations.

Copyright: © 2021 by the authors. Licensee MDPI, Basel, Switzerland. This article is an open access article distributed under the terms and conditions of the Creative Commons Attribution (CC BY) license (https://creativecommons.org/licenses/by/4.0/).

1. Introduction

Radon is a radioactive noble gas with an atomic number of 86. Although there are many isotopes of radon, only three occur in the natural environment: ^{222}Rn, ^{220}Rn (Thoron), and ^{219}Rn (Actinon), with half-lives of 3.8 d, 55.6 s, and 3.9 s, respectively. ^{222}Rn is the most frequently used radon isotope due to its relatively long half-life compared to thoron and actinon. Hereinafter, "radon" refers to ^{222}Rn. Radon is a natural radionuclide belonging to the uranium (^{238}U) decay series, with radium (^{226}Ra) as a parent nuclide. The ^{238}U decay series ends with ^{206}Pb, a stable isotope of lead. Inhalation of radon and its decay products is believed to increase the risk of lung cancer [1]. Most radon in the environment is produced by the alpha decay of radium in the soil and rocks. Since radon is extremely soluble in water (e.g., 0.295 cm^3 kg^{-1} at 15 °C), there may be an exchange and equilibrium between pore-water and pore-gas when the soil is unsaturated [2]. In addition, radon is chemically inert. Therefore, if it is dissipated from soil grains into pore water or voids, it can migrate relatively far from where it is produced by advection or diffusion [2]. Eventually, some of the radon dissipated in the pore water migrates to the groundwater and is dissolved in spring or hot spring water. Radon, which is widely distributed in the natural environment, is commonly used to study atmospheric transport processes and groundwater flow systems such as groundwater recharge, flow, and discharge [3,4].

Radon can be used as a hydrological tracer for estimating the residence time of groundwater under very special boundary conditions (e.g., in limestone areas or for submarine groundwater discharge in the coastal zone) [5–7]. In karst aquifers, researchers have analyzed radon concentrations to understand the recharge dynamics of water passing through the soil layer to the saturated zone [8]. Additionally, groundwater and soil radon concentrations are measured during irrigated and non-irrigated periods in paddy fields, and the difference in the concentration values between groundwater and surface water is used to evaluate surface water infiltration into the aquifer [9]. Radon can also be used for estimating the probability of geophysical risk events such as volcanic activity and earthquakes [10–12]. Pre-earthquake radon anomalies have been found in soil gases, groundwater, and spring water [13,14]. Radon serves as a useful geochemical tracer for studying the short-term environmental characteristics of cave systems, such as the flow of the atmospheric circulation. Variations in the air density and atmospheric radon concentrations inside and outside caves have been reported for the seasonal natural ventilation in the cave [15–17].

The storage capacity of a limestone layer alone is low due to it being highly permeable and porous. However, when a limestone layer overlies an impermeable layer in a nonconformant way, as is the case on Okinawa Island, the limestone serves as an aquifer. Limestones can serve as excellent natural aquifers and provide drinking water to 25% of the world's population [18]. Moreover, water in limestone aquifers is the only available drinking water in some regions and serves as a valuable water source for agriculture [18].

Okinawa Island, a Japanese island in the East China Sea, is characterized by short and steep river channels. Moreover, because its watershed area is small, the rainfall is discharged directly into the ocean. Okinawa Island experienced a relatively high annual precipitation of 2040 mm during the 1981–2010 period [19]. However, due to significant seasonal and interannual changes, the flow of rivers on the island is unstable and the amount of water available is limited. Therefore, it is difficult to secure stable water resources in Okinawa Island from river water alone and part of the water for agriculture and domestic use is provided by groundwater. To establish a stable supply and ensure the sustainable use of groundwater in the future, it is necessary to determine the groundwater characteristics, such as availability and residence time, in limestone aquifers. However, because of the heterogeneous permeability and complex hydrogeological structure of limestone, it is difficult to understand the behavior of groundwater from existing numerical models. For example, groundwater infiltration and residence time in limestone aquifers vary with each precipitation event.

Characteristics of local groundwater processes can be inferred from radon measurements. Shiroma et al. (2016) intermittently measured the radon concentration in dripping water exuding from the ceiling of a cave and reported that it is a potential source of radon in the cave atmosphere [20]. Although other factors may be involved, by comparing radon concentrations and monthly precipitation, changes in radon concentrations were shown to correspond to precipitation changes after a delay of 60–90 days. Furthermore, groundwater was calculated to percolate through the Ryukyu limestone in 9 to 10 days. However, the radon concentration data were collected intermittently for only one year and only at one site.

The main objective of this study is as attempt to calculate the residence time of groundwater in limestone areas. The study area comprised a limestone cave and two springs in the southern part of Okinawa Island. The residence time of groundwater from the soil to the cave was calculated based on the relationship between the radon concentration of the dripping water from the cave ceiling and the monthly precipitation. Moreover, we sampled two springs in the study area to understand the spatial distribution of radon concentrations in the groundwater.

2. Materials and Methods

2.1. Overview of the Study Site

Okinawa Prefecture, located in southwestern Japan, is the only prefecture in the country with a subtropical climate (Figure 1A). Ryukyu limestone, which originates from coral reef sediments, formed approximately one million to 500,000 years ago [21]. Limestone is widely distributed, and there are numerous limestone caves in Okinawa. The southern part of Okinawa Island consists of the Neogene-Quaternary Shimajiri Group and the Ryukyu Group, with low-lying terrain below 200 m in elevation. The Shimajiri Group of the Neogene Pliocene is predominantly composed of mudstone and is prone to erosion, while the limestone Quaternary Pleistocene Ryukyu Group, which is predominantly composed of limestone, is more resistant to erosion and forms a flat-surfaced topography [22]. The Ryukyu limestone overlies the Shimajiri Group in a non-conformant way. The Ryukyu limestone is permeable, while the Shimajiri Group is impermeable [23]. Therefore, Ryukyu limestones serve as aquifers in Okinawa Island (i.e., Ryukyu aquifer).

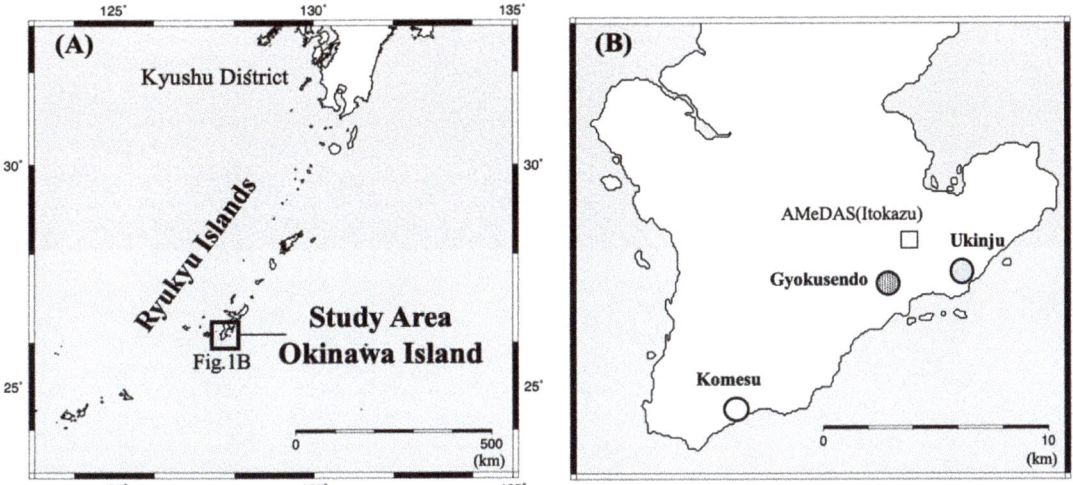

Figure 1. Locations of the study area (**A**) and sampling sites (**B**). The white square shows the Automated Meteorological Data Acquisition System (AMeDAS) situated at Itokazu.

Okinawa Island has three major soil types: Shimajiri Mahji, Kunigami Mahji, and Jahgaru. Shimajiri Mahji is a dark red soil, which is widely distributed in the Ryukyu limestone distribution area [24], with a reddish brown to dark brown color that is neutral to slightly alkaline [25]. Dark red soil is derived from the weathering products of limestone and/or a high-background radiation area, mainly the southeastern part of China [25].

2.2. Sample Collection

Water samples were collected from Gyokusendo cave (26°08′25″N, 127°44′57″W, 46 m altitude, dripping water), Ukinju spring (26°08′15″N, 127°47′35″W, 6.5 m altitude, spring), and Komesu spring (26°05′18″N, 127°42′04″W, 3.2 m altitude, coastal spring), all located in the southern portion of Okinawa Island (Figure 1B). Water samples were collected from October 2016 to October 2020. Sample collection at Ukinju and Komesu started in April 2018 and May 2018, respectively. The collection period in the springs was delayed because it took time to find a location with a high flow rate in the coastal area. However, data for April to June 2020 are missing for each location due to the COVID-19 pandemic.

Gyokusendo cave is a limestone cave situated in a 120-m-thick body of Ryukyu limestone. Shimajiri Mahji soil is distributed on the surrounding ground surface. The total length of Gyokusendo cave reaches 5000 m, and approximately 800 m are open for tourism [26]. A concrete staircase with a height of approximately 30 m serves as an entrance to the main cave. A branch cave in an undisclosed area about 30 m away from the stalagmite named "Shoryu no Kane" was selected as the water sampling point (Figure 2). There are soda-straw stalactites (straws) at this site with a significantly high drip rate. Therefore, it was possible to collect 10 mL of dripping water in approximately 10 min. The Ryukyu limestone is exposed at Ukinju spring and Komesu spring, and Shimajiri Mahji is distributed in the surrounding ground surface at both sites. The Ukinju and Komesu springs are located near the coast, 170 m and 12 m from the coastline, respectively.

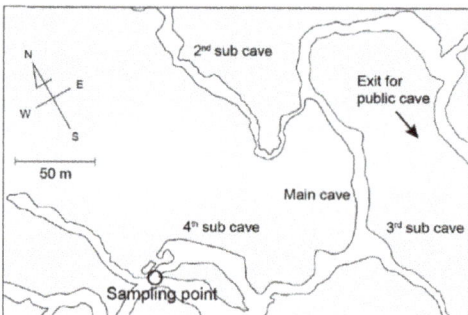

Figure 2. Location of the sampling point in Gyokusendo cave (map from, Shiroma et al. 2016 [20]).

For sample collection, 20 mL high-performance glass vials (PerkinElmer, USA) containing 10 mL of high efficiency mineral oil scintillator (PerkinElmer, USA) were prepared. For each site, 5 samples were collected. The water samples were collected using a syringe with the needle removed. Water samples (12 mL) were collected directly from the straw formed in the cave ceiling in Gyokusendo cave. At the Ukinju and Komesu sites, the same sample amounts were collected near the spring outlets. The syringe was pointed upward, and the plunger was pressed carefully to remove air from the inside. A needle was then attached, and the tip of the needle was positioned just over the bottom of the glass vial, and 10 mL of sample was injected. The time elapsed from water sample injection to the closing of the lid of the glass vial was set as the water sampling time. After water sampling, the samples were shaken for 60 s and left in the dark for 4 h until radiative equilibrium was achieved to extract the radon from the sample water into the mineral oil scintillator.

Temperature and humidity data in the cave were measured using HOBO Pro v2 Loggers (U23–001, ONSET, USA). However, data for December 2016 and February 2017 were missing due equipment failure. Precipitation data outside the cave were obtained from the Automated Meteorological Data Acquisition System (AMeDAS) situated at Itokazu

(Figure 1B). The pH and electrical conductivity (EC) of the water samples were measured using a pH meter (AS-712pH, HORIBA) and an EC meter (B-771COND, HORIBA). To verify the existence of saltwater inflow, the salinity (PSU; Practical Salinity Unit) was also measured at Ukinju and Komesu spring located in the coastal area using a digital salinity meter (HI96822, HANNA instruments).

2.3. Analysis of Radon Concentration in Water

The radon concentrations in water were measured for 60 min per sample using a liquid scintillation counter. The measurements were performed using a Quantulus 1220 (PerkinElmer, USA), at the National Institute for Fusion Science, from October 2016 to February 2019 and a Tri-Carb 2019TR (PerkinElmer, USA), at the University of the Ryukyus Center for Research Advancement and Collaboration, from March 2019 to October 2020. The radon concentration C_R (Bq L^{-1}) was calculated using the following equation:

$$C_R = \frac{(A_0 - B_0)\exp(\lambda T_p)}{f_{Rn} V} \quad (1)$$

where A_0 is the counting rate (cps) of the water sample, B_0 is the counting rate (cps) of the background sample, λ is the radon decay constant (day^{-1}), T_p is the elapsed period (day), which was corrected for radioactive decay to between the sampling time and the middle measurement time, f_{Rn} is the radon conversion factor of 3.24 cps Bq L^{-1} for the Quantulus 1220 and 4.5 cps Bq^{-1} for the Tri-Carb2019TR, and V is the sample volume (0.01 L) [27].

For measurements using the Quantulus 1220, A_0 and B_0 were calculated using the counting rate cps for 600–910 ch. Additionally, for measurements using the Tri-Carb2019TR, A_0 and B_0 were calculated using the counting rate cps for 0–1024 ch using the integral counting method [27–29]. The minimum detected radon concentration MDC (Bq L^{-1}) was calculated using the following equation [30]:

$$N_D = 4.65 \sqrt{\frac{B_0}{t}} + \frac{2.71}{t} \quad (2)$$

$$MDC = \frac{N_D}{f_{Rn} V} \quad (3)$$

where N_D is the minimum value of net count rate (cps), t is the counting time of the sample and the background (sec). The minimum detected radon concentrations by this method were 1.0 Bq L^{-1} for the Quantulus1220 and 0.9 Bq L^{-1} for the Tri-Carb2019TR [30].

Uncertainties were estimated for the following components: the counting rate (cps) of the water sample and background sample, the measurement time (s) of the water sample and background sample, the radon decay constant (s^{-1}), the elapsed period (s), the radon conversion factor (cps Bq L^{-1}), and the sample volume (L). Estimates were also made for each of these components, which were combined to give the expanded uncertainty [31]. By applying a coverage factor of $k = 2$, the expanded uncertainty was evaluated as 10%. In this study, radon concentrations are expressed as the arithmetic mean $\pm$ standard deviation of 5 samples.

3. Results and Discussion

3.1. Physical Parameters and Meteorological Data

The pH and EC of the water samples and the monthly precipitation data are shown in Figure 3. The pH and EC range of the samples from the Gyokusendo cave were 6.8–7.9, 0.76–1.52 mS cm^{-1}. For the Ukinju spring, the pH and EC ranged from 6.7–8.2 and 0.64 and 0.99 mS cm^{-1}. For the Komesu spring, the pH ranged between 6.5–8.1 and the EC measured between 0.55 and 0.96 mS cm^{-1}.

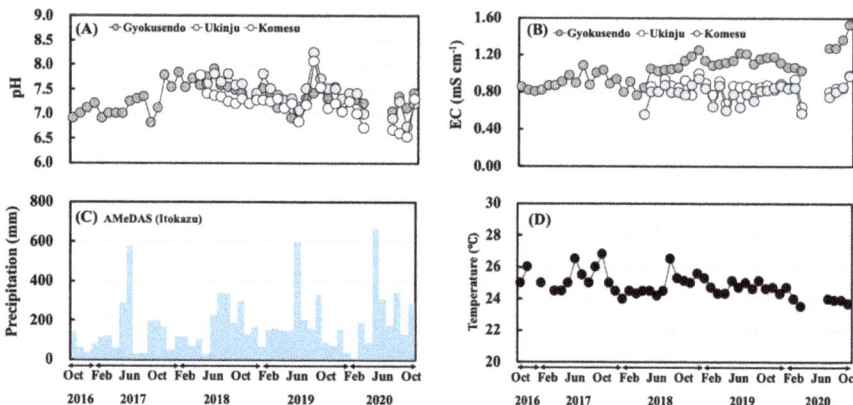

Figure 3. Monthly variations for the October 2016–October 2020 period of pH (**A**), electrical conductivity (**B**), and precipitation (**C**) in the water samples, and temperature (**D**) in the Gyokusendo cave.

The results reveal no significant seasonal variation in pH and EC. The monthly precipitation ranged from 11.50–669.50 mm. The monthly precipitation tended to be higher during the rainy season (May-June) and the typhoon season (August-October) and lower in winter (December–February). The salinity of Ukinju spring and Komesu spring, located near the coast, was in the range of 0–1 PSU, and seawater contamination was not observed. The temperature inside the Gyokusendo cave is shown in Figure 3D. The temperature outside the cave showed a marked seasonal variation (high in summer, low in winter) of 15–27 °C [19], while inside the cave, the temperature varied marginally, ranging from 23–27 °C. The humidity in the cave was generally 100% throughout the measurement period.

3.2. Temporal Variation of Radon Concentrations for the Water Samples

Radon concentrations for the dripping water collected at the Gyokusendo cave ranged from 7.1–13 Bq L^{-1} (Figure 4), with an average of 10 ± 1.3 Bq L^{-1}. The radon concentration for the dripping water collected at the same site between May 2013 and March 2014 was relatively consistent and ranged between 6.4 to 15 Bq L^{-1} [20]. The radon concentration for the dripping water increased gradually from summer (June–August) to autumn (September–November) and then decreased in winter (December–February).

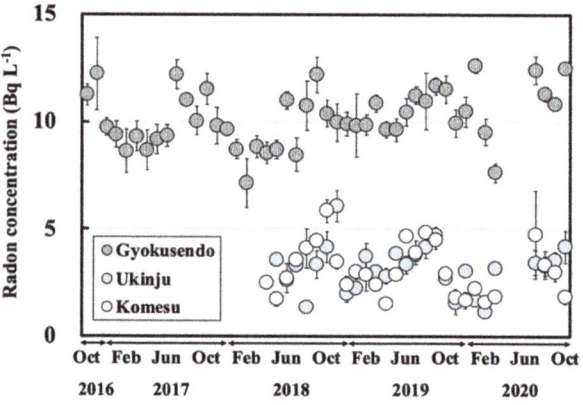

Figure 4. Radon concentration variation for the Gyokusendo cave, Ukinju spring and Komesu spring water samples collected during the October 2016–October 2020 sampling period.

The monthly average radon concentrations of the dripping water for the entire sampling period were the highest (11 ± 0.8 Bq L^{-1}) in October and the lowest (8.8 ± 1.2 Bq L^{-1}) in February (Figure 5). These variations were similar to the seasonal variations in atmospheric radon concentrations in the Gyokusendo cave sample (high in summer and low in winter) observed between July 1990 and January 1993 [15–17]. The radon concentrations for the water collected at Ukinju spring and Komesu spring were 3.2 ± 1.0 Bq L^{-1} (1.1–6.1 Bq L^{-1}) and 3.1 ± 1.1 Bq L^{-1} (1.1–5.8 Bq L^{-1}) (Figure 4). There was a gradual increase in radon concentrations from summer to autumn. However, no clear seasonal variation was apparent (Figure 4).

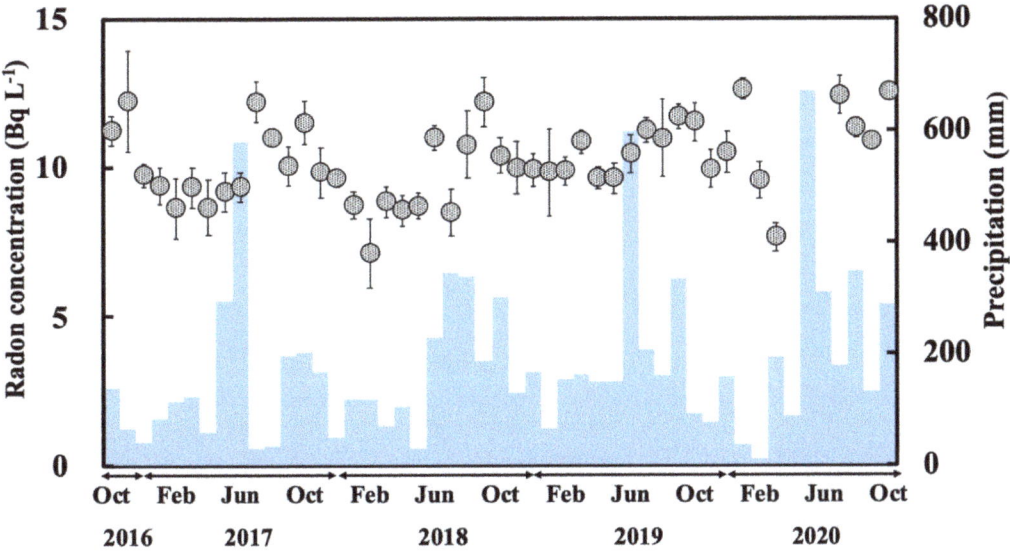

Figure 5. Variation of radon concentrations for the dripping water sample from the Gyokusendo cave compared to the monthly precipitation obtained from AMeDAS (Itokazu) for the study period.

3.3. Relationship between Radon Concentration for Dripping Water and Monthly Precipitation

The temporal variation in the radon concentrations of the dripping water from the Gyokusendo cave and the precipitation recorded for the study period are shown in Figure 5. The monthly precipitation was approximately 500 mm during the rainy season, increased during the typhoon season, and decreased to approximately 100–150 mm during winter.

In May 2017, an anomalously high precipitation amount of 579 mm (equivalent to approximately 30% of the 2017 annual precipitation) was recorded, and the radon concentration of the dripping water in July of that year was 12 Bq L^{-1}, the highest recorded in 2017. The precipitation from May to June 2018 was lower than usual, averaging a monthly amount of 300 mm. However, in September 2018, the radon concentration in the dripping water from the cave was exceptionally high, reaching 12 Bq L^{-1}. In 2019, the highest amount of precipitation for the year (597 mm) was recorded in June, and the maximum radon concentration for the year was recorded in September (12 Bq L^{-1}). More than 600 mm of precipitation was observed in June 2020, and maximum radon concentrations of 12 Bq L^{-1} and 13 Bq L^{-1} were recorded in July and October 2020. Conversely, a decreasing precipitation trend corresponded to a decrease in the radon concentration. Additionally, time series analysis (moving average) of the radon concentrations in dripping water and precipitation showed a correlation between the 2-month moving average ($R = 0.50$) and the 3-month moving average ($R = 0.50$) [32]. Therefore, variations in radon concentrations of the dripping water samples indicated that the radon concentration increased during periods of heavy rainfall, although a delay of around two to three months after a monthly precipitation change was observed. This suggests that precipitation percolates at a rate of 60 to 90 d from the soil to the Ryukyu limestone situated above the Gyokusendo cave and reaches the cave as dripping water.

Radon concentrations in groundwater reflect the inherent ^{226}Ra contents of the host rock or formation [33]. In areas where karst aquifers are distributed, estimated radon concentrations in the soil are higher than the radon concentrations in the groundwater. Therefore, the main source of radon in groundwater has been reported to be soil [8]. Furthermore, the concentrations of the ^{238}U series in the Ryukyu limestone (8.6 Bq kg^{-1}) were reported to be lower than those in Shimajiri red soil (86.0 Bq kg^{-1}) [34], suggesting that the main source of radon in groundwater is the soil deposited in the upper part of the Gyokusendo cave. Additionally, the amount of soil water infiltrating into the aquifer increases with heavy precipitation [7]. In limestone areas, the residence time of soil water was noted to reflect the residence time in the limestone bodies [8]. The flow velocity is proportional to the flow rate and inversely proportional to the cross-sectional area of the channel. The flow velocity is the distance an object moves per unit time, the flow rate is the volume of fluid per unit time flowing past a point through the cross-sectional area. The channel is referring to solution openings through the limestone. The following equations was used to calculate the flow velocity:

$$v = \frac{Q}{A} \quad (4)$$

where v is the flow velocity (m s^{-1}), Q is the flow rate (m^3 s^{-1}), and A is the cross-sectional area of the channel (m^2). It is assumed that the main source of radon in groundwater is the soil deposited in the upper part of the Gyokusendo cave and that the cross-sectional area of the channel does not change significantly. Therefore, radon in the dripping water is derived from radon in the soil pore water, which is governed by the soil ^{226}Ra content and the residence time of groundwater in the Ryukyu limestone. Moreover, the amount of groundwater in the Ryukyu limestone depends on precipitation. High precipitation rates shorten the residence time of groundwater in the Ryukyu limestone by increasing infiltration into the soil, which accelerates the groundwater flow velocity. Low precipitation rates reduce infiltration into the soil, thus, decreasing the groundwater flow velocity and increasing the residence time of groundwater. Attenuation is constant (the half-life, 3.8 day) over time. Therefore, the longer the residence time, the lower the radon concentration and vice versa. In this study, the radon concentration trends correlated with the precipitation trends, suggesting that the soil may be the source of radon in the groundwater. Moreover, the variation in the radon concentration of the dripping water sample may have been due to the residence time of groundwater in the Ryukyu limestone.

3.4. Estimation of Residence Time Using Radon Decay in the Dripping Water

A schematic of a vertical section of the Gyokusendo cave is shown in Figure 6. In the figure, A shows the boundary between the soil and the Ryukyu limestone, and B is a straw stalactite on the cave ceiling where the dripping water is collected. Precipitation percolates through the soil and limestone bodies above the cave and seeps into the cave from the ceiling as dripping water. Since radon is rarely present in precipitation, radon in groundwater is mainly supplied by the soil. The concentration of radon in water infiltrated into the ground increases with time due to the supply of radon produced by soil particles. However, as the concentration increases, the number of decaying radon atoms increases, and eventually, an equilibrium state is reached where supply and decay are equal. Therefore, radon in the soil water and ^{226}Ra in the solid phase are in permanent equilibrium. Additionally, if radon remains in the soil long enough, the concentration of radon in the gas and liquid phases will reach the equilibrium state specific to each soil species. The following equations were used to quantify the radon concentration in soil water and the gas phase at gas-liquid equilibrium:

$$E_w = K_T E_a \quad (5)$$

where E_w is the radon concentration in soil water (kBq m^{-3}), K_T is the radon partition coefficient, and E_a is the radon concentration in the gas phase (kBq m^{-3}). The radon partition coefficient was calculated using the following equation [35]:

$$K_T = \frac{9.12}{17.0 + T} \quad (6)$$

where T is the temperature (°C), and the mean value of the temperature in the cave, 24.9 °C, was used.

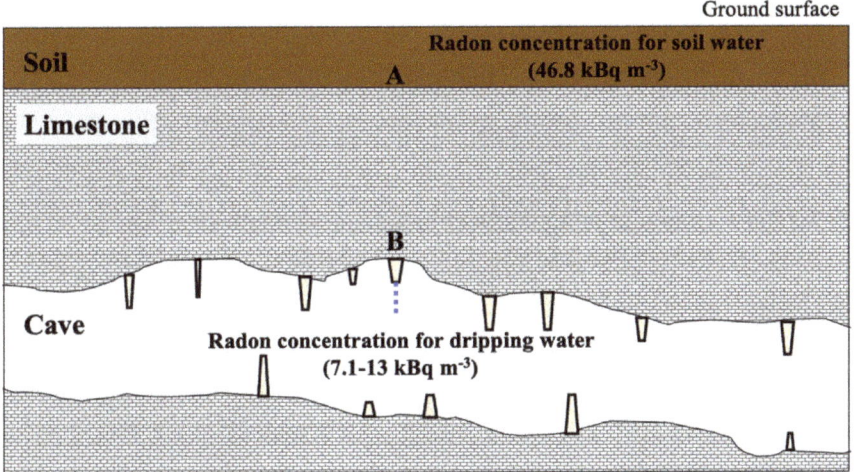

Figure 6. Schematic of the Gyokusendo cave profile, where A is the boundary between the soil and the limestone, and B is the target straw stalactite.

According to the UNSCEAR 2000 (United Nation Scientific Committee on the Effects of Atomic Radiation 2000), the concentration of radon in soil pore gas E_a (Bq m^{-3}) can be calculated using the following equation [36]:

$$E_a = C_{Ra} f \rho_s \varepsilon^{-1} (1 - \varepsilon) [m(K_T - 1) + 1]^{-1} \quad (7)$$

where C_{Ra} is the concentration of ^{226}Ra in the soil (Bq kg^{-1}), f is the radon emanation coefficient, ρ_s is the density of solid particles (kg m^{-3}), ε is the porosity, and m is the water saturation. In this study, based on a previous report [37], the radon emanation coefficient for typical soil on Okinawa Island was set to 0.40, the concentration of ^{226}Ra in soil was set to 106 Bq kg^{-1} dry, the solid particle density was set to 2697 kg m^{-3}, and the porosity was set to 0.67. The water saturation was 0.95, which is representative of the UNSCEAR 2000 [36]. The radon partition coefficient K_T was calculated using Equation (6) [35]. Since we could not directly measure the soil temperature, we used the temperature in the cave (24.9 °C) as approximation of the soil temperature. Radon concentrations (Bq m^{-3}) in soil water were calculated using Equation (5). The above values were defined as the radon concentration in the groundwater at point A (Figure 6).

Because radon was not supplied from the Ryukyu limestone, we assumed that the radon concentration in the groundwater was attenuated by the residence time of the groundwater in the Ryukyu limestone. The estimated radon concentration in the dripping water sample E_d, exuding from point B (Figure 6), was calculated using the estimated radon concentration in soil water from Equation (5) and the following equation.

$$E_d = E_w \exp(-\lambda t) \quad (8)$$

where t is the residence time (days) of groundwater in the Ryukyu limestone.

The estimated radon concentrations in the dripping water sample calculated from Equation (8) were compared with the measured radon concentrations in the dripping water obtained during the study period. The radon concentration in the soil pore gas calculated from Equation (7) was 215 kBq m^{-3}. The radon concentration in the soil pore water calculated from Equation (5) was 46.8 kBq m^{-3}. Radon concentrations for the dripping water sample obtained during the study period ranged from 7.1–13 kBq m^{-3} as shown in Figure 4. Based on the decay of radon (half-life: 3.8 d) from point A (estimated values) to point B (measured values) and the assumption that the residence time of soil and Ryukyu limestone is 60 to 90 d, the residence time of groundwater in the Ryukyu limestone was estimated to be 7 to 10 d. These results are generally consistent with previously reported values (9–10 d) [20]. Moreover, the residence time of groundwater in the soil deposited in the upper part of the Gyokusendo cave was estimated to be approximately 50 to 80 d.

The residence time of groundwater in the Ryukyu limestone at the Ukinju spring and Komesu spring sites was also calculated from Equation (8). For this calculation, we assumed that no radon was supplied from the Ryukyu limestone, the soil was uniformly deposited, and the radon concentration in the soil was in radiative equilibrium. The radon concentrations for the water samples from the Ukinju spring and Komesu spring sites ranged from 3.1–6.1 Bq L^{-1} and 1.1–5.8 Bq L^{-1}, respectively. Based on the radon attenuation between the measured radon concentrations in the water samples and the estimated radon concentrations in the pore water, the residence times in the Ryukyu limestone at Ukinju spring and Komesu spring were estimated to be 12 to 21 d and 12 to 19 d, respectively. Nakaya et al. (2018) reported an average residence time in the Ryukyu limestone aquifer of 14–34 years based on the results of SF$_6$ concentrations in the spring and well water around the Komesu spring site [38]. The residence time estimated in this study is very limited because it was calculated based on observations at only one point in the catchment. Although we were able to calculate the residence time, our results significantly differ from those of previous studies. In the future, it will be necessary to discuss the residence time after considering additional factors such as the frequency of collection, and number of sites, and depth of sampling sites.

4. Conclusions

Radon concentrations for dripping water and spring water samples were collected in the southern part of Okinawa Island from October 2016 to October 2020. The estimated radon concentrations in the dripping water sample were calculated with the measured radon concentrations from the dripping water obtained during the study period. Based on our results, we determined the following:

(1) The radon concentrations in the water samples from the Gyokusendo cave, Ukinju spring, and Komesu spring were 10 ± 1.3 Bq L^{-1}, 3.2 ± 1.0 Bq L^{-1}, and 3.1 ± 1.1 Bq L^{-1}, respectively. Radon concentrations for the water samples showed a gradually increasing trend from summer to autumn and decreased in the winter. This was particularly noticeable in the radon concentrations measured in the dripping water sample from the Gyokusendo cave.

(2) From the variation in the radon concentrations for the dripping water and precipitation, we estimated that the radon concentration changes in the dripping water lags precipitation changes by approximately 2–3 months. These results indicate that precipitation takes 60 to 90 d to percolate into the soil and accumulate in the Ryukyu limestone overlying the Gyokusendo cave. The water then enters the cave as dripping water from the cave ceiling.

(3) From a simple radon behavior model, groundwater in the Gyokusendo cave system was estimated to percolate through the Ryukyu limestone in 7 to 10 d, and the residence time of groundwater in the soil above the Gyokusendo cave was estimated at approximately 50 to 80 d.

(4) The residence times of groundwater in the Ryukyu limestone at the Ukinju spring and Komesu spring sites were calculated to be 12 to 21 d and 12 to 19 d, respectively. However, this estimation was lower than that of previous studies (14–34 years). Therefore, it will be necessary for future studies to discuss the residence time after understanding factors such as the frequency of collection, and the number of sites, and depth of sampling sites. Additionally, to verify the residence time and mixing of groundwater in the area, radioactive isotopes with longer half-lives, such as tritium (half-life: 12.3 y) should be analyzed in the future.

Author Contributions: Conceived and designed the survey: S.N., Y.S., N.A., M.F. Performed experiments: S.N., A.I., S.S., N.M., S.O., K.N., A.K. Analyzed the data: S.N., A.I., S.S., N.M. Wrote the paper: S.N. Acquired the funding: S.N., M.T., N.A., M.H., Y.S. Contributed to discussions: S.N., Y.S., N.A., Y.Y., M.F. All authors have read and agreed to the published version of the manuscript.

Funding: This research was funded by JSPS KAKENHI Grant Number JP20J12397 and 18K14543, the NIFS budget NIFS20KLEA046 and NIFS18KNWA002.

Acknowledgments: The radon concentration analyses were performed at the National Institute for Fusion Science, University of the Ryukyus Center of Research Advancement and Collaboration.

Conflicts of Interest: The authors declare that they have no conflict of interest.

References

1. World Health Organization. *WHO Handbook on Indoor Radon: A Public Health Perspective*; WHO: Geneva, Switzerland, 2009.
2. Nazaroff, W.W. Radon transport from soil to air. *Rev. Geophys.* **1992**, *30*, 137–160. [CrossRef]
3. Hirao, S.; Yamazawa, H.; Moriizumi, J.; Yoshioka, K.; Iida, T. Development and verification of long-range atmospheric radon-222 transport model. *J. Nucl. Sci. Technol.* **2008**, *45*, 166–172. [CrossRef]
4. Csondor, K.; Erőss, A.; Horváth, Á.; Szieberth, D. Radon as a natural tracer for underwater cave exploration. *J. Environ. Radioact.* **2017**, *173*, 51–57. [CrossRef] [PubMed]
5. Hoehn, E.; Von Guten, H.R. Radon in groundwater: A tool to assess infiltration from surface waters to aquifers. *Water Resour. Res.* **1989**, *25*, 1795–1803. [CrossRef]
6. Ellins, K.K.; Roman-mas, A.; Lee, R. Using ^{222}Rn to examine groundwater/surface discharge interaction in the Rio Grande de Manati, Puerto Rico. *J. Hydrol.* **1990**, *115*, 319–341. [CrossRef]
7. Hamada, H. Estimation of groundwater flow rate using the decay of ^{222}Rn in a well. *J. Environ. Radioact.* **2000**, *47*, 1–13. [CrossRef]
8. Savoy, L.; Subeck, H.; Hunkeler, D. Radon and CO_2 as natural tracers to investigate the recharge dynamics of karst aquifers. *J. Hydrol.* **2011**, *406*, 148–157. [CrossRef]
9. Hamada, H.; Komae, T. Analysis of recharge by paddy field irrigation using ^{222}Rn concentration in groundwater as an indicator. *J. Hydrol.* **1998**, *205*, 92–100. [CrossRef]
10. Igarashi, G.; Saeki, S.; Takahata, N.; Sumikawa, K.; Tasaka, S.; Sasaki, Y.; Takahashi, M.; Sano, Y. Ground-water radon anomaly before the Kobe earthquake in Japan. *Science* **1995**, *269*, 60–61. [CrossRef]
11. Yasuoka, Y.; Shinogi, M. Anomaly in atmospheric radon concentration: A possible precursor of the 1995 Kobe, Japan, earthquake. *Health Phys.* **1997**, *72*, 759–761. [CrossRef]
12. Koike, K.; Yoshinaga, T.; Asaue, H. Characterizing long-term radon concentration changes in a geothermal area for correlation with volcanic earthquakes and reservoir temperatures: A case study from Mt. Aso, southwestern Japan. *J. Volcanol. Geotherm. Res.* **2014**, *275*, 85–102. [CrossRef]
13. Oh, H.Y.; Kim, G. A radon-thoron isotope pair as a reliable earthquake precursor. *Sci. Rep.* **2015**, *5*, 13084. [CrossRef] [PubMed]
14. Kuo, T.; Fan, K.; Kuochen, H.; Han, Y.; Chu, H.; Lee, Y. Anomalous decrease in groundwater radon before the Taiwan M6.8 Chengkung earthquake. *J. Environ. Radioact.* **2006**, *88*, 101–106. [CrossRef] [PubMed]
15. Tanahara, A.; Taira, H.; Takemura, M. Radon distribution and the ventilation of a limestone cave on Okinawa. *Geochem. J.* **1997**, *31*, 49–56. [CrossRef]
16. Tanahara, A.; Iha, H.; Taira, H. Factors controlling the changes in ^{222}Rn concentration in Gyokusendo cave on Okinawa Island. *J. Speleol. Soc. Jpn.* **1997**, *22*, 98–105. (In Japanese)
17. Iha, H.; Tanahara, A.; Taira, H. A critical analysis of changing radon concentration patterns on Gyokusendo cave in Okinawa Island. *J. Speleol. Soc. Jpn.* **1999**, *24*, 51–56. (In Japanese)

18. Ford, D.C.; Williams, P.W. *Karst Hydrogeology and Geomorphology*, 1st ed.; Springer: Dordrecht, The Netherlands, 1989; pp. 99–120. ISBN 978–0470849972.
19. Japan Meteorological Agency. Automated Meteorological Data Acquistion System (AMeDAS). Available online: https://www.data.jma.go.jp/obd/stats/etrn/index.php (accessed on 27 November 2020).
20. Shiroma, Y.; Shiroma, M.; Kina, S.; Hosoda, M.; Yasuoka, Y.; Akata, N.; Furukawa, M. Source of atmospheric radon in the Gyokusendo, a limestone cave in Okinawa, Japan. *Jpn. J. Health Phys.* **2016**, *51*, 218–226. (In Japanese) [CrossRef]
21. Iryu, Y.; Matsuda, H.; Machiyama, H.; Piller, E.W.; Quinn, M.T.; Mutti, M. Introductory perspective on the COREF project. *Island Arc* **2006**, *15*, 393–406. (In Japanese) [CrossRef]
22. Furukawa, H. The southern part of Okinawa Island. In *Geological Feature of the Ryukyu Arc*, 1st ed.; Kizaki, K., Ed.; The Okinawa Times Co., Ltd.: Okinawa, Japan, 1985; pp. 107–112. (In Japanese)
23. Kaneko, N.; Ujiie, H. Ryukyu Group. In *Geology of the Itoman and Kudaka Jima District*, 1st ed.; Kaneko, N., Ed.; Geological Survey of Japan, AIST: Ibaraki, Japan, 2006; pp. 16–25. (In Japanese)
24. Hamazaki, T. Parent materials and soils of Nansei-shoto in Japan. *Pedologist* **1979**, *23*, 43–57. (In Japanese) [CrossRef]
25. Tokashiki, Y. The characteristic properties of the Shimajiri Mahji and Jahgaru soils in Okinawa prefecture. *Pedologist* **1993**, *37*, 99–112. [CrossRef]
26. Ishihara, Y.; Yoshimura, K.; Ooka, S.; Sasaki, H. Topography, geology of Sakitarido ruins and ruins formation process. In *Excavation Report of the Sakitari-Do Cave Site, Nanjo City, Okinawa Pref.*, 1st ed.; Yamazaki, S., Ed.; Okinawa Prefectural Museum and Art Museum: Okinawa, Japan, 2018; pp. 221–252. (In Japanese)
27. Tanaka, R.; Araki, S.; Yasuoka, Y.; Mukai, T.; Ohnuma, S.; Ishikawa, T.; Fukuhori, N.; Sanada, T. A simplified method for improved determination of radon concentration in environmental water samples. *Radioisotopes* **2013**, *62*, 423–438. [CrossRef]
28. Yasuoka, Y.; Ishii, T.; Kataoka, Y.; Kubo, T.; Suda, H.; Tokonami, S.; Ishikawa, T.; Shinogi, M. Determination of radon concentration in water using liquid scintillation counter. *Radioisotopes* **2004**, *53*, 123–131. [CrossRef]
29. Yasuoka, Y.; Ishikawa, T.; Fukuhori, N.; Tokonami, S. Comparison of simplified liquid scintillation counter (Triathler) with conventional liquid scintillation counter in the measurement of radon concentration in water. *J. Hot Spring Sci.* **2009**, *59*, 11–21.
30. Knoll, G.F. *Radiation Detection and Measurement*, 4th ed.; Wiley: Hoboken, NJ, USA, 2000; pp. 94–99. ISBN 978-0-470-13148-0.
31. Kraguten, J. Tutorial review. Calculating standard deviations and confidence intervals with a universally applicable spread sheet technique. *Analyst* **1994**, *119*, 2161–2165. [CrossRef]
32. Shumway, R.H.; Stoffer, D.S. *Time Series Analysis and Its Applications with R Examples*, 4th ed.; Springer: New York, NY, USA, 2017; pp. 1–74. ISBN 978-3-319-52452-8.
33. Tenner, A.B. Physical and chemical controls on the distribution of radium-226 and radon-222 in groundwater near Great Salt Lake, Utah. In *The Natural Radiation Environment*, 1st ed.; Actams, J.A.S., Lowder, W.M., Eds.; University of Chicago Press: Chicago, IL, USA, 1964; pp. 253–276. ISBN 978–0080441375.
34. Furukawa, M.; Kina, S.; Shiroma, M.; Shiroma, Y.; Masuda, N.; Motomura, D.; Hiraoka, H.; Fujioka, S.; Kawakami, T.; Yasuda, Y.; et al. Terrestrial gamma radiation dose rate in Ryukyu Islands, subtropical region of Japan. *Radiat. Prot. Dosim.* **2015**, *167*, 223–227. [CrossRef]
35. Noguchi, M. Liquid scintillation counting technique(X), special applications (2), measurements of radon activity. *Radioisotopes* **1975**, *24*, 745–748. [CrossRef]
36. United Nations Scientific Committee on the Effects of Atomic Radiation. Annex B: Exposures from natural radiation sources. In *Sources and Effects of Ionizing Radiation UNSCEAR 2000 Report to the General Assembly, with Scientific Annexes*; United Nations: New York, NY, USA, 2000; Volume 1, pp. 97–108. ISBN 92-1-142238-8.
37. Shiroma, Y.; Hosoda, M.; Ishikawa, T.; Sahoo, S.K.; Tokonami, S.; Furukawa, M. Estimation of radon emanation coefficient for representative soils in Okinawa Japan. *Radiat. Prot. Dosim.* **2015**, *167*, 147–150. [CrossRef]
38. Nakaya, S.; Yasumoto, J.; Ha, M.P.; Aoki, H.; Kohara, F.; Masuda, H.; Masuoka, K. Hydrochemical behavior of an underground dammed limestone aquifer in the subtropics. *Hydrol. Process.* **2018**, *32*, 3529–3546. [CrossRef]

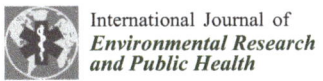

Article

Discriminative Measurement of Absorbed Dose Rates in Air from Natural and Artificial Radionuclides in Namie Town, Fukushima Prefecture

Koya Ogura [1], Masahiro Hosoda [1,2], Yuki Tamakuma [1,2], Takahito Suzuki [1,†], Ryohei Yamada [1,‡], Ryoju Negami [1], Takakiyo Tsujiguchi [1], Masaru Yamaguchi [1], Yoshitaka Shiroma [3], Kazuki Iwaoka [4], Naofumi Akata [2], Mayumi Shimizu [2], Ikuo Kashiwakura [1] and Shinji Tokonami [2,*]

1. Graduate School of Health Sciences, Hirosaki University, 66-1 Hon-cho, Hirosaki, Aomori 036-8564, Japan; kogura@hirosaki-u.ac.jp (K.O.); m_hosoda@hirosaki-u.ac.jp (M.H.); tamakuma@hirosaki-u.ac.jp (Y.T.); suzuki-takahito@fujielectric.com (T.S.); yamada.ryohei@jaea.go.jp (R.Y.); h20gg204@hirosaki-u.ac.jp (R.N.); r.tsuji@hirosaki-u.ac.jp (T.T.); masarun@hirosaki-u.ac.jp (M.Y.); ikashi@hirosaki-u.ac.jp (I.K.)
2. Institute of Radiation Emergency Medicine, Hirosaki University, 66-1 Hon-cho, Hirosaki, Aomori 036-8564, Japan; akata@hirosaki-u.ac.jp (N.A.); mshimizu@hirosaki-u.ac.jp (M.S.)
3. Faculty of Education, University of the Ryukyus, 1 Senbaru, Nishihara-cho, Okinawa 903-0213, Japan; y_shiro@cs.u-ryukyu.ac.jp
4. National Institutes for Quantum and Radiological Science and Technology, 4-9-1 Anagawa, Inage, Chiba 263-0024, Japan; iwaoka.kazuki@qst.go.jp
* Correspondence: tokonami@hirosaki-u.ac.jp
† Present address: Fuji Electric Co., Ltd., 1 Fujimachi, Hino, Tokyo 191-8502, Japan.
‡ Present address: Radiation Protection Department, Nuclear Fuel Cycle Engineering Laboratories, Japan Atomic Energy Agency, 4-33 Muramatsu, Tokai, Ibaraki 319-1194, Japan.

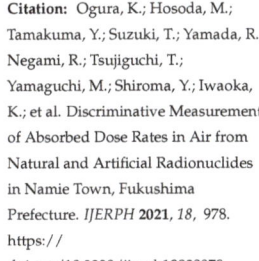

Citation: Ogura, K.; Hosoda, M.; Tamakuma, Y.; Suzuki, T.; Yamada, R.; Negami, R.; Tsujiguchi, T.; Yamaguchi, M.; Shiroma, Y.; Iwaoka, K.; et al. Discriminative Measurement of Absorbed Dose Rates in Air from Natural and Artificial Radionuclides in Namie Town, Fukushima Prefecture. *IJERPH* **2021**, *18*, 978. https://doi.org/10.3390/ijerph18030978

Academic Editor: Paul B. Tchounwou
Received: 28 December 2020
Accepted: 18 January 2021
Published: 22 January 2021

Publisher's Note: MDPI stays neutral with regard to jurisdictional claims in published maps and institutional affiliations.

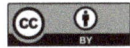

Copyright: © 2021 by the authors. Licensee MDPI, Basel, Switzerland. This article is an open access article distributed under the terms and conditions of the Creative Commons Attribution (CC BY) license (https://creativecommons.org/licenses/by/4.0/).

Abstract: Ten years have elapsed since the accident at the Fukushima Daiichi Nuclear Power Plant in 2011, and the relative contribution of natural radiation is increasing in Fukushima Prefecture due to the reduced dose of artificial radiation. In order to accurately determine the effective dose of exposure to artificial radiation, it is necessary to evaluate the effective dose of natural as well as artificial components. In this study, we measured the gamma-ray pulse-height distribution over the accessible area of Namie Town, Fukushima Prefecture, and evaluated the annual effective dose of external exposure by distinguishing between natural and artificial radionuclides. The estimated median (range) of absorbed dose rates in air from artificial radionuclides as of 1 April 2020, is 133 (67–511) nGy h^{-1} in the evacuation order cancellation zone, and 1306 (892–2081) nGy h^{-1} in the difficult-to-return zone. The median annual effective doses of external exposures from natural and artificial radionuclides were found to be 0.19 and 0.40 mSv in the evacuation order cancellation zone, and 0.25 and 3.9 mSv in the difficult-to-return zone. The latest annual effective dose of external exposure discriminated into natural and artificial radionuclides is expected to be utilized for radiation risk communication.

Keywords: Fukushima Daiichi Nuclear Power Plant; Namie Town; natural radionuclides; artificial radionuclides; cesium-134; cesium-137; external exposure dose evaluation

1. Introduction

On 11 March 2011, a magnitude 9.0 earthquake struck the Tohoku region along the eastern coast of Japan. The earthquake caused a tsunami with a height of more than 15 m, and affected the Fukushima Daiichi Nuclear Power Plant (FDNPP). The FDNPP lost power and the cores of Units 1 to 3 became heated and melted. This caused a hydrogen gas explosion [1]. As a result of the FDNPP accident, ^{132}Te, ^{131}I, ^{134}Cs, ^{137}Cs, and rare gases such as ^{133}Xe, etc., were released into Fukushima Prefecture and other eastern regions of Japan [2]. The radioactivity of radionuclides released into the atmosphere is shown in the UNSCEAR 2013 report (Table 1) [3]. On the day of the accident, the Japanese government issued an indoor evacuation order to residents within 10 km of the FDNPP, and issued an evacuation order to residents within 20 km the next day [4]. Thereafter, the area where the annual cumulative dose may have exceeded 20 mSv, outside the 20 km area from the FDNPP was designated as a "planned evacuation zone". In addition, regardless of the annual cumulative dose, the area within 20 to 30 km of the FDNPP was designated as an "emergency evacuation preparation zone" and the area within 20 km was designated as a "warning zone" [5]. Namie Town, Fukushima Prefecture (The location map that is shown in Figure 1a was made by original maps from d-maps.com), is also one of the areas significantly contaminated by radionuclides due to the FDNPP accident, and because it was a planned evacuation zone, the townspeople living there were forced to evacuate. In 2012, the area where the annual cumulative dose was confirmed to be 20 mSv or less was designated as an "evacuation order cancellation preparation zone". This is the area where temporary return homes, restricted businesses such as shops, hospitals, and farming are permitted. Areas where the annual cumulative dose may exceed 20 mSv but are confirmed to be 50 mSv or less have been designated as a "restricted residence zone" and it has become possible to temporarily return home or enter for road restoration. Areas where the annual cumulative dose exceeds 50 mSv and the annual cumulative dose may not fall below 20 mSv, five years from 2012, has been designated as a "difficult-to-return zone". Figure 1b indicates each area division, and taken from the official website of Fukushima Prefecture [5]. Subsequently, the artificial decontamination of radionuclides was actively promoted, and in 2017, six years after the earthquake, evacuation orders were lifted in some areas of Namie Town [6]. Currently, the return of evacuees is progressing, and by the end of November 2020, more than 1500 people were living in Namie Town [7]. Before the Great East Japan Earthquake, the registered population of Namie Town was 21,434 [8]. Years after the FDNPP accident, the returning residents continue to have a significant amount of radiation anxiety [9]. Experts in radiation science and psychology at each Japanese support organization, including the university of the current authors, have communicated radiation risk, and interacted with residents to reduce anxiety about radiation. In consideration of this, Kudo et al. conducted a questionnaire survey on the basic knowledge of radiation among those who returned to Namie Town. It was found that many Namie townspeople recognize that natural and artificial radiation have different effects on the human body, even if the effective dose is the same [10].

Since the FDNPP accident, national staff and researchers at universities and research institutions have been evaluating artificial radioactive contamination and investigating the distribution of ambient dose equivalent rates [11–13]. In addition, internal and external exposures from artificial radionuclides are being evaluated [14–19], and monitoring posts are installed in various locations to continuously measure the ambient dose equivalent rate [20]. In 2017, Shiroma et al. conducted a car-borne su rvey in Namie Town, Fukushima Prefecture, and reported that the absorbed dose rate in air was 0.041–11 $\mu Gy\ h^{-1}$ [21]. More than nine years have passed since the FDNPP accident, and the relative contribution of natural radiation to ambient dose equivalent rates is increasing because the dose of artificial radiation is decreasing. This means that it is not possible to estimate the effects on the human body due to artificial radionuclides, without correctly evaluating the dose from natural radionuclides. People with a high risk of internal exposure, such as agricultural workers, need information on internal exposure due to inhalation of dust. However, clarifying the actual conditions of external exposure from natural and artificial radionuclides is useful for radiation risk communication for general population, which has a low risk of internal exposure. In this study, the gamma-ray pulse-height distribution was measured and analyzed in Namie Town, which was divided into 1 km × 1 km meshes. An absorbed dose rate map that discriminated between natural and artificial radionuclides was created from the absorbed dose rate in the air, and the annual effective dose to external exposure was calculated.

Table 1. The estimated value of the quantity of typical radionuclides released into the atmosphere by the Fukushima Daiichi Nuclear Power Plant (FDNPP) accident.

The Estimated Value of the Quantity of Radionuclides Released into the Atmosphere (Bq)								
^{132}Te	^{131}I	^{132}I	^{133}I	^{133}Xe	^{134}Cs	^{136}Cs	^{137}Cs	
2.9×10^{16}	1.2×10^{17}	2.9×10^{16}	9.6×10^{15}	7.3×10^{18}	9.0×10^{15}	1.8×10^{15}	8.8×10^{15}	

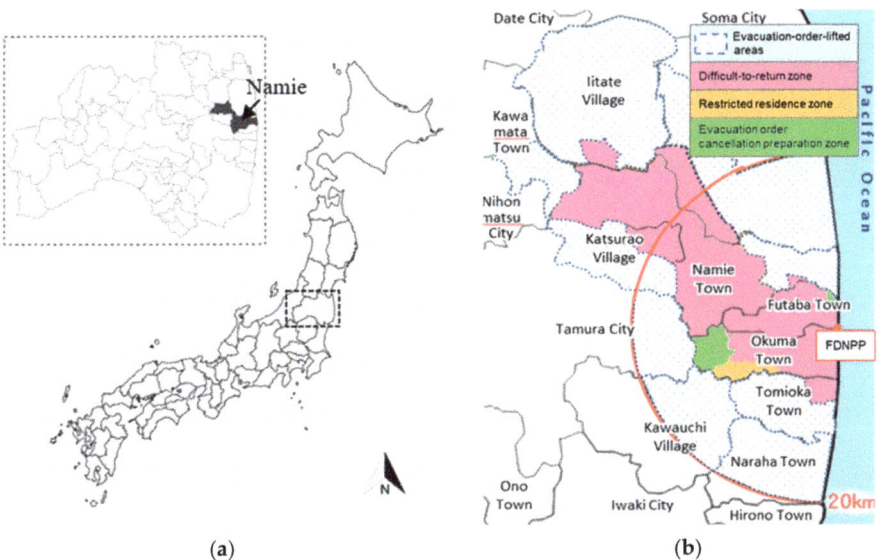

Figure 1. (**a**) Location of Namie Town, Fukushima Prefecture, Japan, and (**b**) officially designed evacuation zones as of 1 April 2017. (**a**) is created by d-maps.com (https://d-maps.com/carte.php?num_car=29487, https://d-maps.com/carte.php?num_car=11273). (**b**) is taken from the official website with permission from the administrative officer in Fukushima Prefecture [5].

2. Materials and Methods

2.1. Measurement Location and Method of γ-Ray Pulse-Height Distribution

From 15 September 2016 to 13 December 2019, gamma-ray pulse-height distributions were obtained at the 130 accessible points that divided the entire area of Namie Town into a mesh of 1 km × 1 km. A 3 × 3-inch NaI(Tl) scintillation spectrometer (EMF-211, EMF Japan Co., Himeji, Japan [22]) was used to obtain the measurements. The detector was installed 1 m above the ground and connected to a control laptop PC. The measurement time was 900 s. Latitude and longitude coordinate data were obtained using a Global Positioning System to create an absorbed dose rate map. Gamma-ray pulse-height distributions at 2–5 points were additionally acquired in six of the 130 meshes, and the fluctuation of the absorbed dose rate in air in the mesh was evaluated.

2.2. Analysis of Gamma-Ray Pulse-Height Distribution and Correction of Absorbed Dose Rate in Air

The gamma-ray pulse-height distributions obtained by the NaI(Tl) scintillation spectrometer is different from the distributions of the gamma-ray energy spectrum. The pulse-height distributions of gamma-ray are unfolded into the energy spectrum by a response matrix of 49 rows × 49 columns, and then the dose contributions for each radionuclide are calculated according to the previous reports to discriminate between natural and artificial radionuclides [23–25]. The absorbed dose rate in air obtained by the analysis needs to be corrected to consider the number of days elapsed from the measured date. Factors that reduce radioactivity in the environment include the physical half-life of radionuclides, diffusion by wind, rain, and infiltration into soil, and the implementation of artificial decontamination of radioactive substances. In order to comprehensively evaluate the factors that affect the attenuation of radioactivity, the apparent half-life was calculated using the data of the air dose rate that is regularly observed at the monitoring posts widely installed in Namie Town. There are 103 monitoring posts in Namie Town, and the measurement data are published on the website [20]. Some of these datasets have long-term data loss within the period in which we measured the gamma-ray pulse-height distribution, and significant dose increases and decreases in a short period of time that are not due to artificial decontamination. It is probable that the data loss could not be measured due to maintenance of the monitoring posts. The short-term significant fluctuation of the ambient dose equivalent rate may be due to a device malfunction, but the specific cause is unknown. These data may affect the appropriate time decay correction of absorbed dose rates in air. Therefore, the apparent half-life was calculated using the data of 55 monitoring posts, and excluding the lossy dataset and coefficient of determination R^2 of less than 0.7 (not due to artificial decontamination) in the exponential approximation of the ambient dose equivalent rate. Equation (1) was used to calculate the apparent half-life (T_a).

$$T_a = t \times \frac{0.693}{\ln\left(\frac{D_1}{D_0}\right)} \tag{1}$$

where D_0 and D_1 are the ambient dose equivalent rates (μSv h^{-1}) as of 1 April 2016, and 1 April 2020, respectively, and t is the elapsed time, which was taken as used four years. The FDNPP accident released short half-life radionuclides such as ^{131}I and ^{133}Xe and long half-life radionuclides such as ^{134}Cs and ^{137}Cs. Originally, it was necessary to calculate the apparent half-life for each of the short-half-life and long-half-life radionuclides, but now that nine years have elapsed since the accident, the contribution from the short-half-life radionuclides can be ignored [26,27]. The apparent half-life was calculated using the simple formula in Equation (1), considering only the contribution from radionuclides with a long half-life. The calculated apparent half-life was divided into an evacuation order cancellation zone and a difficult-to-return zone, and the fluctuation was evaluated to examine the application to the correction of the absorbed dose rate in air.

2.3. Estimating the Effective Dose of External Exposure

The annual effective dose of external exposure in Namie Town was estimated using Equation (2), and the time-corrected absorbed dose rate in air.

$$E = D \times DCF \times T \times (Q_{in} \times R + Q_{out}) \tag{2}$$

where D is the time-corrected absorbed dose rate in air (nGy h^{-1}) and DCF is a dose conversion factor (Sv Gy^{-1}) from the absorbed dose rate in air to the effective dose to external exposure. The natural radionuclide component DCF uses 0.748, as reported by Moriuchi et al., and the artificial radionuclide uses 0.73, as reported by Omori et al. [28,29]. T is the number of hours per year, which is 8766 h (24 h × 365.25 d). Q_{in} is the indoor occupancy factor, Q_{out} is the outdoor occupancy factor, and they are 0.83 and 0.17, respectively, as reported by Ploykrathok et al. [30]. R is a reduction factor, the natural radionuclide is 1, and the artificial radionuclide is 0.43, as reported by Yoshida et al. [31].

3. Results and Discussion

3.1. Absorbed Dose Rate in Air and Dose Rate Map

The gamma-ray pulse-height distribution was measured over the entire accessible area of Namie Town and was developed using a response matrix to determine the absorbed dose rate in air. The absorbed dose rates in air of the natural radionuclides, artificial radionuclides, and their totals are 15–68, 14–11,861, and 47–11,900 nGy h^{-1}, respectively. The total absorbed dose rate in air obtained in this study is almost in agreement with the 0.041–11 µGy h^{-1} measured by Shiroma et al. [21]. The absorbed dose rates in air of natural radionuclides, artificial radionuclides, and their totals in the evacuation order cancellation zone are 19–51, 14–2010, and 47–2040 nGy h^{-1}, respectively. The natural, artificial, and their total absorbed dose rates in air in the difficult-to-return zone are 15–68, 140–11,861, and 186–11,900 nGy h^{-1}, respectively. The radioactivity ratios of cesium (^{134}Cs/^{137}Cs) released from Units 1, 2, and 3 of the FDNPP were reported to be 0.941, 1.082, and 1.046, respectively [32]. This radioactivity ratio is evaluated as the value as of 11 March 2011. As a result of estimating ^{134}Cs/^{137}Cs as of March 2011 for the measured data, the median (range) was 1.07 (1.04–1.09), and it was confirmed that ^{134}Cs and ^{137}Cs were released from FDNPP. The apparent half-life was calculated by analyzing the datasets of 55 monitoring posts installed in Namie Townin order to time-correct the measured absorbed dose rate in air. A total of 32 of them were located in areas exceeding 1.0 µGy h^{-1} as of April 2016. 10 of them were located in areas exceeding 1.0 µGy h^{-1} as of April 2020. The mean ± standard deviation, coefficient of variation, and median (range) of apparent half-lives in the difficult-to-return zone are 4.2 ± 1.4 y, 33%, and 4.7 (4.0–4.8) y, respectively (Appendix A Table A1). Considering that the half-life of ^{137}Cs is approximately 30 years, the reason why the apparent half-life is shortened is seemingly strongly influenced by diffusion due to environmental factors. The mean ± standard deviation, coefficient of variation, and median (range) of the apparent half-life in the evacuation order cancellation zone are 4.8 ± 2.7 y, 56%, and 4.7 (2.3–6.7) y, respectively. It was found that there are variations in the areas where residence is allowed. The apparent half-life was calculated using the data from 1 April 2016 to 1 April 2020. A detailed review of the data for each monitoring post revealed that some areas were decontaminated after April 2016, and some were decontaminated prior to that date [33]. The implementation of artificial decontamination contributes to rapid dose reduction and significantly shortens the apparent half-life. Therefore, the evacuation order cancellation zone was further divided into areas where decontamination was conducted before, and on and after, April 2016, and the apparent half-life was analyzed. Figure 2 indicates the difficult-to-return zone, evacuation order cancellation zone decontaminated before April 2016, and evacuation order cancellation zone decontaminated on, and after, April 2016 areas. The mean ± standard deviation, coefficient of variation, and median (range) of the apparent half-life in the evacuation order cancellation zone are 6.4 ± 2.0 y, 31%, and 6.1 (5.0–7.5) y, respectively (Appendix A Table A2). Conversely, the mean value ± standard deviation, coefficient of variation, and median (range) of the apparent half-life limited to the zones where decontamination was completed after 1 April 2016, are 2.0 ± 0.6 y, 30%, 1.8. (1.6–2.3) y, respectively (Appendix A Table A3). A significant difference test was performed using the Mann–Whitney U test for the apparent half-life of the evacuation order cancellation zone decontaminated before, and on and after, April 2016. It was confirmed there was a significant difference between the two groups (p-value < 3.8 × 10^{-7}). This result demonstrates that the implementation of decontamination significantly contributes to the reduction of the ambient dose equivalent rates from artificial radionuclides. In addition, it was found that the evacuation order cancellation zone can be evaluated with a fluctuation of approximately 30%, by dividing it into two areas for the calculations. This coefficient of variation is significantly lower than when the evacuation order cancellation zone was not divided into two. In addition, a significant difference in apparent half-life was determined using the Mann–Whitney U test for the difficult-to-return zone and evacuation order cancellation zone decontaminated before April 2016, for the difficult-to-return zone and the evacuation order cancellation zone decontaminated on and after April 2016. The p-values are 6.9 × 10^{-4} and 9.5 × 10^{-4}, respectively, confirming that there is a significant difference in distribution. Hayes et al. reported that the effective half-life of radiocesium in the environment was 7.8 years as a theoretical value and 3.2 years as a measured value [34]. Table 2 shows a comparison of the apparent half-life calculated in this study, the previously reported effective half-life, and the theoretical half-life.

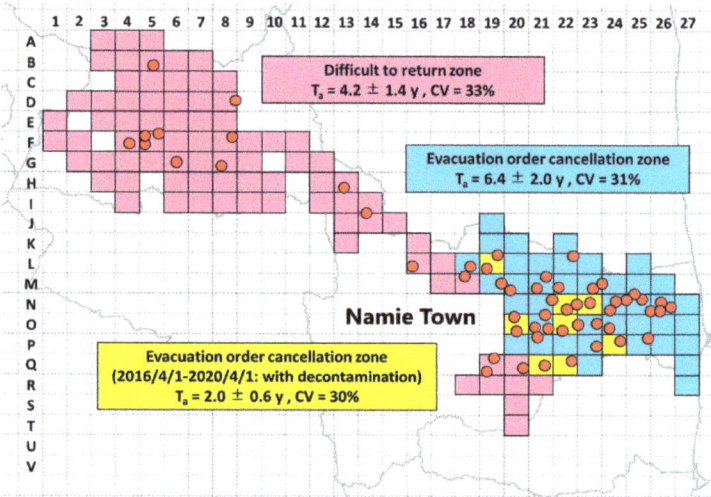

Figure 2. Area classification for which the apparent half-life was calculated, and the location of the monitoring posts. The red circles indicate the location of the monitoring posts used for the analysis, the blue mesh is the difficult-to-return zone, the pink mesh is the evacuation order cancellation zone where the radionuclides decontamination work was carried out before April 2016, and the green mesh is the evacuation order cancellation zone where the radionuclides decontamination work was carried out after April 2016. This map was drawn using a map created by Generic Mapping Tools [35].

Table 2. Comparison of the half-life of radiocesium in the environment.

Apparent Half-Life of Radiocesium in the Environment (y)				
Evacuation Order Cancellation Zone		Difficult-to-Return Zone	Previously Reported Value [34]	Theoretical Value [34]
Decontaminated before April 2016	Decontaminated on and after April 2016			
6.4	2.0	4.2	3.2	7.8

The measured data of absorbed dose rates in air from artificial radionuclides were corrected to the values as of 1 April 2020 using different apparent half-lives for each of the three areas (Appendix B). The median (range) is shown in Table 3, and the distribution of the absorbed dose rate in air of the artificial radionuclides collected as of 1 April 2020 is shown in Figure 3.

Table 3. Median (range) estimated absorbed dose rate in air as of 1 April 2020.

	Absorbed Dose Rate in air as of 1 April 2020 (nGy h^{-1})	
	Evacuation Order Cancellation Zone	Difficult-to-Return Zone
Natural radionuclides	28 (25–35)	37 (30–45)
Artificial radionuclides	133 (67–511)	1306 (892–2081)
Total	161 (995–81)	1340 (921–2124)

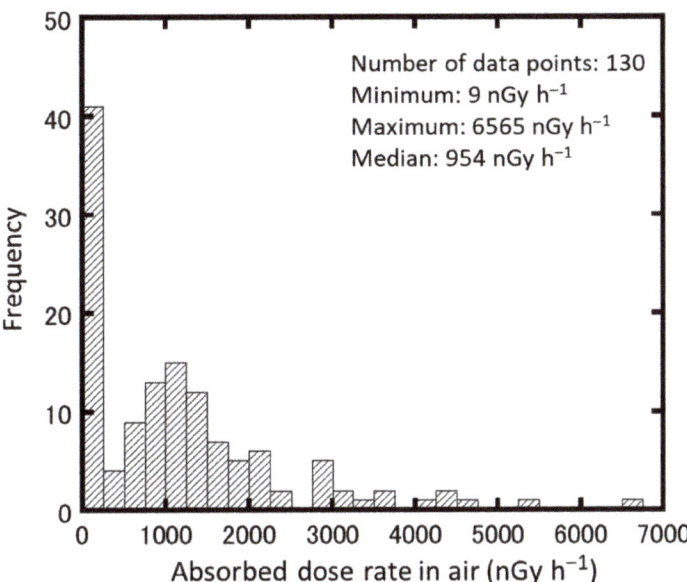

Figure 3. Histogram of absorbed dose rate in air of artificial radionuclides corrected as of 1 April 2020.

A significant difference test was performed using the Mann–Whitney U test on the absorbed dose rates in the air from artificial radionuclides in the evacuation order cancellation zone and the difficult-to-return zone. It was confirmed that the two groups are significantly different (p-value = 6.0×10^{-14}). The evacuation order cancellation zone is an area that the Japanese government has determined people can live in because it has been confirmed that the ambient dose equivalent rate has decreased [6]. In contrast, the difficult-to-return zone is an area where the annual cumulative dose exceeds 50 mSv as of April 2012, and the annual cumulative dose may not fall below 20 mSv after five years have elapsed [5]. It was found that the absorbed dose rate in air remained high in the difficult-to-return zone nine years after the FDNPP accident. The mean ± standard deviation and median (range) of absorbed dose rates in air by natural radionuclides throughout Namie Town are 35 ± 10 and 34 (28–42) nGy h^{-1}, respectively. The national average in Japan is reported to be 50 nGy h^{-1} [36]. It was found that the average value of Namie Town was 70% of the national average value. These data can be used for radiation risk communication. The absorbed dose rate maps (Figure 4a,b) were developed so that the absorbed dose rate in air could be visually understood by dividing it into natural and artificial radionuclides.

The activity concentrations of ^{40}K, ^{232}Th, and ^{238}U are shown in Appendix B. When examining the absorbed dose rate in air from natural radionuclides (Figure 4a), it can be seen that the eastern coastal area of Namie Town is less than 40 nGy h^{-1} in most areas. The range of activity concentrations of ^{40}K, ^{232}Th, and ^{238}U in the evacuation order cancellation zone were 109–444, 9–32, and 9–34 Bq kg^{-1}, respectively. Conversely, in the mountainous areas on the west side, there are many areas of 40 nGy h^{-1} or more. The range of activity concentrations of ^{40}K, ^{232}Th, and ^{238}U in the difficult-to-return zone were 99–1830, 9–46, and 10–161 Bq kg^{-1}, respectively. On the west side of Namie Town, where granite is widely distributed, the activity concentrations of ^{40}K, ^{232}Th, and ^{238}U tended to be high [37]. When examining the absorbed dose rate in air from artificial radionuclides (Figure 4b), it can be seen that there is a clear difference between the coastal areas on the east side and the mountainous areas on the west side. This is a clear result of the evacuation order cancellation zone and the difficult-to-return zone. In the coastal area, decontamination was actively conducted in order to realize the return of evacuees, and the evacuation order was lifted in March 2017 [6]. In contrast, the mountainous area on the west side has many areas exceeding 1.0 µGy h^{-1}, and is remains designated as a difficult-to-return zone. This result indicates that artificial decontamination activities contribute significantly to dose reduction. However, there were two meshes in the evacuation order cancellation area that exceeded 1.0 µGy h^{-1}. Factors that increased the absorbed dose rate in air in this area include the presence of slopes composed of soil and the presence of localized forest areas in the city, such as bamboo groves. Slopes composed of soil have not been actively decontaminated because they may loosen the ground and cause sediment-related disasters. Local forest areas in the city, such as bamboo groves, are difficult to decontaminate by removing the upper part of the soil without cutting, which is a factor that increases the absorbed dose rate in air. However, local forests and slopes composed of soil do not always exist uniformly within a 1 km × 1 km mesh. In order to examine the variation of the measurement data in the mesh, the absorbed dose rate in air was additionally measured at 2–5 points in six out of the 130 meshes (Table 4). Although there are some fluctuations depending on the mesh, it was found that it is possible to evaluate with a volatility of approximately 50% or less. It was also determined that the volatility is not dose-dependent.

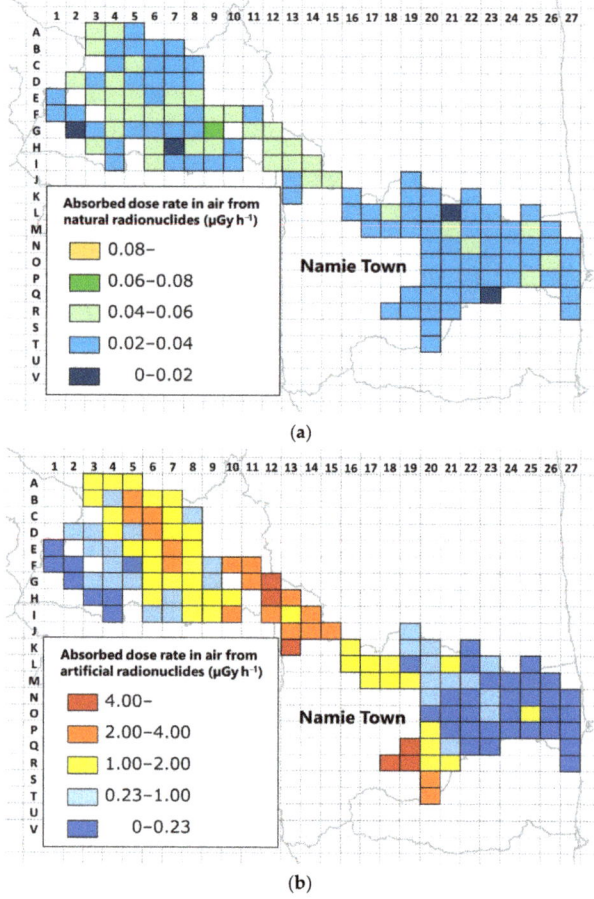

Figure 4. (a) Map of absorbed dose rate in air derived from natural radionuclides and (b) map of absorbed dose rate in air derived from artificial radionuclides. This map was drawn using a map created by Generic Mapping Tools [35].

Table 4. Evaluation of variation of measurements data in a 1 km × 1 km mesh.

Mesh Code	Number of Measurements	Absorbed Dose Rate in Air		
		Average ± Standard Deviation (nGy h^{-1})	Standard Error (nGy h^{-1})	Coefficient of Variation
F5	4	1118 ± 84	42	8%
L22	3	126 ± 33	19	26%
L23	6	312 ± 147	60	47%
M22	5	227 ± 83	37	37%
M24	4	156 ± 14	7	9%
N23	3	147 ± 44	25	30%

3.2. Estimating External Exposure Dose

Table 5 indicates the median (range) of the annual effective dose of external exposure calculated from the absorbed dose rate in the air. The annual effective doses of natural radionuclides in the evacuation order cancellation zone, difficult-to-return zone, and Namie Town as a whole are 0.12–0.33, 0.10–0.45, and 0.10–0.45 mSv, respectively, and their geometric mean (mean ± standard deviation) is 0.20 (0.20 ± 0.05), 0.24 (0.24 ± 0.06), and 0.22 (0.23 ± 0.06), respectively. The national average effective annual dose of ground gamma-rays in Japan is 0.33 mSv. It was found that the average value for the town of Namie is 70% of the national average [38,39]. The annual effective doses of external exposure to artificial radionuclides in the evacuation order cancellation zone, difficult-to-return zone, and entire Namie Town are 0.03–4.6, 0.23–19.6, and 0.03–19.6 mSv, respectively. The median annual external exposure effective dose from artificial radionuclides in the evacuation order cancellation zone (0.40 mSv) is 0.21 mSv, which differs from the median natural radionuclides (0.19 mSv). In contrast, the median annual external exposure effective dose from artificial radionuclides in the difficult-to-return zone (3.9 mSv) is 15.6 times higher than the median from natural radionuclides (0.25 mSv). A significant difference test was performed using the Mann–Whitney U test on the annual effective dose of external exposure from artificial radionuclides in the evacuation order cancellation zone and the difficult-to-return zone. The two groups have a statistically significant difference (p-value $< 6.0 \times 10^{-14}$). This difficult-to-return zone is an area where access to people is restricted. Cars are allowed on some sections, but the general public is still not allowed to stay for a long time [40]. Currently, in difficult-to-return zone, active decontamination is being carried out so that people can live. In the future, this artificial decontamination is expected to reduce the absorbed dose rate in air.

Table 5. Estimated annual external exposure effective dose.

	Median (Range) Annual External Exposure Effective Dose (mSv)	
	Evacuation Order Cancellation Zone	Difficult-to-Return Zone
Natural radionuclides	0.19 (0.16–0.23)	0.25 (0.20–0.29)
Artificial radionuclides	0.40 (0.20–1.5)	3.9 (2.7–6.2)
Total	0.55 (0.39–1.7)	4.1 (2.9–6.5)

4. Conclusions

The absorbed dose rate in air was measured by discriminating between natural and artificial radionuclides in the entire area of Namie Town, an area affected by the FDNPP accident. The following results were obtained from this study:

1. From the measurements of ^{134}Cs and ^{137}Cs concentrations, it was confirmed that Namie Town was radioactively contaminated by artificial radionuclides from the FDNPP accident.
2. From the data of the monitoring posts installed in Namie Town, the median (range) of the apparent half-life of artificial radionuclides in the evacuation order cancellation

zone decontaminated before April 2016, the evacuation order cancellation zone decontaminated after April 2016, and the difficult-to-return zone, is 6.4 ± 2.0, 2.0 ± 0.6, and 4.2 ± 1.4 y, respectively.

3. The median (range) of absorbed dose rates in the air from artificial radionuclides time-corrected as of 1 April 2020, using the apparent half-life are 133 (67–511) and 1306 (892–2081) nGy h^{-1} in the evacuation order cancellation zone and the difficult-to-return zone, respectively.
4. The median annual effective doses of external exposures from natural and artificial radionuclides are 0.19 and 0.40 mSv in the evacuation order cancellation zone and 0.25 and 3.9 mSv in the difficult-to-return zone.

Examination of the absorbed dose rate in the air from artificial radionuclides revealed a clear difference between the eastern coastal area and the western mountainous area. This result suggests that artificial decontamination activities contribute significantly to dose reduction. The distribution map of the absorbed dose rate in air measured in this study, and the information on the annual external exposure effective dose calculated by discriminating between natural and artificial radionuclides, are expected to be utilized for radiation risk communication.

Author Contributions: Conceptualization, M.H. and S.T.; Formal analysis, Y.T., T.S., R.Y., and R.N.; Funding acquisition, S.T.; Investigation, K.O., M.H., Y.T., T.S., T.T., M.Y., Y.S., K.I., and M.S.; Methodology, M.H. and S.T.; Project administration, S.T.; Supervision, M.H. and S.T.; Validation, K.O., M.H. and N.A.; Visualization, K.O.; Writing—original draft, K.O.; Writing—review and editing, M.H., T.T., M.Y., Y.S., I.K., and S.T. All authors have read and agreed to the published version of the manuscript.

Funding: This research was supported by Research on the Health Effects of Radiation, organized by the Ministry of the Environment, Japan.

Conflicts of Interest: The authors declare no conflict of interest.

Appendix A

Table A1. Calculation table of apparent half-life in the difficult-to-return zone.

Mesh Code	Ambient Dose Equivalent Rate (µSv h^{-1})		Apparent Half-Life (y)
	As of 1 April 2016	As of 1 April 2020	
B5	4.2	2.4	4.7
D8	2.4	1.3	4.5
F4	1.2	0.64	4.7
F5	0.96	0.60	5.8
F5	4.9	0.70	1.4
F5	2.1	0.44	1.8
F8	3.6	2.0	4.6
G6	2.3	1.3	5.1
G8	1.7	0.88	4.2
H13	5.4	3.2	5.2
J14	6.4	3.2	4.0
L16	1.0	0.62	5.6
M18	3.6	2.0	4.8
Q19	2.2	1.2	4.7
Q19	11.8	5.7	3.9
Q20	4.7	0.69	1.4

Table A2. Calculation table of apparent half-life in the evacuation order cancellation zone where decontamination was conducted before 1 April 2016.

Mesh Code	Ambient Dose Equivalent Rate (μSv h^{-1})		Apparent Half-Life (y)
	As of 1 April 2016	As of 1 April 2020	
L18	1.5	0.76	3.9
L19	3.2	1.9	5.0
L22	0.40	0.28	8.2
M19	2.2	1.2	4.7
M20	0.59	0.41	7.5
M21	1.1	0.60	4.4
M21	0.38	0.24	6.1
M22	0.41	0.32	10.5
M23	0.25	0.18	8.8
M23	0.16	0.11	8.1
N22	0.88	0.38	3.3
N24	0.22	0.14	5.9
N24	0.19	0.14	10.1
N24	0.12	0.07	5.9
N25	0.25	0.15	5.5
N25	0.08	0.06	7.4
N25	0.10	0.07	6.2
N26	0.21	0.13	6.1
N26	0.13	0.09	6.4
N26	0.09	0.06	7.0
O23	0.46	0.24	4.2
O24	0.23	0.17	9.2
P21	0.64	0.30	3.6
P23	1.6	0.97	5.7
P25	0.16	0.11	7.1

Table A3. Calculation table of apparent half-life in the evacuation order cancellation zone where decontamination was conducted on, and after, 1 April 2016.

Mesh Code	Ambient Dose Equivalent Rate (μSv h^{-1})		Apparent Half-Life (y)
	As of 1 April 2016	As of 1 April 2020	
L19	1.2	0.36	2.3
N21	3.2	0.39	1.3
N22	2.5	0.26	1.2
N23	1.0	0.25	1.9
O20	2.1	0.47	1.8
O20	2.7	0.55	1.7
O21	1.2	0.26	1.8
O21	1.7	0.36	1.8
O21	1.2	0.34	2.3
O22	1.3	0.19	1.4
O22	0.58	0.27	3.6
P24	1.6	0.28	1.6
Q21	1.3	0.38	2.3

Appendix B

Table A4. Measured absorbed dose rate in air from natural and artificial radionuclides, estimated absorbed dose rate in air from artificial radionuclide as of 1 April 2020, and activity concentrations of natural radionuclides.

Mesh Code	Measuring Date	Absorbed Dose Rate in Air (nGy h^{-1})			^{40}K (Bq kg^{-1})	^{232}Th (Bq kg^{-1})	^{238}U (Bq kg^{-1})
		Artificial Radionuclides	Artificial Radionuclides as of 1 April 2020	Natural Radionuclides			
A3	2017/8/23	1620	1048	50	419	32	28
A4	2018/9/10	1320	1017	54	428	39	29
A5	2018/9/10	1600	1233	28	244	21	13
B3	2017/8/23	2230	1442	51	477	27	28
B4	2017/8/23	1370	886	26	248	15	14
B5	2017/11/1	3578	2390	22	273	18	11
B6	2017/8/23	2990	1934	33	262	22	19
B7	2017/11/1	1760	1175	22	178	12	14
C4	2017/8/23	1850	1196	23	139	16	15
C5	2017/8/23	3280	2121	47	431	22	28
C6	2017/11/1	3020	2017	37	354	22	19
C7	2017/11/3	1960	1310	38	286	22	25
C8	2017/11/1	1360	908	28	244	15	17
D2	2017/8/24	1230	796	49	400	28	30
D3	2017/8/24	1240	802	37	382	17	21
D4	2017/11/1	2840	1897	44	382	23	26
D5	2017/8/23	1520	983	39	363	18	23
D6	2017/11/1	3741	2498	29	317	22	15
D7	2017/11/1	2160	1442	32	311	17	17
D8	2017/11/1	1950	1302	30	288	13	18
E1	2017/8/24	239	155	36	314	18	22
E3	2017/8/24	811	525	41	351	25	23
E4	2017/8/24	954	617	41	367	22	24
E5	2017/8/23	2300	1487	45	391	22	28
E6	2017/11/1	2670	1783	35	300	16	23
E7	2017/11/1	3120	2083	43	407	25	22
E8	2017/11/1	2200	1469	50	502	27	25
F1	2017/8/24	305	197	30	302	16	15
F2	2017/8/25	246	159	29	252	17	17
F4	2017/8/24	1200	776	53	419	29	34
F5	2016/9/15	140	77	46	400	19	31
F6	2016/9/15	1980	1095	44	391	20	28
F7	2017/11/3	3010	2012	48	484	22	27
F8	2017/11/3	1770	1183	23	213	13	13
F9	2017/11/3	1060	709	48	428	22	30
F10	2017/11/3	5335	3566	45	545	42	25
F11	2017/11/3	5412	3618	38	530	37	21
G2	2017/8/24	255	165	17	143	10	10
G3	2017/8/24	376	243	31	216	19	20
G4	2017/8/24	891	576	45	407	22	27
G5	2017/8/25	1230	796	30	263	15	18
G6	2017/8/25	2380	1541	28	242	17	16
G7	2017/11/2	1930	1289	36	326	17	22
G8	2017/11/2	2080	1390	37	323	17	23
G9	2017/11/2	913	610	68	628	26	46
G11	2017/11/3	3100	2072	47	477	27	22
G12	2018/5/16	5890	4303	40	545	42	22
H3	2017/8/24	315	204	45	407	26	24
H4	2017/8/24	151	98	36	388	20	17

Table A4. Cont.

Mesh Code	Measuring Date	Absorbed Dose Rate in Air (nGy h^{-1})			^{40}K (Bq kg^{-1})	^{232}Th (Bq kg^{-1})	^{238}U (Bq kg^{-1})
		Artificial Radionuclides	Artificial Radionuclides as of 1 April 2020	Natural Radionuclides			
H6	2018/9/10	1310	1010	42	339	28	23
H7	2017/8/25	1430	926	15	99	11	9
H8	2017/11/2	1690	1129	45	437	16	30
H9	2017/11/2	2090	1396	43	348	22	28
H10	2017/11/2	2360	1577	32	304	18	16
H12	2018/5/16	6466	4723	44	659	45	25
H13	2016/9/16	5306	2935	54	678	45	31
I4	2017/8/24	207	134	28	251	15	16
I6	2018/9/10	1130	871	45	323	35	24
I7	2017/8/25	1220	790	37	330	18	23
I8	2017/11/2	1560	1042	38	348	15	24
I9	2017/11/2	1640	1096	37	333	15	24
I10	2017/11/2	3190	2131	34	407	15	15
I12	2018/5/16	4278	3125	52	582	36	30
I13	2018/9/11	2470	1904	41	354	31	19
I14	2018/5/16	3788	2767	52	447	35	30
J13	2018/5/16	3799	2775	31	336	24	16
J14	2018/5/16	4369	3192	41	459	28	23
J15	2018/5/16	3898	2847	42	394	22	24
J19	2017/12/22	925	724	23	208	15	12
K13	2018/5/16	5721	4179	39	502	39	22
K16	2018/9/10	1570	1210	40	308	33	19
K19	2017/12/22	595	466	21	199	13	10
K20	2017/12/22	1120	876	30	311	16	15
K22	2019/11/14	179	172	26	205	18	14
L16	2018/5/16	2490	1819	37	367	20	19
L17	2018/5/16	2090	1527	40	373	23	21
L18	2018/9/11	1510	1277	46	382	32	24
L19	2017/12/22	231	104	28	290	14	14
L20	2017/12/22	1100	861	24	189	13	15
L21	2017/12/22	1950	1526	19	109	13	13
L22	2017/12/22	147	115	28	258	16	15
L23	2018/12/26	285	249	30	265	20	15
L25	2018/12/26	89	78	22	169	14	13
M17	2018/5/16	1720	1256	24	220	16	11
M18	2018/5/16	2120	1549	33	281	21	18
M19	2016/9/16	1510	1031	26	181	16	16
M20	2017/12/22	1260	986	27	137	21	18
M21	2017/12/22	343	268	44	311	28	27
M22	2016/9/16	423	289	23	222	12	13
M23	2017/12/23	242	189	35	360	17	18
M24	2018/12/26	105	92	32	258	18	20
M25	2018/12/26	35	31	51	339	34	32
M26	2017/12/23	33	26	39	388	17	23
N20	2017/12/22	854	668	24	197	14	14
N21	2017/12/22	174	136	32	305	19	15
N22	2018/5/16	141	73	47	444	20	29
N23	2017/12/22	1460	654	38	413	15	21
N24	2016/9/16	14	9	39	336	20	24
N25	2016/9/15	67	46	28	298	12	16
N26	2018/12/26	76	67	31	244	16	20
N27	2017/12/23	27	21	39	379	18	22
O20	2017/12/22	135	60	26	260	15	12

Table A4. Cont.

Mesh Code	Measuring Date	Absorbed Dose Rate in Air (nGy h^{-1})			^{40}K (Bq kg^{-1})	^{232}Th (Bq kg^{-1})	^{238}U (Bq kg^{-1})
		Artificial Radionuclides	Artificial Radionuclides as of 1 April 2020	Natural Radionuclides			
O21	2017/12/22	120	94	27	272	15	14
O22	2017/12/22	306	137	23	230	12	13
O23	2017/12/23	398	312	34	298	19	19
O24	2017/12/23	231	181	36	388	18	18
O25	2017/12/23	1690	1323	34	257	20	22
O26	2018/12/26	182	159	44	416	22	25
O27	2018/12/26	19	17	32	285	20	17
P20	2017/8/26	2010	1519	25	184	15	16
P21	2017/12/22	100	78	24	242	14	11
P22	2017/12/22	53	41	34	357	19	16
P23	2018/12/26	149	130	21	224	10	11
P24	2016/9/17	563	162	28	236	20	13
P25	2017/12/23	39	30	46	407	31	23
P26	2018/12/26	76	66	40	360	22	22
P27	2018/12/26	20	18	27	254	14	15
Q19	2016/9/17	9604	5316	26	1260	91	13
Q20	2018/9/10	1480	1141	30	257	18	16
Q21	2017/8/26	1620	648	27	260	15	15
Q22	2018/9/11	206	119	28	257	15	15
Q23	2018/9/11	98	83	20	181	14	9
Q27	2018/12/26	61	53	22	225	9	13
R18	2018/9/10	5560	4285	30	416	44	16
R19	2016/9/17	11861	6565	39	1830	161	22
R20	2017/8/26	1650	1069	30	280	18	15
R21	2017/8/26	2390	1548	21	202	15	9
R27	2018/12/26	101	88	30	266	16	18
S20	2017/8/26	5342	3460	28	360	30	15
T20	2017/8/26	4269	2764	21	342	24	11

References

1. Yaneza, J.; Kuznetsova, M.; Souto-Iglesiasb, A. An analysis of the hydrogen explosion in the Fukushima-Daiichi accident. *Int. J. Hydrogen Energy* **2015**, *40*, 8261–8280. [CrossRef]
2. Tominaga, T.; Hachiya, M.; Tatsuzaki, H.; Akashi, M. The Accident at the Fukushima Daiichi Nuclear Power Plant in 2011. *Health Phys.* **2014**, *106*, 630–637. [CrossRef]
3. United Nations Scientific Committee on the Effects of Atomic Radiation. *UNSCEAR 2013 Report Annex A: Levels and Effects of Radiation Exposure Due to the Nuclear Accident after 2011 Great East-Japan Earthquake and Tsunami*; United Nations: New York, NY, USA, 2014.
4. Prime Minister's Office of Japan. Evacuation Order. (Tentative Translation). Available online: http://www.kantei.go.jp/jp/kikikanri/jisin/20110311miyagi/20110312siji11.pdf (accessed on 13 December 2020). (In Japanese)
5. Fukushima Revitalization Station. Transition of Evacuation Designated Zones. Available online: https://www.pref.fukushima.lg.jp/site/portal-english/en03-08.html (accessed on 13 December 2020).
6. Namie Town. About Area Reorganization and Evacuation Order Cancellation. (Tentative Translation). Available online: https://www.town.namie.fukushima.jp/soshiki/2/13457.html (accessed on 13 December 2020). (In Japanese)
7. Namie Town. Now in Namie Town. (Tentative Translation). Available online: https://www.town.namie.fukushima.jp/ (accessed on 13 December 2020). (In Japanese)
8. Fukushima Revitalization Station. The Situation in Namie Town. (Tentative Translation). Available online: https://www.pref.fukushima.lg.jp/site/portal/26-11.html (accessed on 13 December 2020).
9. Takebayashi, Y.; Lyamzina, Y.; Suzuki, Y.; Murakami, M. Risk Perception and Anxiety Regarding Radiation after the 2011 Fukushima Nuclear Power Plant Accident: A Systematic Qualitative Review. *Int. J. Environ. Res. Public Health* **2017**, *14*, 1306. [CrossRef]

10. Kudo, H.; Tokonami, S.; Hosoda, M.; Iwaoka, K.; Kasai, Y. Understanding of Basic Knowledge on Radiation among General Public –Comparison of Residents Participated in the Same Seminar in between Namie Town and Three Cities in Aomori Prefecture–. *Jpn. J. Health Phys.* **2016**, *51*, 92–97. [CrossRef]
11. Saito, K.; Tanihara, I.; Fujiwara, M.; Saito, T.; Simoura, S.; Otsuka, T.; Onda, Y.; Hoshi, M.; Ikeuchi, Y.; Takahashi, F.; et al. Detailed deposition density maps constructed by large-scale soil sampling for gamma-ray emitting radioactive nuclides from the Fukushima Dai-ichi Nuclear Power Plant accident. *J. Environ. Radioact.* **2015**, *139*, 308–319. [CrossRef]
12. Hosoda, M.; Tokonami, S.; Sorimachi, A.; Monzen, S.; Osanai, M.; Yamada, M.; Kashiwakura, I.; Akiba, S. The time variation of dose rate artificially increased by the Fukushima nuclear crisis. *Sci. Rep.* **2011**, *1*, 87. [CrossRef]
13. Andoh, M.; Nakahara, Y.; Tsuda, S.; Yoshida, T.; Takahashi, F.; Mikami, S.; Kinouchi, N.; Sato, T.; Tanigaki, M.; Takemiya, K.; et al. Measurement of air dose rates over a wide area around the Fukushima Dai-ichi Nuclear Power Plant through a series of car-borne surveys. *J. Environ. Radioact.* **2015**, *139*, 266–280. [CrossRef]
14. Akahane, K.; Yonai, S.; Fukuda, S.; Miyahara, N.; Yasuda, H.; Iwaoka, K.; Matsumoto, M.; Fukumura, A.; Akashi, M. NIRS external dose estimation system for Fukushima residents after the Fukushima Dai-ichi NPP accident. *Sci. Rep.* **2013**, *3*, 1670. [CrossRef]
15. Ishikawa, T.; Yasumura, S.; Ozasa, K.; Kobashi, G.; Yasuda, H.; Miyazaki, M.; Akahane, K.; Yonai, S.; Ohtsuru, A.; Sakai, A.; et al. The Fukushima Health Management Survey: Estimation of external doses to residents in Fukushima Prefecture. *Sci. Rep.* **2015**, *5*, 12712. [CrossRef]
16. Tokonami, S.; Hosoda, M.; Akiba, S.; Sorimachi, A.; Kashiwakura, I.; Balonov, M. Thyroid doses for evacuees from the Fukushima nuclear accident. *Sci. Rep.* **2012**, *2*, 507. [CrossRef]
17. Hayano, R.S.; Tsubokura, M.; Miyazaki, M.; Satou, H.; Sato, K.; Masaki, S.; Sakuma, Y. Internal radiocesium contamination of adults and children in Fukushima 7 to 20 months after the Fukushima NPP accident as measured by extensive whole-body-counter surveys. *Proc. Jpn. Acad. Ser. B* **2013**, *89*, 157–163. [CrossRef]
18. Hosoda, M.; Tokonami, S.; Akiba, S.; Kurihara, O.; Sorimachi, A.; Ishikawa, T.; Momose, T.; Nakano, T.; Mariya, Y.; Kashiwakura, I. Estimation of internal exposure of the thyroid to ^{131}I on the basis of ^{134}Cs accumulated in the body among evacuees of the Fukushima Daiichi Nuclear Power Station accident. *Environ. Int.* **2013**, *61*, 73–76. [CrossRef]
19. Kim, E.; Kurihara, O.; Tani, K.; Ohmachi, Y.; Fukutsu, K.; Sakai, K.; Akashi, M. Intake ratio of ^{131}I to ^{137}Cs derived from thyroid and whole-body doses to Fukushima residents. *Radiet. Prot. Dosim.* **2016**, *168*, 408–418.
20. Nuclear Regulation Authority Japan. Monitoring Information of Environmental Radioactivity Level. (Tentative Translation). Available online: http://radioactivity.nsr.go.jp/map/ja/ (accessed on 13 December 2020). (In Japanese)
21. Shiroma, Y.; Hosoda, M.; Iwaoka, K.; Hegedűs, M.; Kudo, H.; Tsujiguchi, T.; Yamaguchi, M.; Akata, N.; Kashiwakura, I.; Tokonami, S. Changes of Absorbed Dose Rate in Air by CAR-BORNE Survey in Namie Town, Fukushima Prefecture After the Fukushima Daiichi Nuclear Power Plant Accident. *Radiet. Prot. Dosim.* **2019**, *184*, 527–530. [CrossRef]
22. EMF Japan Co. Product Overview of EMF211 Type Gamma Ray Spectrometer. (Tentative Translation). Available online: https://www.emf-japan.com/emf/img/PDF/emf211-survey.pdf (accessed on 13 January 2021). (In Japanese)
23. Radiation Earth Science Laboratory. Introduction of 49x49 Response Matrix for Environment Gamma Ray Analysis. (Tentative Translation). Available online: http://www1.s3.starcat.ne.jp/reslnote/YONQ.pdf (accessed on 14 December 2020). (In Japanese)
24. Minato, S. Diagonal elements fitting technique to improve response matrixes for environmental gamma ray spectrum unfolding. *Radioisotopes* **2001**, *50*, 463–471. [CrossRef]
25. International Commission on Radiation Unites and Measurements. *ICRU Report 53: Gamma-Ray Spectrometry in the Environment*; International Commission on Radiation Unites and Measurements: Stockholm, Sweden, 1994.
26. Sanada, Y.; Urabe, Y.; Sasaki, M.; Ochi, K.; Torii, T. Evaluation of ecological half-life of dose rate based on airborne radiation monitoring following the Fukushima Dai-ichi nuclear power plant accident. *J. Environ. Radioact.* **2018**, *192*, 417–425. [CrossRef]
27. Kinase, S.; Takahashi, T.; Saito, K. Long-term predictions of ambient dose equivalent rates after the Fukushima Daiichi nuclear power plant accident. *J. Nucl. Sci. Technol.* **2017**, *54*, 12. [CrossRef]
28. Moriuchi, S.; Tsutsumi, M.; Saito, K. Examination on Conversion Factors to Estimate Effective Dose Equivalent from Absorbed Dose in Air for Natural Gamma Radiations. *Jpn. J. Health Phys.* **1990**, *25*, 121–128. [CrossRef]
29. Omori, Y.; Wakamatsu, H.; Sorimachi, A.; Ishikawa, T. Radiation survey on Fukushima Medical University premises about four years after the Fukushima nuclear disaster. *Fukushima J. Med. Sci.* **2016**, *62*, 1–17. [CrossRef]
30. Ploykrathok, T.; Ogura, K.; Shimizu, M.; Hosoda, M.; Shiroma, Y.; Kudo, H.; Tamakuma, Y.; Tokonami, S. Estimation of annual effective dose in Namie Town, Fukushima Prefecture due to inhalation of radon and thoron progeny. *Radiat. Emer. Med.* **2020**, *10*, 1.
31. Yoshida, H.; Hosoda, M.; Kanagami, T.; Uegaki, M.; Tashima, H. Reduction factors for wooden houses due to external γ-radiation based on in situ measurements after the Fukushima nuclear accident. *Sci. Rep.* **2014**, *4*, 7541. [CrossRef]
32. Nishizawa, Y.; Yoshida, M.; Sanada, Y.; Torii, T. Distribution of the ^{134}Cs/^{137}Cs ratio around the Fukushima Daiichi nuclear power plant using an unmanned helicopter radiation monitoring system. *J. Nucl. Sci. Technol.* **2016**, *53*, 4. [CrossRef]
33. Ministry of the Environment. Decontamination Information Site—Specified Reconstruction and Regeneration Base [Namie Town]-(Tentative Translation). Available online: http://josen.env.go.jp/kyoten/namie/ (accessed on 13 December 2020). (In Japanese)
34. Hayes, J.M.; Johnson, T.E.; Anderson, D.; Nanba, K. Effective Half-life of ^{134}Cs and ^{137}Cs in Fukushima Prefecture When Compared to Theoretical Decay Models. *Health Phys.* **2020**, *118*, 60–64. [CrossRef]

35. Wessel, P.; Smith, W.H.F. Free software helps map and display data. *Trans. Am. Geophys. Union* **1991**, *72*, 441–446. [CrossRef]
36. Furukawa, M.; Shingaki, R. Terrestrial gamma radiation dose rate in Japan estimated before the 2011 Great East Japan Earthquake. *Radiat. Emerg. Med.* **2012**, *1*, 11–16.
37. Geological Survey of Japan. Geology of Namie, Iwaki and Tomioka Areas. (Tentative Translation). Available online: https://www.gsj.jp/data/50KGM/PDF/GSJ_MAP_G050_07046_1994_D.pdf (accessed on 14 December 2020). (In Japanese)
38. Omori, Y.; Hosoda, M.; Takahashi, F.; Sanada, T.; Hirao, S.; Ono, K.; Furukawa, M. Japanese population dose from natural radiation. *J. Radiol. Prot.* **2020**, *40*, 99–140. [CrossRef]
39. Hosoda, M.; Tokonami, S.; Furukawa, M. Dose assessment on natural radiation, natural radionuclide, and artificial radionuclide released by the Fukushima nuclear accident. *Radiat. Biol. Res. Commun.* **2012**, *47*, 22–45.
40. Ministry of Economy, Trade and Industry. Standards for Temporary Entry into Difficult-to-Return Zone. (Tentative Translation). Available online: https://www.meti.go.jp/earthquake/nuclear/kinkyu/hinanshiji/pdf/190905_zissikizyun2.pdf (accessed on 13 December 2020). (In Japanese)

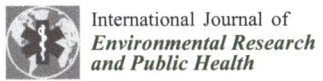

Article

Radon Activity Concentrations in Natural Hot Spring Water: Dose Assessment and Health Perspective

Eka Djatnika Nugraha [1,2], Masahiro Hosoda [2,3], June Mellawati [1], Untara Untara [1], Ilsa Rosianna [4], Yuki Tamakuma [2,3], Oumar Bobbo Modibo [2], Chutima Kranrod [3], Kusdiana Kusdiana [1] and Shinji Tokonami [3,*]

1. Centre for Technology of Radiation Safety and Metrology, National Nuclear Energy Agency of Indonesia (BATAN), Jakarta 12440, Indonesia; eka.dj.n@batan.go.id (E.D.N.); june_mellawati@batan.go.id (J.M.); tara@batan.go.id (U.U.); kusdiana@batan.go.id (K.K.)
2. Department of Radiation Science, Graduate School of Health Sciences, Hirosaki University, Hirosaki 036-8504, Japan; m_hosoda@hirosaki-u.ac.jp (M.H.); tamakuma@hirosaki-u.ac.jp (Y.T.); h19gg701@hirosaki-u.ac.jp (O.B.M.)
3. Institute of Radiation Emergency Medicine, Hirosaki University, Hirosaki 036-8504, Japan; kranrodc@hirosaki-u.ac.jp
4. Centre for Nuclear Minerals Technology, National Nuclear Energy Agency of Indonesia (BATAN), Jakarta 12440, Indonesia; ilsa.r@batan.go.id
* Correspondence: tokonami@hirosaki-u.ac.jp; Tel.: +81-172-39-5404

Abstract: The world community has long used natural hot springs for tourist and medicinal purposes. In Indonesia, the province of West Java, which is naturally surrounded by volcanoes, is the main destination for hot spring tourism. This paper is the first report on radon measurements in tourism natural hot spring water in Indonesia as part of radiation protection for public health. The purpose of this paper is to study the contribution of radon doses from natural hot spring water and thereby facilitate radiation protection for public health. A total of 18 water samples were measured with an electrostatic collection type radon monitor (RAD7, Durridge Co., USA). The concentration of radon in natural hot spring water samples in the West Java region, Indonesia ranges from 0.26 to 31 Bq L^{-1}. An estimate of the annual effective dose in the natural hot spring water area ranges from 0.51 to 0.71 mSv with a mean of 0.60 mSv for workers. Meanwhile, the annual effective dose for the public ranges from 0.10 to 0.14 mSv with an average of 0.12 mSv. This value is within the range of the average committed effective dose from inhalation and terrestrial radiation for the general public, 1.7 mSv annually.

Keywords: radon; hot spring; dose assessment; public health

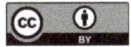

1. Introduction

Odourless and originating from radium-226 (^{226}Ra) decay that naturally occurs in the earth's crust, radon is a radioactive noble gas. According to the United Nations Scientific Committee on the Effects of Atomic Radiation (UNSCEAR), half of the world's mean value of annual effective dose by natural radiation sources is attributed to ^{222}Rn, thoron (^{220}Rn) and their progenies [1]. Radon (^{222}Rn) has been recognised as a carcinogenic gas and is well-known as the second leading health risk factor for lung cancer [1–3]. Radon from water contributes to the total inhalation risk associated with radon in indoor air. In addition to this, drinking water contains dissolved radon and the radiation emitted by radon and its radioactive decay products exposes sensitive cells in the stomach as well as other organs once it is absorbed into the bloodstream. Noting this danger, the United States Environmental Protection Agency (EPA) proposed a maximum contaminant level (MCL) for radon in the water around 11 Bq L^{-1} [4].

Radon dissolves in water that passes through soil and rock containing the natural radioactive substance [5,6]. As a result, water moving deeper through the earth's crust gathers increasing concentrations of radon and other natural radioactive materials. When, during the geothermal process, temperatures and pressures increase enough, some of this water is expelled through faults and cracks, reaching the earth's surface as hot springs. Hot spring water produced under these circumstances usually contains high concentrations of ^{222}Rn. This is due to at least one of two natural processes: ^{226}Ra dissolving in the water after interacting with rock and soil in the earth or ^{222}Rn entering the water from rocks containing ^{226}Ra [6–8].

The world community has long used natural hot springs for tourist and medicinal purposes. In Indonesia, the province of West Java, which is naturally surrounded by volcanoes, is a prime hot spring tourist destination. Approximately 1.8 million tourists visit natural hot springs in the West Java province each year [9–11].

It is, therefore, necessary to study the contribution of ^{222}Rn doses from natural hot spring water as part of radiation protection for public health. This paper is the first report on ^{222}Rn measurements in tourism natural hot spring water in Indonesia. Previous studies related to radon measurements in Indonesia included measurements of air at dwellings [12–15], ^{222}Rn in water samples [15], ^{222}Rn in geothermal and geosciences [16]

2. Materials and Methods

2.1. Study Area

This research was conducted in several districts in West Java, including the Ciater Hot Springs area in Subang; the Ciwidey and Pangalengan Hot Springs areas in Bandung; and the Cipanas and Darajat Hot Springs areas in Garut. Each of these hot springs is a major tourist destination, as shown in Figure 1. Visited by approximately 300,000 tourists each year, the Ciwidey and Pangalengan areas are tourist destinations located on the Patuha volcano. The Ciater Hot Spring, located on the Tangkuban Perahu volcano, is the most popular area for hot spring tourism with approximately 1.3 million visitors annually. Finally, as many as 50,000 tourists visit the Cipanas and Darajat areas every year [9–11]. The Cipanas area is located on the Guntur volcano, and the Darajat area is on the Kamojang volcano, which also has a geothermal power plant.

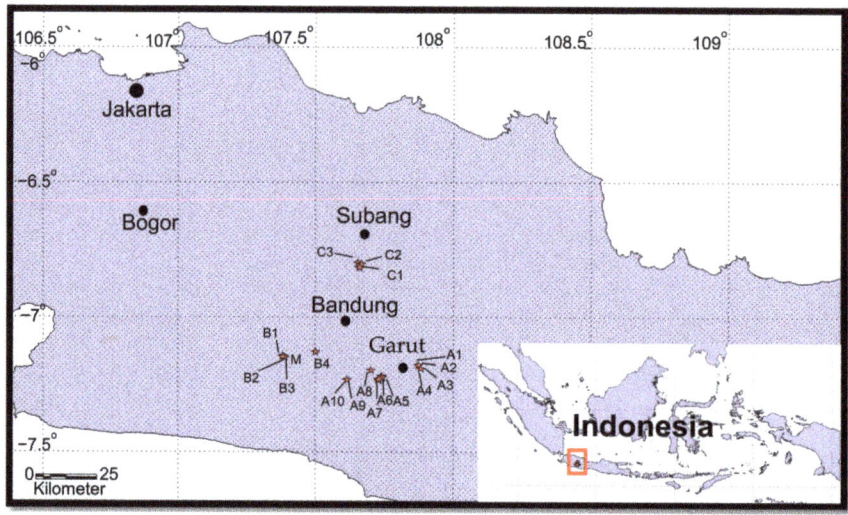

Figure 1. The study area, covering three cities: Bandung, Subang, and Garut. The black dots represent cities, and red asterisks indicate sampling locations.

2.2. Radon Measurement in Water Samples

A total of 18 water samples of 250 mL each were collected using radon-tight reagent bottles as part of the water analysis accessory (RAD-H2O, Durridge Co., USA). This study was conducted in September 2019, which includes the dry season. The samples included 17 natural hot springs water samples and one mineral water sample. The samples were measured for temperature, pH, and electroconductivity (E.C.) (Laquatwin, Horiba, Japan). In addition, the ambient dose equivalent rates (PDR-111, Hitachi, Japan) around the sampling area were measured. An electrostatic collection type ^{222}Rn monitor (RAD7, Durridge Co., USA) connected to a water analysis accessory was used to measure the samples and detect alpha activity. The RAD7 detector connected the monitor with a bubbling kit for degassing of ^{222}Rn in a water sample into the air in a closed circuit, as shown in Figure 2. Before the ^{222}Rn arrived at the detector, it also needed to be dried with a desiccant (CaSO$_4$, Drierite, W A Hammond, USA) to absorb the moisture.

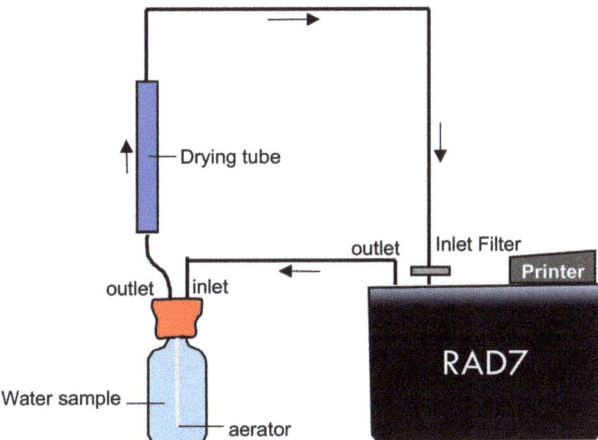

Figure 2. Schematic of experimental setup for measuring dissolved ^{222}Rn measurement

We used the WAT250 protocol in five-minute cycles and five recycles to generate data. In this measurement protocol for grab samples analysis, the pump ran for five minutes, flushing the measurement chamber, and then stopping. The RAD7 waited for five additional minutes at the end of the run before printing a summary. Since the analysis was made more than an hour after the sample was taken, a correction was applied to account for ^{222}Rn decay [17]. The amount of radon loss was calculated using the decay formula, or Equation (1):

$$C'_t = C'_0 A e^{-\lambda t'/60} \qquad (1)$$

where C'_t (Bq m^{-3}) is the ^{222}Rn activity concentration at time t' (min); C'_0 is the ^{222}Rn activity concentration at time $t' = 0$; and λ is the ^{222}Rn decay constant (7.542 × 10^{-3} h^{-1}).

2.3. Radon Measurement in the Air

We measured the ^{222}Rn activity concentration in the air 1 m above the hot spring pool with RAD7 for 8 h. An 'auto' mode was used to obtain this measurement in 60 min cycles, and eight recycles were allowed. ^{222}Rn measurements began with the sniff mode before changing automatically to the normal mode after 3 h 45 min. The results obtained were then averaged. We also measured the ^{222}Rn activity concentration in the dwelling around each natural hot spring area as the background for estimating the transfer coefficient from ^{222}Rn in the water to ^{222}Rn in the air.

2.4. Estimation of Annual Effective Dose

We used Equation (2) to calculate the contribution of ^{222}Rn in the water to ^{222}Rn in the atmosphere. Meanwhile, the internal annual effective dose from ^{222}Rn through inhalation, the annual effective dose from external radiation, and the annual effective dose are shown in Equations (3)–(5), respectively.

$$D_{Rn-w} = C_{Rn-w} \times TF_{Rn-w-a}, \qquad (2)$$

$$E_{in(Rn)} = C_{Rn} \times F \times DCF_{RnP} \times T, \qquad (3)$$

$$E_{ext} = H^* \times CF \times DCF_{H-D} \times T, \qquad (4)$$

$$AED = E_{ext} + E_{in-Rn}. \qquad (5)$$

In Equation (2), D_{Rn-w} is the ^{222}Rn activity concentration contributed from water to the atmosphere (Bq m^{-3}); C_{Rn-w} is the ^{222}Rn activity concentration in the water samples (Bq L^{-1}); and TF_{Rn-w-a} is the transfer coefficient from water to air, which equals 1×10^{-4} [18,19]. In Equation (3), $E_{in(Rn)}$ is the internal annual effective dose from ^{222}Rn through inhalation (mSv); C_{Rn} is the ^{222}Rn activity concentration in the air (Bq m^{-3}); F is the equilibrium factor of ^{222}Rn and radon progeny, which equals 0.4; DCF_{RnP} is the dose conversion factor for ^{222}Rn, which equals 1.7×10^{-5} mSv (Bq h m^{-3})$^{-1}$ [3,20]; and T is the time, which is 2000 h for the worker and 8 h a week, or 384 h annually, for the public. In Equation (4), E_{ext} is the annual effective dose from external radiation; H^* is the ambient dose equivalent rates (nSv h^{-1}); CF is the conversion factor from ambient dose equivalent rates to the absorbed dose in the air, which equals 0.652 (Gy Sv^{-1}) [21]; and DCF_{H-D} is the conversion factor from the absorbed dose in the air to the external effective dose, which equals 0.7 [1]. Finally, AED is the annual effective dose (mSv).

3. Results and Discussion

Natural hot springs are a popular tourist attraction in West Java. Since at least 1980, tourists have enjoyed the natural atmosphere of the area while participating in activities such as swimming, soaking, photographing the scenery, and walking in the park. Many even stay overnight [9–11]. Despite its diverse other uses, natural hot spring water in West Java is not used for drinking. Therefore, we performed dose assessments through inhalation and external dose radiation only.

From a total of 17 natural hot spring water samples and one mineral bottled water sample, the value of electroconductivity ranged from 0.164 to 1.925 mS cm^{-1} with an average value of 1.541 mS cm^{-1}. Meanwhile, the pH ranged from 5 to 7 with an average value of 6. Finally, water temperature, as shown in Table 1, ranged from 36 to 42 °C with an average of 39 °C. According to the regulations of the Indonesian Ministry of Health [22], and the World Health Organisation [23], the E.C. and pH values in natural hot spring water samples in West Java fall above recommended values, which must be below 1.5 mS cm^{-1} and 6.5–8.5 for E.C. and pH, respectively. E.C. is closely related to the content of dissolved solids in the water. Thus, if water with a high E.C. value and pH level is used for drinking, gastrointestinal upset and kidney disease can result. Unlike the natural hot spring water samples, the mineral bottled water is suitable for drinking.

Table 1. The location, physical and chemical properties of the water samples.

Samples	Area	Longitude (E)	Latitude (S)	Elevation (m)	Temperature (°C)	Electroconductivity at 25 °C (mS cm^{-1})	pH
A1	Cipanas	107.8716	−7.17643	1678	38	1.511	6
A2	Cipanas	107.8816	−7.18884	1675	38	1.459	6
A3	Cipanas	107.7016	−7.19645	1668	39	1.485	6
A4	Cipanas	107.5016	−7.19646	1671	39	1.458	6
A5	Darajat	107.7415	−7.21833	1672	37	1.442	6
A6	Darajat	107.7414	−7.21914	1670	38	1.538	6
A7	Darajat	107.7416	−7.22191	1672	37	1.586	6
A8	Darajat	107.7287	−7.22935	1973	42	1.682	5
A9	Darajat	107.7287	−7.22906	1976	42	1.628	5
A10	Darajat	107.7287	−7.22851	1985	42	1.677	5
B1	Ciwidey	107.3843	−7.14416	1779	37	1.425	6
B2	Ciwidey	107.3901	−7.14710	1781	39	1.590	6
B3	Ciwidey	107.3853	−7.14429	1724	36	1.385	6
B4	Pangalengan	107.6148	−7.23211	1450	39	1.925	5
C1	Ciater	107.6544	−6.80861	873	36	1.401	6
C2	Ciater	107.6544	−6.80861	885	38	1.415	6
C3	Ciater	107.6544	−6.80862	897	39	1.598	5
M	Bottled water	-	-	-	25	0.164	7
	min				36	0.164	5
	max				42	1.925	7
	average				39	1.541	6

The dissolved ^{222}Rn in water samples in the natural hot spring area shown in Figure 3 have a range of 1 to 31 Bq L^{-1}. With the exceptions of water samples A1, B4, and C3, these values were all below the maximum concentration limit (MCL), 11 Bq L^{-1}, suggested by the EPA. Water samples from this natural hot spring area contained dissolved ^{222}Rn activity concentrations higher than the MCL but within the limit of the alternative maximum concentration level (AMCL) of 148 Bq L^{-1}, also suggested by the EPA [4]. Based on the UNSCEAR 2000 report, the AMCL of 148 Bq L^{-1} is the limit determining the concentration of ^{222}Rn in the water that will produce an indoor ^{222}Rn increment equal to an outdoor ^{222}Rn activity concentration of 15 Bq m^{-3} with the transfer coefficient from water to indoor air applied as 1×10^{-4} [18]. The ^{222}Rn activity concentration in natural hot spring water in the West Java province will contribute to an ^{222}Rn activity concentration in the air equal to 0.1–3.1 Bq m^{-3} concurrent to the ^{222}Rn activity concentration in air measured in this study as shown in Table 2.

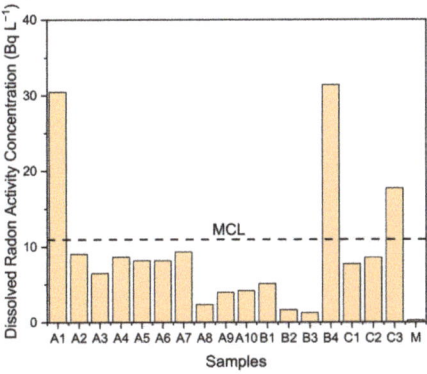

Figure 3. Radon activity concentration in water samples. MCL = maximum contaminant level.

Table 2. Details of measuring result: Dissolved ^{222}Rn in water, ^{222}Rn in air, and calculation of annual effective dose.

Samples	Dissolved Radon in Water	Radon in Air	Ambient Dose Equivalent Rate	Radon Transfer Coefficient from Water to Air	Contributed Dissolved Radon in Water to Radon in Air	Annual Effective Dose due to Ingestion (mSv)		Annual Effective Dose due to External Exposure (mSv)		Total Annual Effective Dose (mSv)	
	Bq L^{-1}	Bq m^{-3}	nSv h^{-1}		Bq m^{-3}	Worker	Public	Worker	Public	Bq L^{-1}	Bq m^{-3}
A1	31 ± 3.4	48 ± 7	43 ± 2	5.9 × 10^{-4}	3.1	0.65	0.13	0.04	0.01	0.69	0.13
A2	9 ± 1.0	49 ± 7	41 ± 2	2.1 × 10^{-3}	0.9	0.67	0.13	0.04	0.01	0.70	0.14
A3	7 ± 0.7	42 ± 6	43 ± 2	1.8 × 10^{-3}	0.7	0.57	0.11	0.04	0.01	0.61	0.12
A4	9 ± 1.0	38 ± 6	41 ± 2	9.3 × 10^{-4}	0.9	0.52	0.10	0.04	0.01	0.55	0.11
A5	8 ± 0.9	39 ± 6	38 ± 2	1.1 × 10^{-3}	0.8	0.53	0.10	0.03	0.01	0.57	0.11
A6	8 ± 0.9	39 ± 6	37 ± 2	1.1 × 10^{-3}	0.8	0.53	0.10	0.03	0.01	0.56	0.11
A7	9 ± 1.0	40 ± 6	36 ± 2	1.1 × 10^{-3}	0.9	0.54	0.10	0.03	0.01	0.58	0.11
A8	2 ± 0.3	38 ± 6	40 ± 2	3.4 × 10^{-3}	0.3	0.52	0.10	0.04	0.01	0.55	0.11
A9	4 ± 0.4	38 ± 6	41 ± 2	2.0 × 10^{-3}	0.4	0.52	0.10	0.04	0.01	0.55	0.11
A10	4 ± 0.5	38 ± 6	40 ± 2	1.9 × 10^{-3}	0.4	0.52	0.10	0.04	0.01	0.55	0.11
B1	5 ± 0.6	38 ± 6	36 ± 2	2.0 × 10^{-3}	0.5	0.52	0.10	0.03	0.01	0.55	0.11
B2	2 ± 0.2	37 ± 6	38 ± 2	5.4 × 10^{-3}	0.2	0.50	0.10	0.03	0.01	0.54	0.10
B3	1 ± 0.1	35 ± 6	35 ± 2	5.5 × 10^{-3}	0.1	0.48	0.09	0.03	0.01	0.51	0.10
B4	31 ± 3.5	42 ± 7	44 ± 2	3.2 × 10^{-4}	3.1	0.57	0.11	0.04	0.01	0.61	0.12
C1	8 ± 0.9	48 ± 7	38 ± 2	1.7 × 10^{-3}	0.8	0.65	0.13	0.03	0.01	0.69	0.13
C2	8 ± 0.9	49 ± 8	37 ± 2	1.6 × 10^{-3}	0.9	0.67	0.13	0.03	0.01	0.70	0.13
C3	18 ± 2.0	50 ± 8	38 ± 2	2.0 × 10^{-3}	1.8	0.68	0.13	0.03	0.01	0.71	0.14
M	0.3 ± 0.1	-	-	-	0.1	-					
Average	9 ± 1.0	42 ± 6	39 ± 2	2.0 × 10^{-3}	0.9	0.53	0.11	0.04	0.01	0.60	0.12
min	1 ± 0.1	35 ± 5	35 ± 2	3.2 × 10^{-4}	0.1	0.48	0.09	0.03	0.01	0.51	0.10
max	31 ± 3.5	50 ± 8	44 ± 2	5.5 × 10^{-3}	3.1	0.68	0.13	0.04	0.01	0.71	0.14

Comparing the values of ^{222}Rn levels in West Java to ^{222}Rn activity concentrations elsewhere reveal that Indonesian levels are rather low. Studies in Slovenia [24], the U.S. [25], Spain [26], Taiwan [27], Hungary [28], Poland [29], Venezuela [30], Germany [31], Croatia [32], Iran [33], and Thailand [6] report ^{222}Rn activity concentrations in hot spring water ranging from 0.2 to 600 Bq L^{-1}. The radon concentration in an area is closely related to geological rock types, which in West Java have andesitic rock types that contain low uranium and radium content [34–36].

The radon activity concentration in the air in the hot spring area of the West Java province ranges from 35 to 50 Bq m^{-3} with an average of 42 Bq m^{-3}. Equation (6) compares the activity value of the ^{222}Rn activity concentration dissolved in water and the ^{222}Rn in the air.

$$\text{Transfer coefficient} = \frac{\overline{\Delta C_a}}{\overline{C_w}}, \tag{6}$$

here, ΔC_a is the average increment of ^{222}Rn activity concentration in the air (Bq m^{-3}). This result is a subtraction of the ^{222}Rn activity concentration in the air around the natural hot spring pool from the ^{222}Rn activity concentration outside of dwellings around the hot spring area. The ^{222}Rn activity concentration outside of dwellings around the hot spring area for Cipanas, Darajat, Ciwidey, Pangalengan and Ciater were 30, 30, 28, 32, and 35 Bq m^{-3}, respectively. C_w is the dissolved ^{222}Rn activity concentration in the water (Bq m^{-3}). The value of ^{222}Rn coefficient transfer from water to air in this study was an average of 2.0×10^{-03}. This value is higher than the value UNSCEAR [18] and Hopke et al. [19] found, possibly due to the effect of water mixing, since tourists were active in the pool while we conducted measurements. Others, including Radolic et al. [32] and Song et al. [37], have reported average transfer coefficients around 4.9×10^{-3} and 1.5×10^{-3}, respectively.

The annual effective dose in the natural hot spring water area ranges from 0.51 to 0.71 mSv with a mean of 0.60 mSv for workers. Meanwhile, the public dose ranges from 0.10 to 0.14 mSv with an average of 0.12 mSv. This value falls within the average committed effective dose from inhalation and terrestrial radiation for the general public, 1.7 mSv annually, determined by UNSCEAR [1].

4. Conclusions

The concentration of ^{222}Rn in natural hot spring water samples in the West Java region of Indonesia has a range of 1 to 31 Bq L^{-1}. An estimate of the annual effective dose in the natural hot spring water area ranges from 0.51 to 0.71 mSv with a mean of 0.60 mSv for workers. Meanwhile, the public is exposed to a range of 0.10 to 0.14 mSv with an average of 0.12 mSv. This value falls within the range of the averaged committed effective dose from inhalation and terrestrial radiation for the general public, 1.7 mSv annually.

Author Contributions: Conceptualisation, E.D.N., M.H. and S.T.; methodology, E.D.N., Y.T., K.K., M.H. and S.T.; validation, E.D.N., M.H, and U.U.; formal analysis, E.D.N., and M.H.; investigation, E.D.N., I.R.; resources, K.K., U.U., M.H. and S.T; data curation, E.D.N.; writing—original draft preparation, E.D.N.; writing—review and editing, E.D.N., M.H., K.K., U.U., I.R., Y.T., O.B.M., C.K., J.M., and S.T.; visualisation, E.D.N.; supervision, M.H., J.M and S.T.; funding acquisition, M.H. and S.T. All authors have read and agreed to the published version of the manuscript.

Funding: This research was partially funded by the Indonesian Government, Japan Society for the Promotion of Science KAKENHI [20H00556, 18KK0261, 16K15368, 16H02667, JP18K10023], and Hirosaki University institutional research grant.

Institutional Review Board Statement: Not applicable.

Informed Consent Statement: Not applicable.

Conflicts of Interest: The authors declare no conflict of interest.

References

1. United Nations Scientific Committee on the Effects of Atomic Radiation. *UNSCEAR 2008 Report, Sources and Effects of Ionising Radiation. Volume I: Annex B Exposures of the Public and Workers from Various Sources of Radiation*; UNSCEAR: New York, NY, USA, 2010.
2. World Health Organization. *WHO Handbook on Indoor Radon: A Public Health Perspective*; WHO: Geneva, Switzerland, 2009.
3. International Commission on Radiological Protection. *Annals of the ICRP: Occupational Intakes of Radionuclides: Part 3*; ICRP: New York, NY, USA, 2017.
4. United State of America Environmental Protection Agency. *USEPA (1991) National Primary Drinking Water Regulations: Radionuclides (Proposed Rule) Federal Register*; U.S. E.P.A.: New York, NY, USA, 1991.
5. Gruber, V.; Maringer, F.J.; Landstetter, C. Radon and other natural radionuclides in drinking water in Austria: Measurement and assessment. *Appl. Radiat. Isot.* **2009**, *67*, 913–917. [CrossRef] [PubMed]
6. Sola, P.; Srisuksawad, K.; Loaharojanaphand, S. Radon activity concentration in air, hot spring water, and bottled mineral water in one hot spring area in Thailand. *J. Radioanal. Nucl. Chem.* **2013**, *297*, 183–187. [CrossRef]
7. Nugraha, E.D.; Hosoda, M.; Kusdiana, I.; Winarni, D.; Prihantoro, A.; Suzuki, T.; Tamakuma, Y.; Akata, N.; Tokonami, S. Dose assessment of radium-226 in drinking water from Mamuju, a high background radiation area of Indonesia. *Radiat. Environ. Med.* **2020**, *9*, 79–83.
8. Patricia, J.E. An assessment of Role of Natural Hot and Mineral Springs in Health, Wellness and Recreational Tourism. Ph.D. Thesis, James Cook University, Douglas, Australia, November 2011.
9. Fitriyani, P.; Waluya, B. The influence of competitive advantage in the tourist area of the hot spring water park, Sabda alam hotels and resorts Cipanas, Garut Regency in increasing visiting decisions (Pengaruh keunggulan bersaing di kawasan wisata air panas taman air sabda alam hotel dan resort cipanas kabupaten garut dalam meningkatkan keputusan berkunjung). *Tour. Hosp. Essent. J.* **2013**, *1*, 483.
10. Ananda, R.P.; Ahman, E.; Riwanudin, O. The effect of physical evidence of Ciwalini hot springs on the decision to visit tourists (Pengaruh physical evidence pemandian air panas ciwalini terhadap keputusan berkunjung wisatawan). *Tour. Hosp. Essent. J.* **2013**, *1*, 461.
11. Arif, M. Limit Proccess Application of Acceptable Change in Sari Ater Hot Spring Resort. Ph.D. Thesis, Tourism University, Hong Kong, January 2016.
12. Nugraha, W.; Kusdiana, E.D.; Iskandar, D. Radon activity concentrations in dwellings in East Kalimantan. In Proceedings of the National Seminar of Sains and Technology 2017, Bandung, Indonesia, 14 November 2017.
13. Nugraha, E.D.; Wahyudi, K.; Iskandar, D. Radon activity concentrations in dwelling of South Kalimantan, Indonesia. *Radiat. Prot. Dosim.* **2019**, *184*, 463–465. [CrossRef]

14. Saputra, M.A.; Nugraha, E.D.; Purwanti, T.; Arifianto, R.; Laksmana, R.I.; Hutabarat, R.P.; Hosoda, M.; Tokonami, S. Exposures from radon, thoron, and thoron progeny in high background radiation area in Takandeang, Mamuju, Indonesia. *Nukleonika* **2020**, *65*, 89–94. [CrossRef]
15. Hosoda, M.; Nugraha, E.D.; Akata, N.; Yamada, R.; Tamakuma, Y.; Sasaki, M.; Kelleher, K.; Yoshinaga, S.; Suzuki, T.; Rattanapongs, C.P.; et al. A unique high natural background radiation area—Dose assessment and perspectives. *Sci. Total Environ.* **2021**, *750*, 142346. [CrossRef]
16. Iskandar, I.; Dermawan, F.A.; Sianipar, J.; Suryantini, Y.; Notosiswoyo, S. Characteristic and Mixing Mechanisms of Thermal Fluid at the Tampomas Volcano, West Java, Using Hydrogeochemistry, Stable Isotope and 222Rn Analyses. *Geosciences* **2018**, *8*, 103. [CrossRef]
17. Durridge. *Manual Book of RAD7*; Durridge Company Inc.: Billerica, MA, USA, 2018.
18. United Nations Scientific Committee on the Effects of Atomic Radiation. *UNSCEAR 2000 Report, Sources and Effects of Ionising Radiation. Volume I: Annex B Exposures from Natural Radiation Sources*; UNSCEAR: New York, NY, USA, 2000.
19. Hopke, P.K.; Borak, T.B.; Doull, J.; Cleaver, J.E.; Eckerman, K.F.; Gundersen, L.C.S.; Harley, N.H.; Hess, C.T.; Kinner, N.E.; Kopecky, K.J.; et al. Health risks due radon in drinking water. *J. Environ Sci. Technol.* **2000**, *34*, 921–926. [CrossRef]
20. Tokonami, S. Some thought on new dose conversion factors for radon progeny inhalation. *Jpn J. Health Phys.* **2018**, *53*, 282–293. [CrossRef]
21. Hosoda, M.; Fukui, Y.; Pornnumpa, C.; Sorimachi, S.; Ishikawa, T.; Yachi, M.; Nara, A.; Yokota, H.; Tokonami, S. Absorbed dose rate in air at the Bunkyo-cho Campus of Hirosaki University. *Radiat. Environ. Med.* **2014**, *3*, 59–62.
22. Ministry of Health of Indonesia. *Drinking Water Quality Reference Level*; Ministry of Health of Indonesia: Jakarta, Indonesia, 2002.
23. World Health Organization. *WHO Guidelines for Drinking Water Quality, Vol. 1. Recommendations*; WHO: Geneva, Switzerland, 2017.
24. Kobal, I.; Krista, J.; Ancik, M.; Jerencic, S.; Skofljanec, M. Radioactivity of thermal and mineral springs in Slovenia. *Health Phys.* **1979**, *37*, 239–242. [PubMed]
25. Nazaroff, W.; Nero, A. *Radon and Its Decay Products in Air*; John Wiley & Sons: New York, NY, USA, 1988.
26. Soto, J.; Fernández, P.; Quindos, L.; Gomezarozamena, J. Radioactivity in Spanish spas. *Sci. Total Environ.* **1995**, *162*, 187–192. [CrossRef]
27. Sabol, J.; Weng, P.-S.; Mao, C.-H. Monitoring of ^{222}Rn in Taiwanese Hot Spring SPA Waters Using a Modified Electret Ion Chamber Method. *Health Phys.* **1995**, *68*, 100–104. [CrossRef]
28. Szerbin, P. Natural radioactivity of certain spas and caves in Hungary. *Environ. Int.* **1996**, *22*, 389–398. [CrossRef]
29. Przylibski, T. ^{222}Rn concentration changes in medicinal groundwaters of Lądek Zdrój (Sudety Mountains, SW Poland). *J. Environ. Radioact.* **2000**, *48*, 327–347. [CrossRef]
30. Horvath, A.; Bohus, L.O.; Urbani, F.; Marx, G.; Piroth, A.; Greaves, E.D. Radon activity concentration in hot spring waters in northern Venezuela. *J. Environ. Radioact.* **2000**, *47*, 127–133. [CrossRef]
31. Trautmannsheimer, M.; Schindlmeier, W.; Boerner, K. Radon activity concentration measurements and personnel exposure levels in Bavarian water supply facilities. *Health Phys.* **2003**, *84*, 100–110. [CrossRef]
32. Radolić, V.; Vuković, B.; Smit, G.; Stanic, D.; Planinić, J. Radon in the spas of Croatia. *J. Environ. Radioact.* **2005**, *83*, 191–198. [CrossRef]
33. Jalili-Majareshin, A.; Behtash, A.; Rezaei-Ochbelagh, D. Radon activity concentration in hot springs of the touristic city of Sarein and methods to reduce radon in water. *Radiat. Phys. Chem.* **2012**, *81*, 749–757. [CrossRef]
34. Utami, P. Characteristics of the Kamojang geothermal reservoir (West Java) as revealed by its hydrothermal alteration mineralogy. In Proceedings of the World Geothermal Congress 2000, Sendai, Japan, 28 May–10 June 2000.
35. Sunarwan, B. Physical characterization of groundwater and identification of springs in the volcanic sediment aquifer (case study: Tangkuban perahu volcanic sediment in the Bandung basin) (karakterisasi phisik air tanah dan identifikasi pemunculan mata air pada akuifer endapan gunung api (studi kasus: Endapan gunungapi Tangkuban perahu di cekungan Bandung). *Technol. J. Sci. Mag. Unpak.* **2014**, *15*, 16–26.
36. Hidayat, M.R.; Mardiana, U.; Suganda, B.R.; Hadian, M.S.D. Geometry activities of Bandung area and surroundings, West Java Province (geometri akifer daerah Bandung dan sekitarnya, Provinsi Jawa Barat). *Padjajaran Univ. Geom. Sci. J.* **2017**, *1*, 86–97.
37. Song, G.; Zhang, B.; Wang, X.; Gong, J.; Chan, D.; Bernett, J.; Lee, S.C. Indoor radon levels in selected hot spring hotels in Guangdong, China. *Sci. Total Environ.* **2005**, *339*, 63–70. [CrossRef]

Radiological Assessment of Indoor Radon and Thoron Concentrations and Indoor Radon Map of Dwellings in Mashhad, Iran

Mohammademad Adelikhah [1], Amin Shahrokhi [1], Morteza Imani [2], Stanislaw Chalupnik [3] and Tibor Kovács [1,*]

1. Institute of Radiochemistry and Radioecology, University of Pannonia, 8200 Veszprém, Hungary; emad@mk.uni-pannon.hu (M.A.); ashahrokhi@almos.uni-pannon.hu (A.S.)
2. Materials and Nuclear Fuel Research School, Nuclear Science and Technology Research Institute, Tehran 11365-8486, Iran; imani.mrt@gmail.com
3. Silesian Centre for Environmental Radioactivity, Central Mining Institute, plac Gwarków 1, 40-166 Katowice, Poland; schalupnik@gig.eu
* Correspondence: kt@almos.uni-pannon.hu; Tel.: +36-88-624-178

Abstract: A comprehensive study was carried out to measure indoor radon/thoron concentrations in 78 dwellings and soil-gas radon in the city of Mashhad, Iran during two seasons, using two common radon monitoring devices (NRPB and RADUET). In the winter, indoor radon concentrations measured between 75 ± 11 to 376 ± 24 Bq·m^{-3} (mean: 150 ± 19 Bq·m^{-3}), whereas indoor thoron concentrations ranged from below the Lower Limit of Detection (LLD) to 166 ± 10 Bq·m^{-3} (mean: 66 ± 8 Bq m^{-3}), while radon and thoron concentrations in summer fell between 50 ± 11 and 305 ± 24 Bq·m^{-3} (mean 115 ± 18 Bq·m^{-3}) and from below the LLD to 122 ± 10 Bq m^{-3} (mean 48 ± 6 Bq·m^{-3}), respectively. The annual average effective dose was estimated to be 3.7 ± 0.5 mSv yr^{-1}. The soil-gas radon concentrations fell within the range from 1.07 ± 0.28 to 8.02 ± 0.65 kBq·m^{-3} (mean 3.07 ± 1.09 kBq·m^{-3}). Finally, indoor radon maps were generated by ArcGIS software over a grid of 1×1 km^2 using three different interpolation techniques. In grid cells where no data was observed, the arithmetic mean was used to predict a mean indoor radon concentration. Accordingly, inverse distance weighting (IDW) was proven to be more suitable for predicting mean indoor radon concentrations due to the lower mean absolute error (MAE) and root mean square error (RMSE). Meanwhile, the radiation health risk due to the residential exposure to radon and indoor gamma radiation exposure was also assessed.

Keywords: residential exposure; dose; gamma radiation; health risk; radon mapping; CR-39

1. Introduction

In general, people are exposed to ionizing radiation from various natural and artificial sources. Radon (^{222}Rn), thoron (^{220}Rn), and the progeny of both can be regarded as the largest contributor to the annual effective dose for the public in the world (50% of the total public dose) [1,2]; however, public exposure to ionizing radiation can be higher due to a new dose conversion factor [3]. Exposure to radon and its decay products is the second most common cause of lung cancer after tobacco smoking [4]. The health risks related to radon exposure primarily arise in indoor environments, while outdoor radon levels are generally low. The most important source of indoor radon is soil gas infiltration, and the intensity of this source relies on the composition of the ground, i.e., granite, tile, clay, etc. Soil gas infiltration is produced in mineral grains by the radioactive decay of ^{226}Ra, emanated into the void spaces between the grains, transported by diffusion and advection/convection, and eventually exhaled from the soil into boreholes where it is detected. Moreover, cracks in concrete floors and walls, drainage pipes, connecting parts of buildings, heating, ventilation, and air conditioning ducts are the possible routes through which radon can enter into indoor environments [5].

Measuring indoor radon and thoron concentrations and radon mapping was considered for years and several papers were published on the topic around the world [6–17], including in many Iranian cities [18–27] to increase public awareness of environmental radioactivity and to predict radon-prone areas, which would help authorities with regard to the development of an appropriate strategy to reduce public exposure to radon and thoron. This reduced exposure would increase the quality of life and improve public long-term health. Due to the lack of data concerning indoor radon and thoron concentrations in houses in the city of Mashhad, an attempt was made to measure indoor radon and thoron concentrations in 78 houses to calculate the annual committed effective dose caused by the inhalation of radon and thoron. The measurements were taken during two seasons, summer (July–September 2019) and winter (December 2019–February 2020). The annual average radon and thoron concentrations were estimated by averaging measured concentrations during these periods. Subsequently, a radon map was produced using ArcGIS software and three different interpolation techniques, within a grid with the dimensions of 1 km × 1km. Meanwhile, the soil gas radon concentrations (as the major source of indoor radon) in different districts of Mashhad were also measured using a passive method based on CR-39 detectors during the summer when soil moisture and precipitation is low. Moreover, external exposure rates for terrestrial gamma radiation in Iran from 36 to 130 nGy h^{-1} with an average of 71 nGy h^{-1} have been reported [1,2]. In 2015, Sohrabi et al. also measured the indoors and outdoors gamma dose rates for about 1000 houses in 36 cities in Iran and the national mean background outdoor gamma dose rates were reported as being 70.2 nGy h^{-1} [28]. Therefore, to assess the radiation health risk, the public indoor doses from radon gas and indoor gamma radiation were compared and assessed.

2. Materials and Methods

2.1. Study Area

Mashhad is the second largest metropolis in Iran and is the capital of Razavi Khorasan Province in northeastern Iran. It has an area of 351 km^2 and its population is more than 3 million people according to the last census (Statistical Centre of Iran, 2016). It has witnessed rapid growth over the last two decades, mostly as a result of its economic, social, and religious attractions. The city is 985 m above sea level with the geographic coordinates of 36°17′45″ N, 59°36′43″ E. Geologically, the Kalaj mountains, which consist of granitic hills covered by silty deposits, are situated to the south of Mashhad, towards the northwest is Kale Ghaemabad that is comprised of more sandy soil, and in all other directions is a plateau with a mix of clay loam and soft sandy soils. Figure 1 shows the location of Mashhad in Iran.

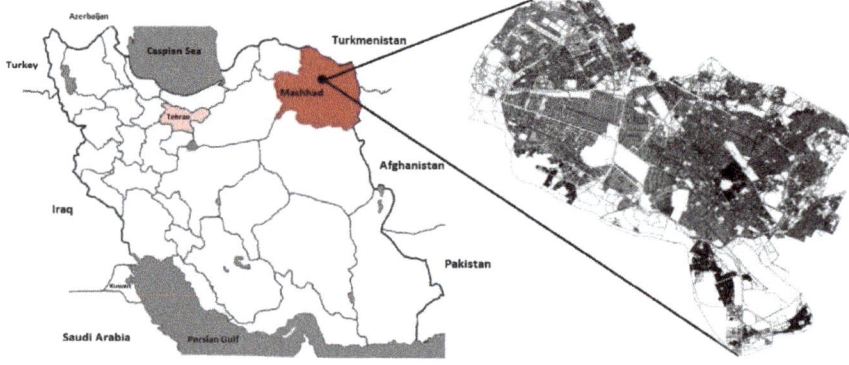

Figure 1. Location of the city of Mashhad in Razavi Khorasan Province, Iran.

2.2. Measuring Techniques

Indoor radon and thoron concentrations are measured in the living rooms of houses at ground level. Regarding the recruited of participants, the priority was given to the older houses by selecting 3 to 5 dwellings from each district randomly depending on the size of the residential area. The majority of the houses examined were built 15 to 45 years ago using bricks composed of sand and cement along with cemented floors. The indoor measurements were conducted over a period of 90 days in total during the summer (July–September 2019) and winter (December 2019–February 2020). To determine the indoor radon and thoron concentrations, RADUET, a commercially available passive integrated radon–thoron discriminative detector, was used. These detectors consist of two diffusion chambers with different ventilation rates, and each chamber contains a CR-39 chip with the dimensions of 10 × 10 mm^2 (RADUET, Radosys Ltd., Budapest, Hungary) for detecting the alpha particles emitted from radon and thoron as well as their progenies [29,30]. All detectors were hung at a height of 1–2 m above the ground using hard wire and positioned at least 20 cm away from any of the wall surfaces in the living rooms of the houses.

In addition, a solid-state nuclear track detector (SSNTD), CR-39, was used to measure radon concentrations in soil gas. In this regard, a hole was dug in the soil of about 11 cm in diameter and 50–60 cm in depth. Then, a long PVC tube was fixed into the hole with the covered top end of the tube protruding from the ground by about 5 cm. At the bottom of each tube, a NRBP radon dosimeter [31] was placed for a period of 45 days between July and September 2019.

After exposure, all detectors were wrapped in protective aluminum foil and returned for processing at the Institute. In the laboratory, they washed with distilled water and dried and then chemically etched. The etching condition for CR-39 was as follows: Solution: 6.0 M NaOH; Temperature: 90 °C; Time: 3 h. The track densities were counted using an optical transmission microscope and image analysis software. The calibration factors were determined as a result of exposure tests using radon and thoron calibration chambers at the Institute of Radiochemistry and Radioecology of the University of Pannonia, Hungary, and is comprehensively described in [30–32].

2.3. Annual Effective Dose, Excess Lifetime Cancer Risk (ELCR) and Lung Cancer Cases (LCC) Associated with Radon/Thoron Exposure

The annual committed effective doses originating from the inhalation of indoor radon or thoron were calculated using the following equation provided by [1]:

$$E_{(Rn/Tn)} = C_{(Rn/Tn)} \times F_{(Rn/Tn)} \times t \times K_{(Rn/Tn)} \qquad (1)$$

where $E_{Rn/Tn}$ denotes the annual committed effective dose from exposure to radon or thoron (mSv yr^{-1}); $C_{Rn/Tn}$ stands for the annual average radon or thoron concentrations in houses (Bq m^{-3}); $F_{(Rn/Tn)}$ represents the indoor equilibrium factors for radon or thoron and their respective progenies. The following values were provided by United Nations Scientific Committee on the Effects of Atomic Radiation (UNSCEAR) in 2000 [1]: $F = 0.40$ and $F = 0.02$ for radon and thoron, respectively; t is the number of hours spent inside annually (7000 h). Also, $K_{(Rn/Tn)}$ denotes the following dose conversion factors recommended by UNSCEAR in 2000 [1]: $K_{Rn} = 9$ nSv and $K_{Tn} = 40$ nSv per unit of integrated radon and thoron concentrations (Bq h m^{-3}), respectively.

In this survey, the average of the radon concentrations in the summer and winter represents the annual radon concentration. Furthermore, between December and February is regarded as the winter season when people tend to close windows because of the cold weather. The total exposure time was 90 days over the two seasons assessed. The Excess Lifetime Cancer Risk (*ELCR*) per 100,000 people was calculated using the following equation [33]:

$$ELCR = E_{(Rn/Tn)} \times D_L \times R_F \qquad (2)$$

where D_L represents the life expectancy, estimated to be 70 years; and R_F stands for the risk of fatal cancer per Sievert of $5.5 \times 10^{-2}\,\text{Sv}^{-1}$ as recommended by International Commission on Radiological Protection (ICRP) Publication 103. Finally, the Lung Cancer Cases per year per million people (LCC) was estimated by using the risk factor lung cancer induction $18 \times 10^{-6}\,\text{mSv}^{-1}$ and calculated by the following equation [34]:

$$LCC = E_{(Rn/Tn)} \times 18 \times 10^{-6}. \tag{3}$$

2.4. Statistical Analysis

The statistical analysis was carried out using IBM SPSS Statistics 21 (Armonk, NY, USA). The Kolmogorov-Smirnov test was applied to test the null hypothesis for the homogeneous distribution of the datasets. The Kruskal–Wallis non-parametric test with the Dunn's post-hoc analysis was also used to test whether the samples originated from the same distribution based on the comparison of medians.

2.5. Radon Mapping and Cross-Validation

Radon mapping has great economic and social consequences; moreover, a high-resolution, accurate, and statistically powerful radon map is necessary to increase public awareness of environmental radioactivity and influence government policy with the purpose of reducing radon exposure in the general population. Depending on the datasets applied, two types of maps can be used: 1. Indoor Radon Maps which are based on indoor radon measurements (as applied in this study); and 2. Geogenic Radon Maps which are based on geological information [35]. The major merit of indoor radon maps is that radon concentrations are directly measured at the exposure point.

In this study, an indoor radon map was generated by using ArcGIS software version 10.7 (GDi Esri Hungary Ltd., Budapest, Hungary) over a grid with the dimensions of 1 km × 1 km; moreover, three interpolation methods were tested: inverse distance weighting (IDW), ordinary kriging (OK), and Empirical Bayesian kriging (EBK). The arithmetic mean (AM) was used over grid cells with the dimensions of 1 km × 1 km to predict the mean indoor radon concentration on the ground floor of buildings in the grid cells where no data was available. It is important to keep in mind that radon maps are only a probabilistic tool to make policy decisions such as prioritization; they cannot be used to derive radon concentrations for an individual dwelling. By using some indexes, namely the mean absolute error (MAE), root mean square error (RMSE), root mean squared logarithmic error (RMSLE), percentage bias (PB), and coefficient of determination (R^2), the accuracy of the different techniques was also examined, as presented in Equations (4)–(8):

$$\text{MAE} = \frac{1}{n}\sum_{i=1}^{n}|Z_i - X_i| \tag{4}$$

$$\text{RMSE} = \sqrt{\frac{1}{n}\sum_{i=1}^{n}(Z_i - X_i)^2} \tag{5}$$

$$\text{RMSLE} = \frac{1}{n}\sum_{i=1}^{n}(log(Z_i+1) - log(X_i+1))^2 \tag{6}$$

$$\text{PB} = 100\frac{\sum_{i=1}^{n}(Z_i - X_i)}{\sum_{i=1}^{n}X_i} \tag{7}$$

$$R^2 = 1 - \frac{\sum_{i=1}^{n}(Z_i - X_i)^2}{\sum_{i=1}^{n}(|X_i - \overline{X}|)^2} \tag{8}$$

where X_i and Z_i denote the measured and predicted values in the location, n stands for the number of points in the validation group, and $\overline{X}$ represents the mean of X_i. MAE and RMSE are often applied to assess the performance of models. The model fits properly if the aforementioned indicators approach zero when calculated. PB (%) is the mean of the tendency in larger/smaller predicted values than those observed [36]. R^2 is the fit line explaining to which degree the model is going to fit to the dataset [37].

3. Results and Discussion
3.1. Activity Measurements

Within this study, the radon and thoron concentrations in 78 houses were surveyed over a total exposure time of 90 days (45 days in both the summer and the winter) by using a RADUET detector. The frequency distribution of the indoor radon and thoron for the 78 houses assessed in Mashhad over the two seasons are shown in Figure 2. In addition, a comparison among normal distribution and log-normal distribution of data is also illustrated in Figure 3. The indoor ^{222}Rn and ^{220}Rn concentrations in the winter ranged from 75 ± 11 to 376 ± 24 Bq·m^{-3} with a mean value of 150 ± 19 Bq·m^{-3} and from below the Lower Limit of Detection (LLD) to 166 ± 10 Bq·m^{-3} with a mean value of 66 ± 8 Bq m^{-3}, respectively. In the case of the summer, the indoor ^{222}Rn and ^{220}Rn concentrations ranged from 50 ± 11 to 305 ± 24 Bq·m^{-3} with a mean value of 114 ± 18 Bq·m^{-3} and from below the LLD to 122 ± 10 Bq·m^{-3} with a mean value of 48 ± 6 Bq m^{-3}, respectively. In addition, the annual average indoor ^{222}Rn and ^{220}Rn concentrations in the studied areas were 132 ± 19 Bq·m^{-3} and 58 ± 7 Bq m^{-3}, respectively. The main source of indoor ^{222}Rn originates from soil gas infiltration, building materials, and ventilation [4]. Meanwhile, during cold winters, residents use natural gas and close all vents, causing the radon accumulation found in houses.

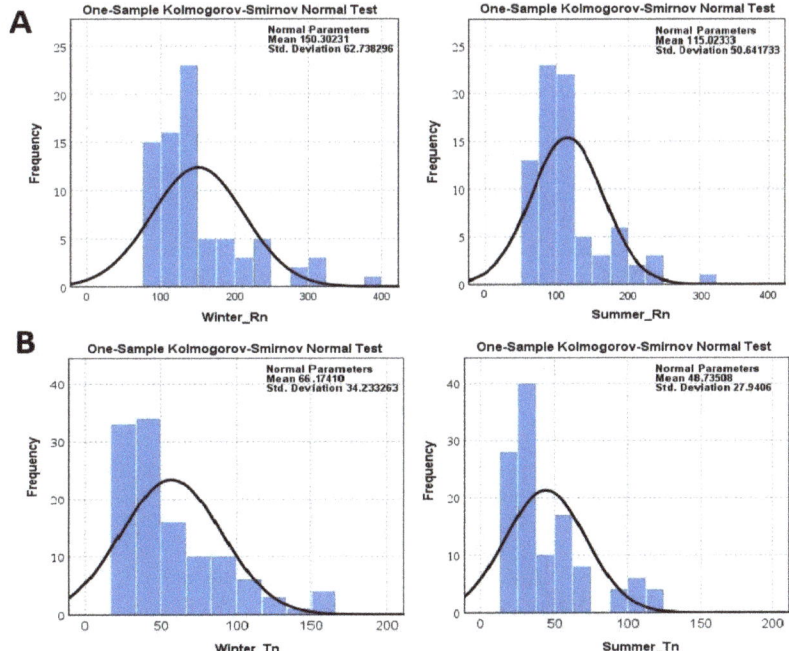

Figure 2. Normal Distribution of indoor (**A**) radon and (**B**) thoron concentrations (Bq m^{-3}) over the two seasons at the ground level of dwellings examined in Mashhad.

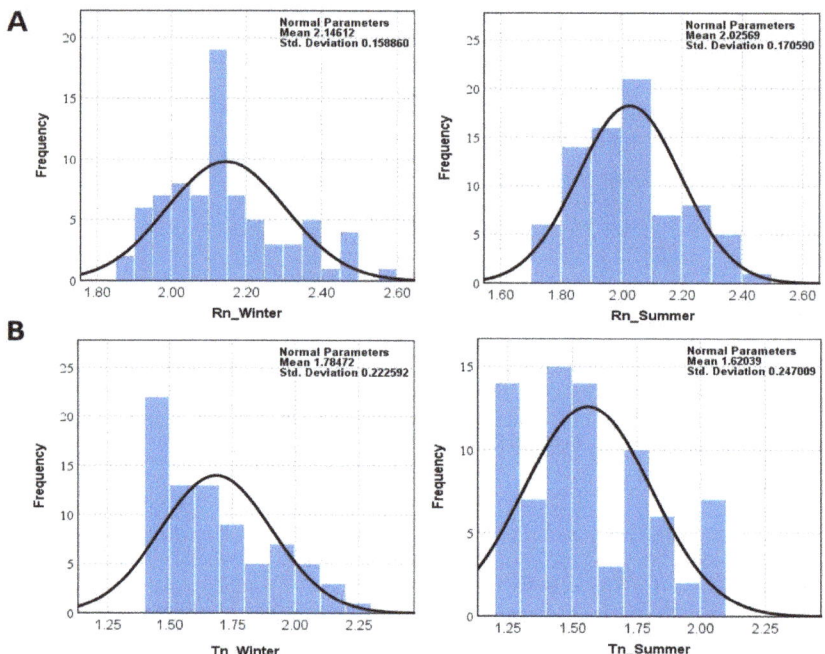

Figure 3. Log-Normal Distribution of indoor (**A**) radon and (**B**) thoron concentrations (Bq m^{-3}) over the two seasons at the ground level of dwellings examined in Mashhad.

World organizations such as ICRP, WHO, and U.S. Environmental Protection Agency (EPA) have recommended various guidelines for radon exposure [1,4,33,38,39]. The annual average indoor radon concentration is below the recommendation values (300 Bq m^{-3}) provided by the ICRP in 2010. The results concerning the annual average radon concentration exceed the action level (100 Bq m^{-3}) recommended by the WHO in 2009. When compared to the worldwide geometric mean (GM) of 37 Bq·m^{-3} (geometric standard deviation (GSD) = 2.2) reported by UNSCEAR in 2000, the indoor radon in the city of Mashhad is almost 4 times (139.68 Bq m^{-3}) and approximately 3 times (105.8 Bq m^{-3}) higher than the world average in the winter and summer, respectively. It was also found that during the winter and summer, the indoor radon concentrations in 31% and 20% of the dwellings were higher than the reference level of 148 Bq·m^{-3} recommended by the US EPA in 2003.

The graph in Figure 4 shows the correlation between indoor ^{222}Rn and ^{220}Rn concentrations for the dwellings examined in Mashhad. Regarding the relationship between radon and thoron concentrations, no clear and strong correlation between was observed and thoron concentrations could not be predicted from widely available information concerning radon. However, indoor radon and thoron concentration might directly depend on the activity of ^{226}Ra and ^{232}Th (^{228}Th) in building materials, ground is the main entry path of radon at dwellings; therefore, it could say that the content of both ^{222}Rn and ^{220}Rn depends on the building materials and soil composition.

As previously discussed, the main source of indoor ^{222}Rn originates from soil gas infiltration, ^{222}Rn concentrations in the soil gas of different districts in Mashhad were measured by using a passive method based on CR-39 detectors in the summer when soil moisture and precipitation are low. In order to determine soil gas radon concentrations, only 36 NRPB dosimeters were retrieved from where they were set up, while the remaining 6 dosimeters were considered lost. Figure 5 shows a histogram of soil gas radon concentrations in Mashhad during the summer. The soil gas radon concentrations recorded in the studied area fell within the range of 1.07 ± 0.28 to 8.02 ± 0.65 kBq·m^{-3} with a mean value of 3.07 ± 1.09 kBq m^{-3}. As is shown in Figure 4, the activity concentrations of ^{222}Rn vary from location to location, possibly because of the physic geological properties of the types of soil studied, topographic differences, as well as geomorphology and meteorological conditions of the region. The average radon concentrations in both soil gas and indoor environments are approximately the minimum and maximum values in the same region, respectively. Moreover, the correlation between indoor radon and soil gas radon concentrations for the districts studied is shown in Figure 6. The correlation analysis yielded a positive correlation (R^2 = 0.361) between average indoor radon and soil-gas radon concentrations.

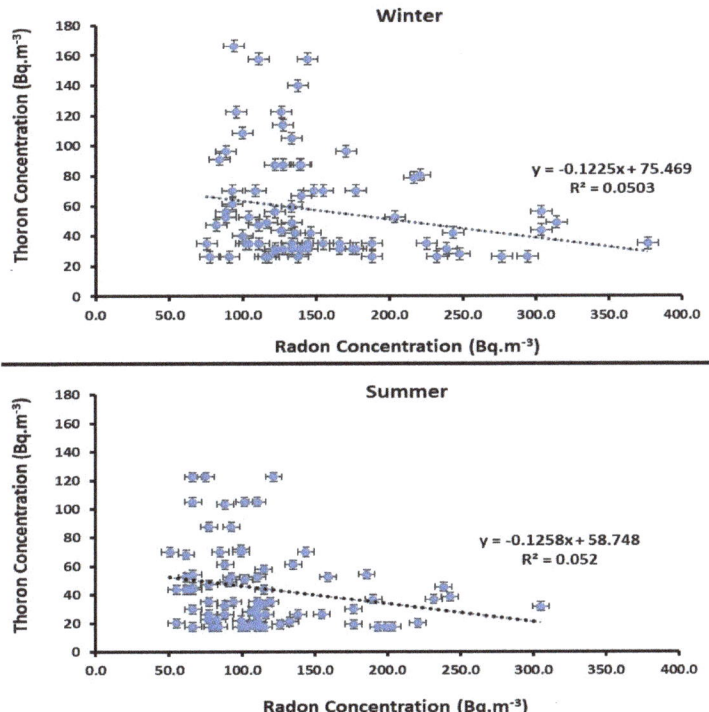

Figure 4. Correlation between the indoor radon and thoron concentrations of the 78 houses examined in Mashhad over two seasons.

The normality distribution of data was checked using the Kolmogorov–Smirnov test. Considering the normality assumption in the null hypothesis of the Kolmogorov–Smirnov test, the probability value (p-value) in all tests was less than 1%; therefore, the normality distribution of radon and thoron concentrations in any of the following subfactors was rejected. In this study, by applying the Kruskal–Wallis nonparametric test with Dunn's post hoc analysis, the null hypothesis, due to the absence of a statistically significant difference in the average gas concentration, was rejected; therefore, the season and type of gas affect the gas concentration (p-value < 0.05). The difference in radon concentrations between well-ventilated and poorly ventilated dwellings was statistically significant ($p < 0.05$). It was assumed that houses with natural ventilation are poorly ventilated and houses mechanical ventilation systems are well-ventilated houses. The finding indicates that the radon concentration is lower for well-ventilated dwellings compared to poorly ventilated ones. The results of this study are consistent with others that have been conducted concerning this topic [40–42]. Because the level of indoor radon concentration depends on the degree of indoor ventilation, moreover, in well-ventilated dwellings, radon can easily escape and does not accumulate inside, meaning indoor radon concentrations are less high in well-ventilated dwellings compared to in poorly ventilated ones [40].

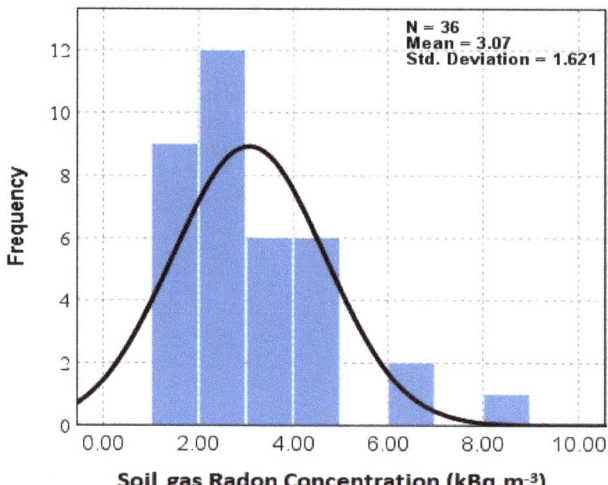

Figure 5. The soil-gas radon concentrations (kBq m^{-3}) in the studied area.

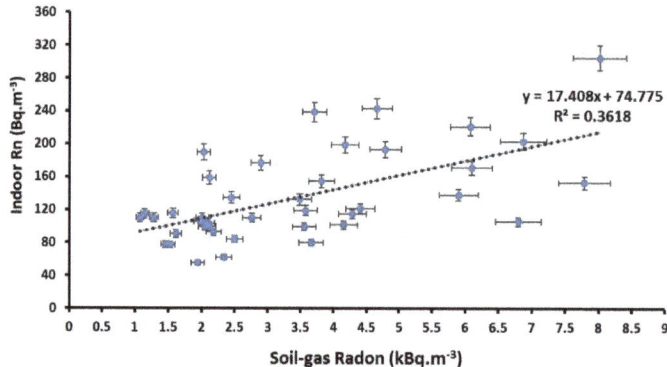

Figure 6. The correlation between indoor radon and soil-gas radon concentrations.

Table 1 shows descriptive statistics that resulted from the measurement of the indoor radon and thoron concentrations in the 78 houses studied in Mashhad during the two seasons considered. Furthermore, the results reveal a seasonal variation in indoor radon and thoron concentrations, which were higher in the winter than in the summer. This is because the doors and windows of dwellings remain closed most of the time in the winter compared to in the summer, hence ventilation is poorer in the winter. The ratio of winter to summer concerning indoor radon and thoron concentrations was also established for all 78 dwellings studied. This ratio of indoor radon concentrations ranged from 1.23 to 1.48 with an average value of 1.31. With regard to the indoor thoron concentration, the average of this ratio was similar, at 1.36. The reason of heterogeneous behavior of seasonal variations in ^{222}Rn and ^{220}Rn concentrations might be that the source of ^{220}Rn is mainly limited to the concentration of ^{232}Th (^{228}Th) in building materials, while in case of radon, the ground's concentration is additionally considered. Therefore, in summer due to a high air exchange rate, e.g., using a ventilator or opening windows, the concentration of both ^{220}Rn and ^{222}Rn goes down, while in winter since the air exchange rate is lower than summer, the concentration of ^{220}Rn and ^{222}Rn build up but as the source of indoor ^{222}Rn is both ground and building material rather than the only source of ^{220}Rn as building materials, the seasonal change of indoor thoron concentration is less than that of indoor radon.

Table 1. Basic Statistics of indoor and soil gas ^{222}Rn and ^{220}Rn concentrations in samples from Mashhad.

Season	Parameter	A.M [1]	G.M [2]	S.D [3]	Min	Max	Winter/Summer Ratio (Mean)	
							^{222}Rn	^{220}Rn
Summer	Indoor air radon (Bq m^{-3})	115.02	105.8	50.64	50.8	305.2	1.31	1.36
	Indoor air thoron (Bq m^{-3})	48.73	37.4	27.95	<LLD	122.5		
	Soil-gas radon (kBq m^{-3})	3.07	2.71	1.621	1.078	8.021		
Winter	Indoor air radon (Bq m^{-3})	150.3	139.68	62.74	75.3	376.6		
	Indoor air thoron (Bq m^{-3})	66.17	49.41	34.24	<LLD	166.3		

[1] A.M = Arithmetical mean, [2] G.M = Geometrical mean, [3] S.D = Standard deviation.

A comparison of radon concentration in the soil gas under investigation with those reported in other countries is also given in Table 2. It can clearly be seen that the radon concentration in soil samples from the Sri Ganganagar district and the northern state of Rajasthan in India, the city of Najaf in Iraq, and Yemen are in close agreement with the present work. It can be concluded that the soil in Mashhad is suitable for construction without posing any health hazards.

Table 2. Comparison of soil-gas radon concentrations under investigation with those in other countries using different methods and sampling depths.

Region	Radon in Soil-Gas (KBq m^{-3})	Measurement Method	Sampling Depth (cm)	Reference
Băita-Stei, Romania	5.5–512	Lucas Cell	40–80	[43]
Bolsena, Italy	7–176	RAD 7	60–70	[14]
Bulgaria	3–97	AlphaGuard	100	[44]
Hungary	1–47.1	RAD 7	80	[45]
Najaf, Iraq	0.009–9.29	RAD 7	5–60	[46]
Rajasthan, India	0.94–10.05	RAD 7	100	[47]
Sharr-Korabi, Kosovo	0.295–32	SSNTDs (CR-39)	80	[48]
Slovenia	0.9–32.9	AlphaGuard	100	[49]
Sri Ganganagar, India	0.9–10.10	RAD 7	10–100	[50]
Yemen	0.15–13.56	SSNTDs (CR-39)	0–150	[51]
Mashhad, Iran	1.07–8.02	SSNTDs (CR-39)	50–60	Present study

3.2. Radiation Dose and Risk Assessment

In this study, the average of the radon concentrations in the summer and winter was assumed to be the annual average radon concentration. The corresponding annual effective dose from the inhalation of radon and thoron was calculated as 3.7 ± 0.5 mSv yr^{-1}. The committed effective dose from indoor radon and thoron was found to vary from 2.11 to 9.73 mSv yr^{-1} with a mean value of 4.22 mSv yr^{-1} for the winter, and 1.51 to 7.92 mSv yr^{-1} with a mean value of 3.14 mSv yr^{-1} for the summer. It can be seen that the committed effective doses were higher in the winter compared to the summer. The excess lifetime cancer risk and lung cancer cases per year per million people were also calculated to be 14.1 and 65.4, respectively.

According to the WHO in 2009, the risk of lung cancer increases by 16% per a 100 Bq·m^{-3} increase in radon concentration (long-time average) [4]. Therefore, the dose-response relation is linear, i.e., the risk of lung cancer is proportional to radon exposure [4]. Nevertheless, based on a report produced by the Ministry of Health's Center for Disease Management in Iran, cancer is the third most significant cause of death after road traffic accidents and cardiovascular mortality. In 2019, Roshandel et al. reported that the age-standardized rates (ASR) of lung cancer were 127 and 52.1 per 100,000 Iranian males and females, respectively [52]. In the case of Razavi Khorasan Province, the ASR was 121.2 and 54.0 per 100,000 Iranian males and females, respectively. Therefore, the annual average excess risk due to radon inhalation in Mashhad is 14/100,000, i.e., less than the age-standardized death rate from cancer in Mashhad. Hence, indoor radon exposure is responsible for approximately 12% of lung cancer deaths in this city, which is close to the estimates by WHO in 2009 of the worldwide proportion of lung cancer due to radon (3–14%).

Given the annual average excess risk values by comparing local radiological risks with national cancer incidence data, it can be concluded that the local risks are raised but are not necessarily representative of the city as a whole. This radiation risk assessment should be considered with caution as the radon measurements are not sufficiently representative of the investigated area; moreover, calculations made using ICRP data only provide a broad overview of the risk and comparison with the national cancer incidence rate. Therefore, extensive measurements are needed for a reliable comparison.

It is also essential to measure the amount of natural radiation in each area as this can determine the suitability of the environment for a healthy lifestyle. The indoor and outdoor gamma exposure rates in the air 1 m above the ground from terrestrial radionuclides and cosmic rays in Mashhad are 155.73 ± 13.92 nGy h^{-1} and 126.15 ± 15.66 nGy h^{-1}, respectively [28]. Using a determined conversion factor as 0.7 Sv Gy^{-1}, converting the absorbed doses to effective doses [1], the annual indoor and outdoor effective dose rates of the public from gamma exposure were found to be 0.95 ± 0.08 and 0.77 ± 0.09 mSv yr^{-1}. Therefore, by comparing these values with the corresponding annual effective doses from the inhalation of radon and thoron (3.7 ± 0.5 mSv yr^{-1}), it could be concluded that most of the doses received indoors in the dwellings studied in Mashhad city are from the inhalation of radon and thoron (about 79 % of the total dose). A comparison of the indoor radon concentration and radiation risk assessment under investigation, with those reported in other Iranian cities also provided in Table 3.

Table 3. Studies on indoor radon concentration (Bq m^{-3}) and radiation health risk in various Iranian cities.

Region	Number of Dwelling	Mean Radon Concentration (SD [1])	Mean Effective Dose (mSv yr^{-1})	ELCR [2]	LCC [3] × 10^{-6}	Excessive Rate (%)	Reference
Isfahan	51	28.57 (39.38)	0.72	2.7×10^{-1}	12.96	4% > 100 Bq m^{-3}	[26]
Lahijan	400	163 (57)	3.43	1.3×10^{-2}	61.74	In most dwellings > 100 Bq m^{-3}	[19]
Mashhad	148	31.9	(0.25–3.78)	-	-	5.3% of apartments > 100 Bq m^{-3}	[22]
Qom	123	95.83	2.41	9.2×10^{-3}	43.38	24.3% > 100 Bq m^{-3}	[23]
Ramsar	500	Autumn: 355 Winter: 476	Autumn: 8.95 Winter: 12	3.44×10^{-2} 4.6×10^{-2}	161.11 216	-	[18]
Shiraz	185	57.6 (33.06)	1.45	5.6×10^{-3}	26.1	5.4% > 100 Bq m^{-3}	[24]
Tehran	30	104	2.62	1×10^{-2}	47.16	38% > 100 Bq m^{-3}	[25]
Yazd	84	137.4 (149.5)	3.46	1.3×10^{-2}	62.28	30% of basements > 148 Bq m^{-3}	[21]
Mashhad	78	Summer: 115(51) Winter: 150 (62)	Summer: 3.1 Winter: 4.2	(12.3×10^{-3}) (15.9×10^{-3})	(56.7) (74.1)	Summer: 20% > 148 Bq m^{-3} Winter: 31% > 148 Bq m^{-3}	Current study

[1] SD = Standard deviation, [2] ELCR = Excess Lifetime Cancer Risk, [3] LCC = Lung Cancer Cases.

3.3. Spatial Distribution Map of Indoor Radon Concentrations

The Distance Weighting (IDW) and Ordinary Kriging (OK) techniques, known as Kriging techniques, depend on the distance between two points, namely those of observation and estimation in the interpolation. IDW weighted the contribution of the observed points on the estimated interpolation with regard to this distance alone. On the other hand, OK also considers the correlation between the points and forms an initial function, i.e., covariance or variogram, which can iteratively be updated.

The spatial distribution map of indoor radon concentrations in Mashhad dwellings were plotted in Figure 7 by various interpolation techniques, e.g., IDW, OK, and Empirical Bayesian Kriging (EBK) over a grid with the dimensions of 1 km × 1 km using ArcGIS software version 10.7. Accordingly, radon concentrations were lower than standard values in eastern residential areas and were higher in central as well as southern districts. Nevertheless, when the spatial autocorrelation between cells was considered, predictions about radon concentrations using different methods range from 65 to 260 Bq m^{-3}. These values may be more realistic and similar to average values found in some dwellings in the region.

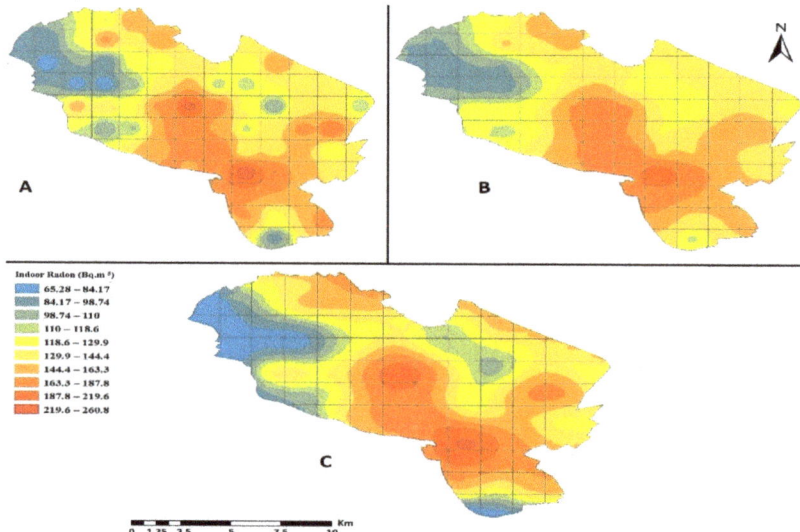

Figure 7. Predicted Indoor Radon Map of Mashhad dwellings over a grid with the dimensions of 1 km × 1 km using the (**A**) Inverse distance weighting, (**B**) Empirical Bayesian Kriging, and (**C**) Ordinary Kriging interpolation techniques.

Moreover, the accuracies of the various techniques applied according to five indicators are given in Table 4. IDW, which predicts unknown values using known values concerning their distance, was proven to be more suitable for predicting mean indoor radon concentrations over grids with the dimensions of 1 km × 1 km (i.e., arithmetic mean, ground floor), due to the lower MAE and RMSLE values of 28.159 and 0.01210, respectively, in addition to a lower bias, 20.069 to be exact. However, all mentioned models have a tendency to overestimate bias (PB > 0). In addition, the model with the higher R^2 is IDW, which indicates that this model fits the data better.

Table 4. Summary of the cross-validation results.

Method	MAE [1]	RMSE [2]	RMSLE [3]	PB [4]	R^2
Inverse distance weighting	28.159	34.931	0.01210	20.069	0.234
Empirical Bayesian Kriging	28.235	35.148	0.01218	20.123	0.224
Ordinary Kriging	28.424	36.364	0.01346	20.268	0.169

[1] MAE = mean absolute error, [2] RMSE = root mean square error, [3] RMSLE = root mean squared logarithmic error, [4] PB= percentage bias.

4. Conclusions

To estimate the impact of indoor radon and thoron on residentials as well as develop and implement the most economical method to reduce radon exposure using a radon map, this paper presents the measured indoor radon and thoron concentrations in 78 dwellings as well as soil gas radon concentrations in different districts of Mashhad, Iran during summer and winter. As the average of the radon concentrations in the summer and winter were assumed to be the annual average radon concentration in this study, the annual average indoor radon and thoron concentrations were calculated as being 132 ± 19 and 58 ± 7 Bq m^{-3}, respectively. Soil gas radon concentrations also ranged from 1.07 ± 0.28 to 8.02 ± 0.65 kBq·m^{-3} with a mean value of 3.07 ± 1.09 kBq·m^{-3} during the summer.

The corresponding annual effective dose from the inhalation of radon and thoron was calculated as being 3.7 ± 0.5 mSv yr^{-1}. Subsequently, the excess lifetime cancer risk was calculated as 14.13. Hence, exposure to indoor radon is responsible for approximately 12% of lung cancer deaths in Mashhad, which is close to the WHO estimates of the worldwide proportion of lung cancer due to radon (3–14%). By comparing the annual indoor effective dose rate from gamma exposure with the annual effective dose from the inhalation of radon and thoron, it was concluded that most of the dose received inside the dwellings studied in Mashhad, approximately 79% of the total dose, originates from the inhalation of radon and thoron.

Since high-risk areas can be recognized on radon maps, which are useful for targeting landlords and the building industry, an indoor radon map was generated by using ArcGIS software over a grid with the dimensions of 1 km × 1 km using three interpolation techniques. The arithmetic mean was used over the grid cells to predict a mean indoor radon concentration on the ground-floor level of buildings in the grid cells where no data was available. The IDW technique was proven to be most suitable one for predicting mean indoor radon concentrations over grids with the dimensions of 1 km × 1 km.

In addition to the results and given the significant health impacts of radon and thoron, it is hoped that both radon and thorn gases will be studied more seriously in Iran and that these techniques as well as complementary procedures will be used to minimize its concentration. It is recommended that radon gas concentrations should be measured in all regions of the country by numerous devices supplied by the Atomic Energy Organization of Iran (AEOI). As a result, it would be possible to compile a radon map of Iran to estimate the concentration and number of radon-induced incidences of cancer, as well as decide how to distribute the population. This would aid to reduce the number of cases of lung cancer and other radon-induced human health problems.

Author Contributions: Conceptualization, M.A., A.S., and T.K.; methodology, M.A., A.S., and T.K.; software, M.A. and M.I.; validation, M.A., A.S., T.K., and S.C.; formal analysis, M.A., A.S.; investigation, M.A., A.S., and T.K.; resources, T.K.; data curation, T.K. and S.C.; writing—original draft preparation, M.A.; writing—review and editing, M.A., A.S., S.C., and T.K.; visualization, M.A. and A.S.; supervision, T.K.; project administration, T.K.; funding acquisition, T.K. All authors have read and agreed to the published version of the manuscript.

Funding: This work was supported by the TKP2020-IKA-07 project financed under the 2020-4.1.1-TKP2020 Thematic Excellence Programme by the National Research, Development and Innovation Fund of Hungary and by the Hungarian National Research OKTA grant No. K128805 and K128818.

Institutional Review Board Statement: Not applicable for studies not involving humans or animals.

Informed Consent Statement: Not applicable for studies not involving humans.

Data Availability Statement: The data presented in this study are available on request from the corresponding author.

Conflicts of Interest: The authors declare no conflict of interest.

References

1. United Nations Scientific Committee on the Effects of Atomic Radiation. *UNSCEAR 2000 Report, Sources 473 and Effects of Ionizing Radiation*; Annex B Exposures from Natural Radiation Sources; UNSCEAR: New York, NY, USA, 2000; Volume 1.
2. United Nations Scientific Committee on the Effects of Atomic Radiation. *UNSCEAR 2008 Report, Sources and Effects of Ionizing Radiation*; Annex B Exposures of the Public and Workers from Various Sources of Radiation; UNSCEAR: New York, NY, USA, 2010; Volume 1.
3. Shahrokhi, A. Application of the European Basic Safety Standards Directive in Underground Mines: A Comprehensive Radioecology Study in a Hungarian Manganese Mine. Ph.D. Thesis, Pannon Egyetem, Veszprem, Hungary, 2018.
4. World Health Organization. *WHO Handbook on Indoor Radon: A Public Health Perspective*; WHO: Geneva, Switzerland, 2009.
5. United States Environmental Protection Agency. *EPA Protocol for Conducting Radon and Radon Decay Product Measurements in Multifamily Buildings*; Environmental Protection Agency: Washington, DC, USA, 2017.
6. Dubois, G. *An Overview of Radon Surveys in Europe*; European Commission, Ed.; EUR 21892 EN; Publications Office of the European Union: Luxembourg, 2005.
7. Rahman, S.; Mati, N.; Ghauri, B.M. Seasonal indoor radon concentration in the North West Frontier Province and federally administered tribal areas—Pakistan. *Radiat. Meas.* **2007**, *42*, 1715–1722. [CrossRef]
8. Rafique, M.; Rahman, S.U.; Mahmood, T.; Rahman, S.; Matiullah. Assessment of seasonal variation of indoor radon level in dwellings of some districts of Azad Kashmir, Pakistan. *Indoor Built Environ.* **2011**, *20*, 354–361. [CrossRef]
9. Kim, Y.; Chang, B.U.; Park, H.M.; Kim, C.K.; Tokonami, S. National radon survey in Korea. *Radiat. Prot. Dosim.* **2011**, *146*, 6–10. [CrossRef]
10. Szeiler, G.; Somlai, J.; Ishikawa, T.; Omori, Y.; Mishra, R.; Sapra, B.K.; Mayya, Y.S.; Tokonami, S.; Csordás, A.; Kovács, T. Preliminary results from an indoor radon thoron survey in Hungary. *Radiat. Prot. Dosim.* **2012**, *152*, 243–246. [CrossRef]
11. Sainz-Fernandez, C.; Fernandez-Villar, A.; Fuente-Merino, I.; Gutierrez-Villanueva, J.L.; Martin-Matarranz, J.L.; Garcia-Talavera, M.; Casal-Ordas, S.; Quindós-Poncela, L.S. The Spanish indoor radon mapping strategy. *Radiat. Prot. Dosim.* **2014**, *162*, 58–62. [CrossRef]
12. Shahrokhi, A.; Shokraee, F.; Reza, A.; Rahimi, H. Health risk assessment of household exposure to indoor radon in association with the dwelling's age. *J. Radiat. Prot. Res.* **2015**, *40*, 155–161. [CrossRef]
13. Singh, P.; Singh, P.; Singh, S.; Sahoo, B.K.; Sapra, B.K.; Bajwa, B.S. A study of indoor radon, thoron and their progeny measurement in Tosham region Haryana, India. *J. Radiat. Res. Appl. Sci.* **2015**, *8*, 226–233. [CrossRef]
14. Cinelli, G.; Tositti, L.; Capaccioni, B.; Brattich, E.; Mostacci, D. Soil gas radon assessment and development of a radon risk map in Bolsena, Central Italy. *Environ. Geochem. Health* **2015**, *37*, 305–319. [CrossRef]
15. Elío, J.; Crowley, Q.; Scanlon, R.; Hodgson, J.; Long, S. Logistic regression model for detecting radon prone areas in Ireland. *Sci. Total Environ.* **2017**, *599*, 1317–1329. [CrossRef]
16. Hoffmann, M.; Aliyev, C.S.; Feyzullayev, A.A.; Baghirli, R.J.; Veliyeva, F.F.; Pampuri, L.; Valsangiacomo, C.; Tollefsen, T.; Cinelli, G. First map of residential indoor radon measurements in Azerbaijan. *Radiat. Prot. Dosim.* **2017**, *175*, 186–193. [CrossRef]
17. Park, J.H.; Lee, C.M.; Lee, H.Y.; Kang, D.R. Estimation of seasonal correction factors for indoor radon concentrations in Korea. *Int. J. Environ. Res. Public Health* **2018**, *15*, 2251. [CrossRef]
18. Sohrabi, M.; Babapouran, M. New public dose assessment from internal and external exposures in low and elevated-level natural radiation areas of Ramsar, Iran. *Int. Congr. Ser.* **2005**, *1276*, 169–174. [CrossRef]
19. Hadad, K.; Doulatdar, R.; Mehdizadeh, S. Indoor radon monitoring in northern Iran using passive and active measurements. *J. Environ. Radioact.* **2007**, *95*, 39–52. [CrossRef]
20. Hadad, K.; Mokhtari, J. Indoor radon variations in central Iran and its geostatistical map. *Atmos. Environ.* **2015**, *102*, 220–227. [CrossRef]
21. Bouzarjomehri, F.; Ehrampoosh, M.H. Radon level in dwellings basement of Yazd-Iran. *Iran. J. Radiat. Res.* **2008**, *6*, 141–144.
22. Mowlavi, A.A.; Fornasier, M.R.; Binesh, A.; De Denaro, M. Indoor radon measurement and effective dose assessment of 150 apartments in Mashhad, Iran. *Environ. Monit Assess.* **2012**, *184*, 1085–1088. [CrossRef]
23. Fahiminia, M.; Fard, R.F.; Ardani, R.; Naddafi, K.; Hassanvand, M.S.; Mohammadbeigi, A. Indoor radon measurements in residential dwellings in Qom, Iran. *Int. J. Radiat Res.* **2016**, *14*, 331–339. [CrossRef]
24. Yarahmadi, M.; Shahsavani, A.; Mahmoudian, M.H.; Shamsedini, N.; Rastkari, N.; Kermani, M. Estimation of the residential radon levels and the annual effective dose in dwellings of Shiraz, Iran, in 2015. *Electron. Phys.* **2016**, *8*, 2497–2505. [CrossRef]
25. Shahbazi Sehrani, M.; Boudaqpoor, S.; Mirmohammadi, M. Measurement of indoor radon gas concentration and assessment of health risk in Tehran, Iran. *Int. J. Environ. Sci. Technol.* **2019**, *16*, 2619–2626. [CrossRef]
26. Mirbag, A.; Shokati Poursani, A. Indoor radon measurement in residential/commercial buildings in Isfahan city. *J. Air Pollut. Health* **2019**, *3*, 209–218. [CrossRef]

27. Shahrokhi, A.; Adelikhah, M.; Chalupnik, S.; Kocsis, E.; Toth-Bodrogi, E.; Kovács, T. Radioactivity of building materials in Mahallat, Iran–an area exposed to a high level of natural background radiation–attenuation of external radiation doses. *Materiales de Construcción* **2020**, *70*, e233. [CrossRef]
28. Sohrabi, M.; Roositalab, J.; Mohammadi, J. Public effective doses from environmental natural gamma exposures indoors and outdoors in Iran. *Radiat. Prot. Dosim.* **2015**, *167*, 633–641. [CrossRef] [PubMed]
29. Tokonami, S.; Takahashi, H.; Kobayashi, Y.; Zhuo, W.; Hulber, E. Up-to-date radon-thoron discriminative detector for a large-scale survey. *Rev. Sci. Instrum.* **2005**, *76*, 113505. [CrossRef]
30. Adelikhah, M.E.; Shahrokhi, A.; Chalupnik, S.; Toth-Bodrogi, E.; Kovács, T. High level of natural ionizing radiation at a thermal bath in Dehloran, Iran. *Heliyon* **2020**, *6*, e04297. [CrossRef]
31. Shahrokhi, A.; Nagy, E.; Csordás, A.; Somlai, J.; Kovács, T. Distribution of indoor radon concentrations between selected Hungarian thermal baths. *Nukleonika* **2016**, *61*, 333–336. [CrossRef]
32. Csordás, A.; Fábián, F.; Shahrokhi, A.; Somlai, J.; Kovács, T. Calibration of CR-39-based thoron progeny device. *Radiat. Prot. Dosim.* **2014**, *160*, 169–172.
33. International Commission on Radiological Protection. *Lung Cancer Risk from radon and Progeny and Statement on Radon*; Annals of the ICRP: New York, NY, USA, 2010.
34. Özen, S.; Celik, N.; Dursun, E.; Taşkın, H. Indoor and outdoor radon measurements at lung cancer patients' homes in the dwellings of Rize Province in Turkey. *Environ. Geochem. Health* **2018**, *40*, 1111–1125. [CrossRef]
35. Bossew, P.; Tollefsen, T.; Gruber, V.; De Cort, M. The European radon mapping project. In Proceedings of the IX Latin American IRPA Regional Congress on Radiation Protection and Safety, IRP, Rio de Janeiro, Brazil, 14–19 April 2013.
36. Janik, M.; Bossew, P.; Kurihara, O. Machine learning methods as a tool to analyse incomplete or irregularly sampled radon time series data. *Sci. Total Environ.* **2018**, *630*, 1155–1167. [CrossRef]
37. Alexander, D.L.; Tropsha, A.; Winkler, D.A. Beware of R2: Simple, unambiguous assessment of the prediction accuracy of QSAR and QSPR models. *J. Chem. Inf. Model.* **2015**, *55*, 1316–1322. [CrossRef]
38. International Commission on Radiological Protection. *Protection Against Radon-222 at Home and at Work*; Annals of the ICRP: New York, NY, USA, 1993.
39. United States Environmental Protection Agency. *Assessment of Risk from Radon in Homes*; Environmental Protection Agency: Washington, DC, USA, 2003.
40. Mehra, R.; Badhan, K.; Kansal, S.; Sonkawade, R.G. Assessment of seasonal indoor radon concentration in dwellings of Western Haryana. *Radiat. Meas.* **2011**, *46*, 1803–1806. [CrossRef]
41. Dey, G.K.; Das, P.K. Estimation of radon concentration in dwellings in and around Guwahati. *J. Earth Syst. Sci.* **2012**, *121*, 237–240. [CrossRef]
42. Kapdan, E.; Altinsoy, N. A comparative study of indoor radon concentrations between dwellings and schools. *Radiat Phys. Chem.* **2012**, *81*, 383–386. [CrossRef]
43. Cosma, C.; Cucoş-Dinu, A.; Papp, B.; Begy, R.; Sainz, C. Soil and building material as main sources of indoor radon in Băiţa-Ştei radon prone area (Romania). *J. Environ. Radioact.* **2013**, *116*, 174–179. [CrossRef]
44. Kunovska, B.; Ivanova, K.; Stojanovska, Z.; Vuchkov, D.; Zaneva, N. Measurements of radon concentration in soil gas of urban areas, Bulgaria. *Rom. J. Phys.* **2013**, *58*, S172–S179.
45. Szabó, K.Z.; Jordan, G.; Horváth, Á.; Szabó, C. Mapping the geogenic radon potential: Methodology and spatial analysis for central Hungary. *J. Environ. Radioact.* **2014**, *129*, 107–120. [CrossRef]
46. Hasan, A.K.; Subber, A.R.; Shaltakh, A.R. Measurement of radon concentration in soil gas using RAD7 in the environs of Al-Najaf Al-Ashraf City-Iraq. *Adv. Appl. Sci. Res.* **2011**, *2*, 273–278.
47. Mittal, S.; Rani, A.; Mehra, R. Estimation of radon concentration in soil and groundwater samples of Northern Rajasthan, India. *J. Radiat. Res. Appl. Sci.* **2016**, *9*, 125–130. [CrossRef]
48. Kikaj, D.; Jeran, Z.; Bahtijari, M.; Stegnar, P. Radon in soil gas in Kosovo. *J. Environ. Radioact.* **2016**, *164*, 245–252. [CrossRef]
49. Vaupotič, J.; Gregorič, A.; Kobal, I.; Žvab, P.; Kozak, K.; Mazur, J.; Kochowska, E.; Grządziel, D. Radon concentration in soil gas and radon exhalation rate at the Ravne Fault in NW Slovenia. *Nat. Hazard. Earth Sys.* **2010**, *10*, 895–899. [CrossRef]
50. Duggal, V.; Rani, A.; Mehra, R. Measurement of soil-gas radon in some areas of northern Rajasthan, India. *J. Earth Syst Sci.* **2014**, *123*, 1241–1247. [CrossRef]
51. Al Mugahed, M.; Bentayeb, F. Studying of Radon Gas Concentrations in Soil Qaa Al-Hakel Agricultural Area, Ibb, Yemen. *Mater. Today Proc.* **2019**, *13*, 525–529. [CrossRef]
52. Roshandel, G.; Ghanbari-Motlagh, A.; Partovipour, E.; Salavati, F.; Hasanpour-Heidari, S.; Mohammadi, G.; Khoshaabi, M.; Sadjadi, A.; Davanlou, M.; Tavangar, S.M.; et al. Cancer incidence in Iran in 2014: Results of the Iranian National Population-based Cancer Registry. *Cancer Epidemiol.* **2019**, *61*, 50–58. [CrossRef]

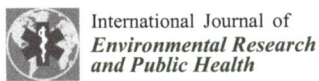 

Article

An Improved Passive CR-39-Based Direct ^{222}Rn/^{220}Rn Progeny Detector

Jun Hu [1], Guosheng Yang [2], Chutima Kranrod [1], Kazuki Iwaoka [2], Masahiro Hosoda [1,3] and Shinji Tokonami [1,*]

1. Institute of Radiation Emergency Medicine, Hirosaki University, 66-1 Hon-cho, Hirosaki 036-8564, Japan; hujun@hirosaki-u.ac.jp (J.H.); kranrodc@hirosaki-u.ac.jp (C.K.); m_hosoda@hirosaki-u.ac.jp (M.H.)
2. National Institutes for Quantum and Radiological Science and Technology, 4-9-1 Anagawa, Inage, Chiba 263-8555, Japan; yang.guosheng@qst.go.jp (G.Y.); iwaoka.kazuki@qst.go.jp (K.I.)
3. Graduate School of Health Sciences, Hirosaki University, 66-1 Hon-cho, Hirosaki 036-8564, Japan
* Correspondence: tokonami@hirosaki-u.ac.jp; Tel.: +81-172-39-5404

Received: 23 October 2020; Accepted: 16 November 2020; Published: 18 November 2020

Abstract: An improved passive CR-39-based direct ^{222}Rn/^{220}Rn progeny detector with 3 detection channels was designed and tested in this study to measure and calculate equilibrium equivalent concentration (EEC) of both ^{222}Rn and ^{220}Rn without the equilibrium factor. A theoretical model was established to calculate the EEC with optimization. Subsequently, an exposure experiment was carried out to test the performance of this detector, and we compared the chamber experiment and the theoretical model by estimating and measuring various parameters. The deposition flux of progeny derived from the prediction agreed well with the value measured in the exposure chamber. The energy-weighted net track density (NTD) measured by this detector is much more reliable to reflect the linear relation between NTD and time-integrated EEC. Since the detector is sensitive to the exposure environmental condition, it is recommended to apply the detector to measure the EEC after its calibration in a typical indoor environment.

Keywords: ^{222}Rn progeny; ^{220}Rn progeny; CR-39; equilibrium equivalent concentration; deposition velocity

1. Introduction

In the conventional integrating measurements for ^{222}Rn and ^{220}Rn activity concentrations in a large-scale survey, the solid-state nuclear track detector (SSNTD) technique is usually used. Several designs of measuring devices using SSNTD have been used for indoor ^{222}Rn and ^{220}Rn surveys, such as RADUET [1], Pin-hole dosimeter [2–4], and so on. In the two different diffusion rate chambers of these measuring devices, because there is a diffusion barrier against ^{220}Rn based on its quite short half-life, the low diffusion rate chamber detects mainly ^{222}Rn and the high diffusion rate chamber detects both ^{222}Rn and ^{220}Rn. However, evaluation of the internal exposure to ^{222}Rn and ^{220}Rn does not directly use the activity concentration of ^{222}Rn and ^{220}Rn gas instead of the equilibrium equivalent concentration (EEC). It should be noted that the equilibrium factor depends on various parameters, such as the radioactive decay, ventilation, and reactions with the structure and the surface of furnishing. Because of the short half-life of ^{220}Rn (55.6 s), the indoor ^{220}Rn concentration distributes heterogeneously, decreasing with distance from the source [5,6]. Therefore, it is not feasible to use the ^{220}Rn concentration directly measured by the integrating detectors to evaluate its internal exposure. Otherwise, study of the behavior of ^{222}Rn and ^{220}Rn decay products indoors is important for assessing the natural background radiation exposures on the public through the inhalation route. Therefore, the direct measurement technique of ^{222}Rn and ^{220}Rn progeny is desirable and necessary for the evaluation of internal indoor ^{222}Rn and ^{220}Rn exposure.

In the recent 20 years, a direct ^{220}Rn progeny measurement technique based on CR-39 detector for EEC of ^{220}Rn was developed and used by Zhuo and Iida [7], Tokonami et al. [8], Zhuo and Tokonami [9], Tokonami [10], Sorimach et al. [11], and Hu et al. [12]. Mishra and Mayya [13] were the first to develop the direct ^{222}Rn and ^{220}Rn progeny measurement techniques using LR-115 detector. CR-39 is the most sensitive and popular detector for recording α-particles [14] and performs stable results; no direct ^{222}Rn and ^{220}Rn progeny detector using CR-39 was developed and applied because its energy windows for recording α-particles is quite wide, and it is unable to distinguish alpha energy directly, although some researchers make great efforts to develop dedicated tools based on the track geometrical characteristics to measure alpha particles. Moreover, the application of the direct measurement technique for determining their progeny concentrations depends on estimation of the effective deposition velocities of combinations of ^{222}Rn and ^{220}Rn progenies in a typical indoor environment. Some researchers [11,15] used the experimental method to estimate the geometric mean deposition velocity and applied the data to actual measurement in an indoor environment. However, the experimental conditions had a lot of limitations on environmental parameters for estimating the deposition velocity. In this study, we developed a passive CR-39-based direct ^{222}Rn/^{220}Rn progeny detector. The ^{222}Rn and ^{220}Rn behavior model and particle deposition model were used to estimate the concentration of each ^{222}Rn and ^{220}Rn progeny as well as the EEC.

2. Materials and Methods

2.1. The Passive CR-39-Based Direct ^{222}Rn/^{220}Rn Progeny Detector

The structure of the detector is shown in Figure 1. The piece of commercially available ally diglycol carbonate (CR-39) (the BARYOTRAK, produced by Fukuvi Chemical Industry Co., Ltd., Fukui, Japan) was used as a detecting material to measure alpha particles emitted from ^{222}Rn and ^{220}Rn progeny. Each detection channel was mounted with a different thickness of aluminum-vaporized polyethylene films (Mylar films), which can only detect the alpha particles emitted from corresponding progeny radionuclides and ensure that lower energy alpha emissions (from the gases and other airborne alpha emitters) do not pass through the absorber. In the conventional passive direct ^{222}Rn/^{220}Rn progeny detector, there are only 2 detecting channels: the ^{220}Rn progeny (TnP) channel and the ^{222}Rn progeny (RnPII) channel. The TnP channel can only detect the 8.78 MeV alpha particles emitted from ^{212}Po atoms, which are formed from the decay of ^{212}Pb and ^{212}Bi atoms deposited on the film surface without any interference from other alpha emissions of natural radioactivity decay series. The RnPII channel selectively detects ^{212}Po and ^{214}Po (7.69 MeV) from the decay of surface deposited ^{222}Rn and ^{220}Rn progeny. In the improved passive detector, we added one more detecting channel RnPI to detect the alpha emission energy higher than that of ^{218}Po (6.0 MeV). The design information is present in Table 1. Since the RnPI and RnPII cthannels are in a mixed ^{222}Rn and ^{220}Rn progeny environment, there are interferences from the high energy alpha particles, which could be subtracted using the tracks on the TnP channel. Therefore, 4 slices of CR-39 detector are used on the TnP channel instead of 2 slices on the other channels to decrease the error.

Table 1. The design information of each detector channel.

Channel	Membrane Thickness (mg cm^{-2})	Nuclide	Energy of α-Particle (MeV)	Track Registration Efficiency, η	Deposited Atoms
TnP	7.10	^{212}Po	8.785	0.063	^{212}Pb, ^{212}Bi
RnPII	5.05	^{212}Po	8.785	0.212	^{212}Pb, ^{212}Bi
		^{214}Po	7.687	0.182	^{218}Po, ^{214}Pb, ^{214}Bi
RnPI	3.25	^{212}Po and ^{212}Bi	8.785 and 6.051	0.152	^{212}Pb, ^{212}Bi
		^{214}Po	7.687	0.249	^{218}Po, ^{214}Pb, ^{214}Bi
		^{218}Po	6.003	0.135	^{218}Po

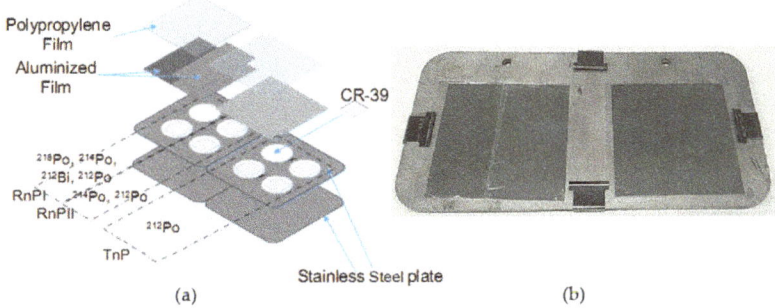

Figure 1. The passive CR-39-based direct ^{222}Rn/^{220}Rn progeny detector: (**a**) a schematic diagram of the progeny detector showing the detectable radionuclides of each channel and (**b**) a photo of the actual setup of the progeny detector.

2.2. The Theoretical Model and Parameters

2.2.1. Theoretical Model

Among the several aspects of indoor behaviors of ^{222}Rn and ^{220}Rn, apart from the decay losses, deposition and ventilation are two major mechanisms to remove the decay products from indoor air. Unlike the removal process by ventilation which depends essentially on the air exchange rate in a given room environment, the removal by deposition depends on the activity size distribution and the structure of turbulence at the air–surface interface. Since this detector is designed using the deposition mode, it is necessary to avoid uncontrolled static charges from affecting the deposition rates. Hence, the aluminized side of the Mylar is chosen to act as the deposition surface.

To describe the behavior of ^{222}Rn and ^{220}Rn progeny, the relationship between the attached ^{222}Rn and ^{220}Rn progeny deposition flux, J (atom cm^{-2} s^{-1}), and track density, N (tracks cm^{-2}) can be expressed as follows:

$$J = \frac{N}{\eta t} \tag{1}$$

where η is the track registration efficiency, which is the multiplier of the branching ratio of its progeny, the geometric efficiency, and etching efficiency. For each channel, the geometric efficiency depends on the energies of incident α-particle, incident angles against the absorbers, and the thickness of the absorbers. The track registration efficiency measured in this study is present in Table 1, which corresponds to the etching condition using 6 N NaOH solutions at 60 °C for 24 h without stirring. t is the exposure period (s).

The effective deposition velocity of the progeny, V_e (cm s^{-1}), is defined as follows:

$$V_e = \frac{J}{C} \tag{2}$$

where C is the atom concentration of the progeny (atom cm^{-3}).

To determine the deposited progeny atoms from the alpha tracks registered in CR-39, we need to check the progeny atoms' ultimate decay on the surface of the detector, which causes the alpha track to the CR-39. In the case of ^{222}Rn progeny, a fraction of all the alpha particles emitted from the atoms of ^{218}Po, ^{214}Pb, and ^{214}Bi deposited on the absorber can form tracks on the CR-39. Therefore, the tracks counted at the end can be directly proportional to the sum of the ^{218}Po, ^{214}Pb, and ^{214}Bi atoms deposited. Similarly, the total tracks registered by the ^{220}Rn progeny will be proportional to the sum of the ^{212}Pb and ^{212}Bi atoms deposited. Accordingly, we can define the following:

$$N_{Tn} = \eta_{Tn,Po212} \cdot V_{e,Tn} \cdot (C_{Pb212} + C_{Bi212}) \cdot t \tag{3}$$

$$N_{Rn2} = \eta_{Rn2,Po212} \cdot V_{e,Tn} \cdot (C_{Pb212} + C_{Bi212}) \cdot t + \eta_{Rn2,Po214} \cdot V_{e,Rn} \cdot (C_{Po218} + C_{Pb214} + C_{Bi214}) \cdot t \quad (4)$$

$$\begin{aligned}N_{Rn1} &= \eta_{Rn1,Po212} \cdot V_{e,Tn} \cdot (C_{Pb212} + C_{Bi212}) \cdot t + \eta_{Rn1,Po214} \cdot V_{e,Rn} \cdot (C_{Po218} + C_{Pb214} + C_{Bi214}) \cdot t \\ &+ \eta_{Rn1,Bi212} \cdot V_{e,Tn} \cdot (C_{Pb212} + C_{Bi212}) \cdot t + \eta_{Rn1,Po218} \cdot V_{e,Rn,Po218} \cdot C_{Po218} \cdot t\end{aligned} \quad (5)$$

where the subscripts of Tn, $Rn1$, and $Rn2$ mean the parameters of the TnP channel, RnPI channel, and RnPII channel, respectively, and the subscript of each radionuclide means the corresponding parameter. Some of the parameters used in this study are shown in Table 1. $V_{e,Tn}$ is the effective deposition velocity of ^{220}Rn progeny, which is a combination of deposition velocities of ^{212}Pb and ^{212}Bi. $V_{e,Rn}$ is a combination of deposition velocities of ^{218}Po, ^{214}Pb, and ^{214}Bi. $V_{e,Rn,Po218}$ is the only effective deposition velocity of ^{218}Po.

In the mixed ^{222}Rn and ^{220}Rn environment, we can easily count the registered tracks on the TnP channel from ^{212}Po decay, which come from the decay of the deposition flux of ^{212}Pb and ^{212}Bi, as shown in Equation (6). Accordingly, from Equations (3)–(5), we can also calculate the counts of registered tracks from ^{214}Po on the RnPII channel and ^{218}Po on the RnPI channel as in Equations (7) and (8).

$$N^{TnP}_{Po212} = \eta_{Tn,Po212} \cdot V_{e,Tn} \cdot (C_{Pb212} + C_{Bi212}) \cdot t = N_{Tn} \quad (6)$$

$$\begin{aligned}N^{RnP2}_{Po214} &= \eta_{Rn2,Po214} \cdot V_{e,Rn} \cdot (C_{Po218} + C_{Pb214} + C_{Bi214}) \cdot t \\ &= N_{Rn2} - \frac{\eta_{Rn2,Po212}}{\eta_{Tn,Po212}} N_{Tn}\end{aligned} \quad (7)$$

$$\begin{aligned}N^{RnP1}_{Po218} &= \eta_{Rn1,Po218} \cdot V_{e,Rn,Po218} \cdot C_{Po218} \cdot t \\ &= N_{Rn1} - \frac{(\eta_{Rn1,Po212} + \eta_{Rn1,Bi212})}{\eta_{Tn,Po212}} N_{Tn} - \frac{\eta_{Rn1,Po214}}{\eta_{Rn2,Po214}} N^{RnP2}_{Po214}\end{aligned} \quad (8)$$

In the atmosphere, a large fraction of ^{218}Po and ^{212}Pb can react with the ions in the air and form clusters in a short time by the neutralization process. Due to the larger diffusion coefficient of these cluster particles, ^{222}Rn and ^{220}Rn progenies can attach themselves to various surfaces, such as the surfaces of aerosol particles and droplets in the atmosphere, thereby giving rise to a consecutive activity size distribution. This distribution is broadly classified into two groups: the unattached fraction and the attached fraction. The effective deposition velocities combine the contribution from both the unattached and attached fractions of each progeny species. Considering the contributions of these two fractions, the deposition velocity of each radionuclide can be demonstrated as follows:

$$V_i = p_i \cdot V^u_d + (1 - p_i) \cdot V^a_d \quad (9)$$

where p_i denotes the unattached fraction of radionuclide i, and V^u_d and V^a_d denote the deposition velocities of the unattached and attached fraction of airborne particles, respectively, which are dependent on the aerodynamic factors instead of the radionuclides themselves.

Since the registered tracks from ^{212}Po decay come from the decay of the deposition flux of ^{212}Pb and ^{212}Bi, according to the concept of the effective deposition velocity, the deposition velocity of TnP channel could be written as follows:

$$V_{e,Tn} = \frac{V_{Pb212} \cdot C_{Pb212} + V_{Bi212} \cdot C_{Bi212}}{C_{Pb212} + C_{Bi212}} \quad (10)$$

Similarly, the deposition velocity of the RnPII and RnPI channels could be written as follows:

$$V_{e,Rn} = \frac{V_{Po218} \cdot C_{Po218} + V_{Pb214} \cdot C_{Pb214} + V_{Bi214} \cdot C_{Bi214}}{C_{Po218} + C_{Pb214} + C_{Bi214}} \quad (11)$$

$$V_{e,Rn,Po218} = V_{Po218} \quad (12)$$

The atom concentrations in these equations could also be reexpressed in terms of the activity concentrations (A_i, Bq m^{-3}) by using the decay constant λ_i, s^{-1}. Subsequently, Equations (6)–(8) could be modified as follows:

$$N_{Po212}^{TnP} = \eta_{Tn,Po212} \cdot \frac{V_{Pb212} \cdot \lambda_{Bi212} + V_{Bi212} \cdot \lambda_{Pb212} \cdot r_3}{\lambda_{Bi212} + \lambda_{Pb212}} \cdot \left(\frac{1}{\lambda_{Pb212}} + \frac{r_3}{\lambda_{Bi212}}\right) \cdot A_{Pb212} \cdot t \quad (13)$$

where $r_3 = A_{Bi212}/A_{Pb212}$.

$$N_{Po214}^{RnP2} = \eta_{Rn2,Po214} \cdot \frac{V_{Po218} \cdot \lambda_{Pb214} \cdot \lambda_{Bi214} + V_{Pb214} \cdot \lambda_{Po218} \cdot \lambda_{Bi214} \cdot r_1 + V_{Bi214} \cdot \lambda_{Po218} \cdot \lambda_{Pb214} \cdot r_2}{\lambda_{Pb214} \cdot \lambda_{Bi214} + \lambda_{Po218} \cdot \lambda_{Bi214} \cdot r_1 + \lambda_{Po218} \cdot \lambda_{Pb214} \cdot r_2}$$
$$\cdot \left(\frac{1}{\lambda_{Po218}} + \frac{r_1}{\lambda_{Pb214}} + \frac{r_2}{\lambda_{Bi214}}\right) \cdot A_{Po218} \cdot t \quad (14)$$

where $r_1 = A_{Pb214}/A_{Po218}$ and $r_2 = A_{Bi214}/A_{Po218}$.

$$N_{Po218}^{RnP1} = \eta_{Rn1,Po218} \cdot V_{Po218} \cdot \frac{A_{Po218}}{\lambda_{Po218}} \cdot t \quad (15)$$

To solve these equations above, we introduced the Jacobi room model [16] for both ^{222}Rn and ^{220}Rn. Because the steady-state Jacobi room model is a system of linear equations, the number of unknowns, such as the unattached fractions of each progeny radionuclide and the ratios of the progeny concentration, is less than the number of equations. The solutions of the unknowns could be deduced by the parameters in the Jacobi room model, which are the attachment rate constant, λ_a (s^{-1}); the rate constant for deposition of unattached progeny, λ_d^u (s^{-1}); the rate constant for deposition of attached progeny, λ_d^a (s^{-1}); and the ventilation rate constant, λ_v (s^{-1}). The details of the equations of the Jacobi room model for both ^{222}Rn and ^{220}Rn behaviors could be found elsewhere [6]. Finally, the A_{Pb212} can be solved by the data of the TnP channel and A_{Po218} can be solved by both the RnPI channel and RnPII channel in the equations.

2.2.2. Parameters Estimation

Deposition Velocity

In the theoretical model, Lai and Nazaroff's [17] three-layer model was adopted to simulate the particle deposition. Compared to the other existing formulations of such models based on the pioneering work of Corner and Pendlebury [18], lacking a thorough physical foundation, the proposed model involves three mechanisms of particle transport: Brownian diffusion, turbulent diffusion, and gravitational settling. It predicts deposition to smooth surfaces as a function of particle size and density. Therefore, the only required input parameters are enclosure geometry and friction velocity. This deposition velocity estimation method has already been applied for deposition particles in a room and experimentally verified by Mishra et al. [15].

Parameters in the Jacobi Room Model

In practice, the indoor rooms can be regarded as a rectangular cavity. The rate constant for deposition in the Jacobi room model is estimated by using the deposition velocity calculated by Lai and Nazaroff's three-layer model [17]. For the rectangular cavity, the rate constant for deposition can be written as follows:

$$\lambda_d^i = n_c \cdot \frac{v_{d,u}^i S_u + v_{d,v}^i S_v + v_{d,d}^i S_d}{V} \quad (16)$$

where the superscript i, with the allowed values a and u, allows us to distinguish the two important states of ^{222}Rn and ^{220}Rn progeny: attached and unattached. S_u, S_v, and S_d are the areas of upward-facing surfaces, vertical surfaces, and downward-facing surfaces, respectively; and n_c is the correction coefficient of the surface area [19], which can be used to correct the changes of ratio caused by the increased furnishing surface area in practical application. The deposition velocity of the unattached fraction was interpolated by the result of the numerical integration for fine particles in the reference [17].

The rate constant for attachment in the Jacobi room model reflects the attachment velocity of the unattached ^{222}Rn and ^{220}Rn progeny to the ambient aerosol. The charging process depends on the electric charge distribution of an aerosol in steady state. In most used theories, attachment is diffusion-controlled as a result of electrostatic attraction and follows the gas kinetic laws [20–22]. The expression of the rate constant for attachment can be written as follows:

$$\lambda_a = \overline{\beta} \cdot N_o \tag{17}$$

$$\overline{\beta} = \int_0^\infty \beta(d_p) Z(d_p) \mathrm{d}d_p \tag{18}$$

where N_o is the aerosol concentration, reflecting the concentration of condensation nuclei and where $Z(d_p)$ is the number size distribution of aerosol for unit aerosols concentration and can be described as a frequency function of the lognormal distribution with the count median diameter (CMD) and geometric standard deviation (GSD, σ_g). $\beta(d_p)$ is the attachment coefficient. The rate constant for attachment was estimated by the compound trapezoid formula with the Latin-hypercube sampling method.

3. Results and Discussion

3.1. The Comparison of Chamber Test with a Theoretical Model

To verify the feasibility of measuring the EEC, a verification experiment was conducted in ^{222}Rn and ^{220}Rn exposure chambers located in Hirosaki University, Japan. The chamber verification system includes 4 function cells, as shown in Figure 2. (1) The source generation cell is a ^{222}Rn gas and ^{220}Rn gas generation system, which employs the natural uranium rock and commercially available lantern mantles as the ^{222}Rn and ^{220}Rn sources, respectively, to generate and import ^{222}Rn and ^{220}Rn to the mix chamber. The humidifier in this cell is responsible for maintaining the stability of the inlet gas concentration. (2) The aerosol generation cell contains 3 components, a compressor, a constant output atomizer (TSI, Inc., Aerosol Generator Model 3076), and a diffusion dryer filled with silica gel. The 5000 µg mL^{-1} NaCl solution is employed to generate droplets with the median diameter of 0.3 µm (GSD < 2.0) to mix with ^{222}Rn gas or ^{220}Rn gas in the mix chamber. (3) The exposure cell includes two chambers: a mix chamber and an exposure chamber. The volumes of the mix chamber and exposure chamber are 150 L and 3.24 m^3 (dimensions of 2.25 × 1.2 × 1.2 m^3, L × W × H), respectively. The mix chamber provides a buffer to create more chances for the aerosol particles and gas to form a stable progeny flux to the exposure chamber. To maintain stable concentration in the exposure chamber, the experiment adopted a circulating connection that applies the outlet of the exposure chamber as the inlet of the source generation cell with an airflow rate of 3 L min^{-1}. (4) The measurement cell is responsible for measuring progeny concentrations and environmental parameters in the verification experiment. The portable Si-photodiode detector with a sampling flow rate of 0.5 L min^{-1} and an EMD Millipore MF-Millipore AAWG02500 Mixed Cellulose Ester Filter Membrane were used to measure the EEC of ^{222}Rn in real-time. The details of the Si-photodiode detector can be found elsewhere [23,24]. The periodic grab sampling method was carried out to replace the portable Si-photodiode detector to measure the EEC of ^{220}Rn. The Model 3034 SMPS^{TM} Scanning Mobility Particle Sizer produced by TSI® was adopted to measure the concentration of condensation nuclei, CMD, and its GSD (σ_g). The concentration of condensation nuclei in the exposure chamber ranged from 2.05 × 10^4 to 4.32 × 10^4 particles per cm^3. The CMD of the aerosol in the exposure chamber ranged from 0.187 to 0.218 µm. The friction velocity was calculated using a fan-turbulence model [11,25], as follows:

$$u^* = \frac{N_s d_t^2}{V^{1/3}} \tag{19}$$

where N_s is the rotation speed of the fan (2300 rotation min^{-1}), d_t is the blade length for rotation (5 cm), and V is the volume of the exposure chamber. In this exposure chamber, we set two fans in opposite directions; as a result, we obtained u^* as 23.53 cm s^{-1}. In the verification experiment, each channel had 4 slices of CR-39 in the vertical and upward orientations as one group. For the total verification experiment, each exposure period had 3 groups of progeny detectors in the front, middle, and back of the bottom of the exposure chamber. In the theoretical model, the genetic algorithm is adopted to optimize the parameters in the calculation process. The measured values of the concentration of nuclei condensation number, CMD and its GSD, estimated friction velocity, and ventilation rate are the input parameters. Since the friction velocity, ventilation rate, and particle distribution fluctuate and change all the time, the equilibrium value of each parameter during the exposure period should be optimized depending on the different circumstances for each survey.

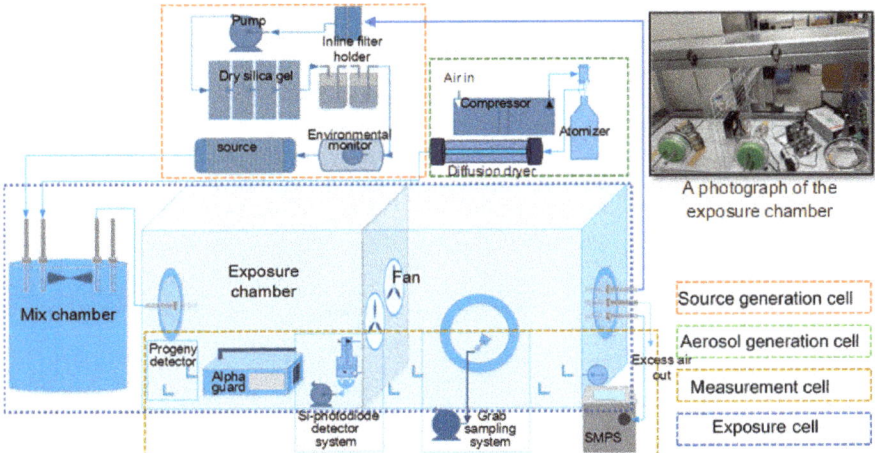

Figure 2. A schematic diagram of the chamber verification system.

A genetic algorithm with an improved goodness-of-fit objective function was adopted to optimize the results of the theoretical method [26]. The improved genetic algorithm was used to maximize the goodness-of-fit objective function $f(x)$ as follows:

$$f(x) = \frac{\sum_{i=1}^{n} \omega_i}{\sum_{i=1}^{n} \frac{|x_{1,i}-x_{2,i}|}{x_i} \cdot \omega_i} \tag{20}$$

where n is the number of objects of the model; $x_{1,i}$ and $x_{2,i}$ are the measured data from actual measurement of EEC; and ω_i is the weight. The measured ranges of the concentration of nuclei condensation number, CMD, and its GSD are the optimized parameters, and the goodness-of-fit function is carried out to decrease the error of the average EEC of ^{222}Rn calculated by the calibrated portable Si-photodiode detector and the CR-39-based progeny detector. The average track density of detectors deployed in the upward and vertical orientations was used to calculate the EEC of ^{222}Rn by the progeny detector, which is in the same orientation as that placed in use. The same verification experiment was also conducted for ^{220}Rn progeny except for the measurement method for the EEC of ^{220}Rn, which used the periodic grab sampling method to replace the portable Si-photodiode detector. The comparison results of the progeny detector and experiment are shown in Tables 2 and 3. In the calculation, we estimated the deposition velocity of total condensation nuclei in the vertical and upward orientations, which were in the same orientation as the setting in the experiment, and the total deposition velocity and deposition flux of each channel. As shown in Table 2, for the ^{220}Rn progeny with an exposure time of 36.9 h, the average experimentally estimated deposition velocities in the upward and vertical orientations were 0.193 ± 0.067 and 0.217 ± 0.045 m h^{-1}, respectively. Additionally, the model-simulated deposition velocities were 0.243 and 0.238 m h^{-1}, respectively, which were located in the ranges of the experimental data. In the experiment, the deposition velocity in the upward orientation presented insignificant variation with that of the vertical orientation. The exposure time also presented an insignificant influence on the deposition velocity between 25.5 and 36.9 h. For deposition flux, the variation of deposition flux on the TnP channel estimated by the model showed excellent agreement with experimental values. As shown in Table 3, for the ^{222}Rn progeny, among distinct exposure times of 30, 70, and 102 h, the calibrated deposition velocities varied narrowly in the upward and vertical orientations, with the ranges of 0.123–0.136 and 0.117–0.131 m h^{-1}, respectively. The average deposition fluxes in the theoretical model of ^{222}Rn progeny on the RnPII channel and of ^{218}Po on the RnPI channel were located in the ranges of the experimental values in most cases. The deposition flux was calculated by the net track density (NTD). The calculation process of NTD itself has uncertainty, especially caused by the sensitivity of the CR-39 detector, read-out of the tracks, counting statistics, and assumed background of the CR-39 detectors [11], except for the exposure environment. Additionally, from Equations (6)–(8), the calculation of the tracks registered by lower alpha-energy progeny should exclude the tracks registered by higher alpha-energy progeny on the channel. Therefore, with a thinner absorber filter, a higher uncertainty of the measured deposition flux is present due to propagations of the uncertainty during the calculation of the NTD.

Table 2. The comparison results of the progeny detector and experiment in a ^{220}Rn chamber verification system.

		Model	Experiment	Model	Experiment
Exposure time (h)		25.5		36.9	
The number concentration (N cm^{-3})		27,297		30,417	
GSD, σ_g		1.506		1.613	
CMD (μm)		0.203		0.203	
Track density (tr mm^{-2})	Upward	3.9		2.9	
	Vertical	4.3		4.8	
Deposition velocity (m h^{-1})	Upward	0.185	0.143 ± 0.029	0.243	0.193 ± 0.067
	Vertical	0.169	0.158 ± 0.040	0.238	0.217 ± 0.045
	^{212}Pb	0.185	——	0.219	——
	^{212}Bi	0.132	——	0.183	——
Deposition flux (atoms cm^{-2} s^{-1})	Upward	0.081	0.081	0.055	0.069
	Vertical	0.090	0.090	0.042	0.042
EEC of ^{220}Rn (Bq m^{-3})	Upward	237 ± 88	244 ± 108 [1]	148 ± 38	155 ± 67 [1]
	Vertical	263 ± 88		188 ± 50	

[1] The value was calculated by the average equilibrium equivalent concentration (EEC) of ^{220}Rn over the whole exposure period by grab sampling method.

Table 3. The comparison results of the progeny detector and experiment in a ^{222}Rn chamber verification system.

		Model	Experiment	Model	Experiment	Model	Experiment
Exposure time (h)		30	30	70	70	102	102
Concentration of nuclei number (N cm^{-3})		34,528		33,833		33,278	
GSD, σ_g		1.714		1.761		1.768	
CMD (μm)		0.233		0.200		0.191	
Track density (tr mm^{-2})	Upward RnPI	6.3 ± 1.3		16.4 ± 2.5		14.9 ± 2.3	
	Upward RnPII	4.5 ± 1.2		6.2 ± 1.6		4.9 ± 1.1	
	Vertical RnPI	7.4 ± 1.5		13.6 ± 2.1		17.2 ± 2.7	
	Vertical RnPII	1.1 ± 0.8		7.1 ± 1.8		5.9 ± 1.3	
Deposition velocity (m h^{-1})	Upward	0.136	—	0.123	—	0.125	—
	Vertical	0.131	—	0.117	—	0.119	—
	^{218}Po	0.290	—	0.248	—	0.230	—
	^{214}Pb	0.155	—	0.135	—	0.112	—
	^{214}Bi	0.101	—	0.091	—	0.092	—
Deposition flux (atoms cm^{-2} s^{-1})	^{218}Po to RnPI Upward	0.041	0.051 ± 0.010	0.022	0.048 ± 0.017	0.018	0.030 ± 0.016
	^{218}Po to RnPI Vertical		0.043 ± 0.009		0.040 ± 0.014		0.035 ± 0.019
	^{218}Po, ^{214}Pb, ^{214}Bi to RnPII Upward	0.014	0.005 ± 0.004	0.011	0.014 ± 0.008	0.008	0.007 ± 0.006
	^{218}Po, ^{214}Pb, ^{214}Bi to RnPII Vertical		0.023 ± 0.006		0.016 ± 0.009		0.009 ± 0.007
EEC of ^{222}Rn (Bq m^{-3})	Upward	1214 ± 322	740 ± 27 [1]	730 ± 290	693 ± 16 [1]	758 ± 370	686 ± 31 [1]
	Vertical	267 ± 187		603 ± 312		630 ± 375	

[1] The value was calculated by the average EEC of ^{222}Rn over the whole exposure period by the continuous portable Si-photodiode detector.

3.2. Comparison of the Estimated Deposition Velocities with Previous Studies

Compared with the deposition velocities of the total ^{222}Rn and ^{220}Rn progeny of the other researchers [7,11,15,27], as shown in Table 4, these values varied widely from 0.117 to 8.64 m h^{-1} and 0.072 to 19.08 m h^{-1}, respectively. To analyze the impact factors of the deposition velocity of ^{222}Rn and ^{220}Rn progenies, except the deposition velocities measured by Bigu [25], other deposition velocities measured in small-size chambers are much higher than that measured in the test rooms, dwellings, or large-size chambers. This can be explained by the turbulence, caused by the surface roughness, friction velocity, and airflow rate on the surface in a small-size chamber, being much more intense than that in a large room. Similarly, in Bigu's research, the mixing fan was operated to investigate the effect of strong airflow and turbulence on the deposition velocity [24]. When the fan is on, the surface airflow and turbulence would be more intense, accompanying the increasing deposition velocity of the ^{222}Rn and ^{220}Rn progenies.

Table 4. Summary of the deposition velocities of ^{222}Rn and ^{220}Rn progenies in previous studies.

Reference	Deposition Velocity (m h^{-1})		Remark
	RnP Detector	TnP Detector	
[27]	8.64	19.08	Fan on, 26 m^3 test facility
	3.24	2.16	Fan off, 26 m^3 test facility
[7]		0.19 ± 0.04	Dwelling, the same structure of TnP detector as this study
[15]	0.132 ± 0.0036	0.075 ± 0.0072	22.5 m^3 test room
	2.37 ± 0.785		0.5 m^3 chamber
	0.117	0.072	Dwelling
[11]		0.828 ± 0.072	150 L chamber, same TnP detector as this study
This study	0.125 ± 0.007	0.178 ± 0.045	3.24 m^3 chamber

The design of TnP detectors from Zhuo and Iida [7] and Sorimachi et al. [11] are the same as that in the present study, and only the measuring environmental conditions are different. The deposition velocity measured in the small-size chamber [11] is significantly higher than that measured in dwellings [7] and the present study. It should be noted that the deposition velocity measured in this study agreed well with that measured in dwellings. Besides, the deposition velocities of the RnP detector measured by Marsh et al. [15] in the test room and dwelling were also comparable to that of the present study. Therefore, the deposition velocities estimated by both experiments and theoretical models are acceptable in this study. Furthermore, the calibration results from this study are suitable to assess the ^{222}Rn and ^{220}Rn progeny exposure in test rooms and dwellings.

3.3. The Relationship between NTD and Time-Integrated EEC

The relationship between the NTD and the time-integrated EEC of ^{222}Rn and ^{220}Rn is shown in Figure 3. Based on the concept of the potential alpha energy concentration of ^{222}Rn and ^{220}Rn progeny, the NTD caused by ^{212}Po on the TnP channel can be used to estimate the total potential alpha energy of ^{212}Po emitted by the deposited ^{212}Pb and ^{212}Bi. The detectors were exposed to a total of ^{220}Rn progeny concentration of 83 ± 20 Bq m^{-3} during the exposure period from 0.2 to 2.5 d. The time-integrated EEC of ^{220}Rn ranged from approximately 16 to 168 Bq m^{-3} d, which corresponded to the time-integrated EEC of ^{220}Rn in an exposure period between 1 week to 3 months with the average EEC of ca. 2 Bq m^{-3} per day indoors [5]. The result demonstrated that the values of NTD increased linearly with an increase of time-integrated EEC of ^{220}Rn. Accordingly, the NTD caused by ^{218}Po on channel RnPI can be used to estimate the atom number of the deposited ^{218}Po on the detector firstly decaying to ^{214}Pb. Furthermore, the NTD of ^{214}Po can be used to calculate the total potential alpha energy of ^{214}Po emitted by the deposited ^{218}Po, ^{214}Pb, and ^{214}Bi during the decay. Therefore, in Figure 3a, the energy-weighted NTD was calculated as follows:

$$\text{Energy weighted NTD} = \frac{\left(\varepsilon(^{218}\text{Po}) \cdot \text{NTD of } ^{218}\text{Po} + \varepsilon(^{214}\text{Po}) \cdot \text{NTD of } ^{214}\text{Po}\right)}{(\varepsilon(^{218}\text{Po}) + \varepsilon(^{214}\text{Po}))} \quad (21)$$

where ε (i) is the alpha energy of the radionuclide i emitted during the decay. $\varepsilon(^{218}\text{Po})$ is 6.0 MeV, and $\varepsilon(^{214}\text{Po})$ is 7.7 MeV. The progeny detectors were exposed to an average EEC of ^{222}Rn of 685 ± 6 Bq m^{-3} during the exposure period. The time-integrated EEC of ^{222}Rn ranged from approximately 863 to 2839 Bq m^{-3} d, which corresponds to the time-integrated EEC of ^{222}Rn in an exposure period from 1 month to 3 months with an average EEC of ^{222}Rn of ca. 30 Bq m^{-3} per day. As a result, the values of the three NTDs increased linearly with the increase of the time-integrated EEC of ^{222}Rn. Thus, it is possible to estimate the EEC of ^{222}Rn indoors during a certain period. To compare the three NTDs as a function of the time-integrated EEC of ^{222}Rn, the R^2 of NTD of ^{218}Po, energy-weighted NTD, and NTD of ^{214}Pb were successively decreased from 0.9861 to 0.5625. Therefore, compared to the other deposition-based passive ^{222}Rn progeny detectors which only measure the NTD contributed by ^{214}Po, the detector with two channels is much more reliable. Besides, the progeny detector with 4 slices of CR-39 for the TnP channel designed rather than the same slices of CR-39 for each channel is recommended to decrease the error in calculation.

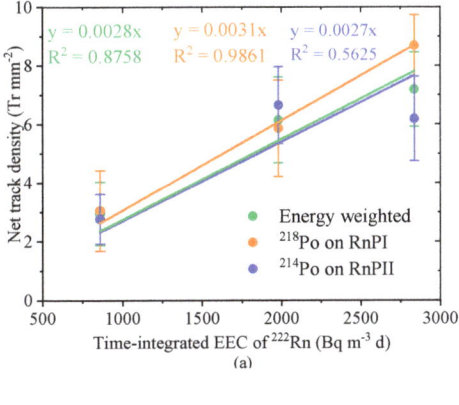

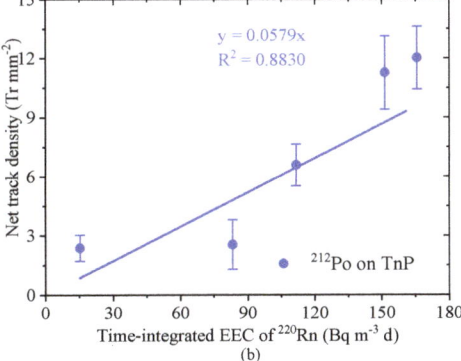

Figure 3. The net track density (NTD) as a function of time-integrated equilibrium equivalent concentration (EEC): (**a**) the NTD as a function of time-integrated EEC of ^{222}Rn, where the NTD has excluded the contribution of other radionuclides on the CR-39, and (**b**) the NTD as a function of time-integrated EEC of ^{220}Rn.

4. Conclusions

In this study, a 3-channel passive CR-39-based direct ^{222}Rn/^{220}Rn progeny detector was developed and tested to measure and calculate the EEC of both ^{222}Rn and ^{220}Rn without the equilibrium factor. In the verification chamber experiment, the genetic algorithm was implemented to optimize the estimation result of the theoretical model. The optimized deposition fluxes of ^{220}Rn progeny on the TnP channel, the ^{222}Rn progeny on the RnPII channel, and ^{218}Po on the RnPI channel agreed well with the experimental measurements. The EEC of ^{220}Rn and ^{222}Rn measured by the calibrated devices are comparable to the estimated value of the detector. Compared with the two channels' detectors, the energy-weighted NTD is much more reliable to estimate the EEC of ^{222}Rn rather than only measuring the NTD contributed by ^{214}Po. Moreover, because the exposure conditions, especially the airflow and turbulence in the room, are smaller than that in the small-size chamber, the deposition velocity measured in this study is close to the value measured in the room. Therefore, a detector calibrated in a similar size to the chamber test as in this study is more reliable for assessment of ^{220}Rn and ^{222}Rn progeny exposure. At last, since the detector is sensitive to the exposure environmental condition, in the site survey, it is recommended to use the improved passive CR-39-based direct progeny detector after its calibration in a typical indoor environment.

Author Contributions: Conceptualization, J.H. and S.T.; data curation, J.H. and G.Y.; formal analysis, J.H. and G.Y.; funding acquisition, J.H. and S.T.; investigation, J.H.; methodology, J.H., C.K., and K.I.; project administration, S.T.; resources, M.H.; supervision, S.T.; writing—original draft, J.H.; writing—review and editing, G.Y. and S.T. All authors have read and agreed to the published version of the manuscript.

Funding: This research was funded by JSPS KAKENHI, grant numbers 16K15368, 18KK0261, 19J14291, and 20H00556.

Conflicts of Interest: The authors declare no conflict of interest.

References

1. Tokonami, S.; Takahashi, H.; Kobayashi, Y.; Zhuo, W.; Hulber, E. Up-to-date radon-thoron discriminative detector for a large scale survey. *Rev. Sci. Instrum.* **2005**, *76*, 113505. [CrossRef]
2. Eappen, K.; Mayya, Y. Calibration factors for LR-115 (type-II) based radon thoron discriminating dosimeter. *Radiat. Meas.* **2004**, *38*, 5–17. [CrossRef]
3. Sciocchetti, G.; Sciocchetti, A.; Giovannoli, P.; DeFelice, P.; Cardellini, F.; Cotellessa, G.; Pagliari, M. A new passive radon-thoron discriminative measurement system. *Radiat. Prot. Dosim.* **2010**, *141*, 462–467. [CrossRef] [PubMed]
4. Sahoo, B.; Sapra, B.; Kanse, S.; Gaware, J.; Mayya, Y. A new pin-hole discriminated 222Rn/220Rn passive measurement device with single entry face. *Radiat. Meas.* **2013**, *58*, 52–60. [CrossRef]
5. Guo, Q.; Iida, T.; Okamoto, K.; Yamasaki, T. Measurements of thoron concentration by passive cup method and its application to dose assessment. *J. Nucl. Sci. Technol.* **1995**, *32*, 794–803. [CrossRef]
6. Hu, J.; Yang, G.; Hegedűs, M.; Iwaoka, K.; Hosoda, M.; Tokonami, S. Numerical modeling of the sources and behaviors of 222 Rn, 220 Rn and their progenies in the indoor environment—A review. *J. Environ. Radioact.* **2018**, *189*, 40–47. [CrossRef]
7. Zhuo, W.; Iida, T. Estimation of thoron progeny concentrations in dwellings with their deposition rate measurements. *Jpn. J. Health Phys.* **2000**, *35*, 365–370. [CrossRef]
8. Tokonami, S.; Sun, Q.; Yonehara, H.; Yamada, Y. A Simple Measurement Technique of the Equilibrium Equivalent Thoron Concentration with a CR-39 Detector. *Jpn. J. Health Phys.* **2002**, *37*, 59–63. [CrossRef]
9. Zhuo, W.; Tokonami, S. Convenient methods for evaluation of indoor thoron progeny concentrations. *Int. Congr. Ser.* **2005**, *1276*, 219–220. [CrossRef]
10. Tokonami, S. Why is ^{220}Rn (thoron) measurement important? *Radiat. Prot. Dosim.* **2010**, *141*, 335–339. [CrossRef]
11. Sorimachi, A.; Tokonami, S.; Kranrod, C.; Ishikawa, T. Preliminary Experiments Using a Passive Detector for Measuring Indoor 220Rn Progeny Concentrations with an Aerosol Chamber. *Health Phys.* **2015**, *108*, 597–606. [CrossRef] [PubMed]

12. Hu, J.; Hosoda, M.; Tokonami, S. Parameter sensitivity analysis of the theoretical model of a CR-39-based direct ^{222}Rn/^{220}Rn progeny monitor. *Nukleonika* **2020**, *65*, 95–98. [CrossRef]
13. Mishra, R.; Mayya, Y.S. Study of a deposition-based direct thoron progeny sensor (DTPS) technique for estimating equilibrium equivalent thoron concentration (EETC) in indoor environment. *Radiat. Meas.* **2008**, *43*, 1408–1416. [CrossRef]
14. L'Annunziata, M.F. *Handbook of Radioactivity Analysis: Radiation Physics and Detectors*, 4th ed.; Academic Press: Cambridge, MA, USA, 2020; pp. 318–332.
15. Mishra, R.; Mayya, Y.; Kushwaha, H. Measurement of 220Rn/222Rn progeny deposition velocities on surfaces and their comparison with theoretical models. *J. Aerosol Sci.* **2009**, *40*, 1–15. [CrossRef]
16. Jacobi, W. Activity and potential α-energy of ^{222}Rn and ^{220}Rn-daughters in different air atmospheres. *Health Phys.* **1972**, *22*, 441–450. [CrossRef] [PubMed]
17. Lai, A.C.K.; Nazaroff, W.W. Modeling indoor particle deposition from turbulent flow onto smooth surfaces. *J. Aerosol Sci.* **2000**, *31*, 463–476. [CrossRef]
18. Corner, J.; Pendlebury, E.D. The coagulation and deposition of a stirred aerosol. *Proc. Phys. Soc. B* **1951**, *64*, 645–654. [CrossRef]
19. Porstendörfer, J. Behaviour of radon daughter products in indoor air. *Radiat. Prot. Dosim.* **1984**, *7*, 107–113. [CrossRef]
20. Porstendörfer, J.; Röbig, G.; Ahmed, A. Experimental determination of the attachment coefficients of atoms and ions on monodisperse. *J. Aerosol Sci.* **1979**, *10*, 21–28. [CrossRef]
21. Porstendörfer, J. Radon: Measurements related to dose. *Environ. Int.* **1996**, *22*, 563–583. [CrossRef]
22. Stevanovic, N.; Markovic, V.M.; Nikezic, D. Relationship between deposition and attachment rates in Jacobi room model. *J. Environ. Radioact.* **2010**, *101*, 349–352. [CrossRef] [PubMed]
23. Tokonami, S.; Ichiji, T.; Iimoto, T.; Kurosawa, R. Calculation procedure of potential alpha energy concentration with continuous air sampling. *Health Phys.* **1996**, *71*, 937–943. [CrossRef] [PubMed]
24. Tamakuma, Y.; Yamada, R.; Iwaoka, K.; Hosoda, M.; Kuroki, T.; Mizuno, H.; Yamada, K.; Furukawa, M.; Tokonami, S. A portable radioactive plume monitor using a silicon photodiode. *Perspect. Sci.* **2019**, *12*, 100414. [CrossRef]
25. Shimada, M.; Okuyama, K.; Kousaka, Y.; Seinfeld, J.H. A model calculation of particle deposition onto a rough wall by Brownian and turbulent diffusion. *J. Colloid Interface Sci.* **1988**, *125*, 198–211. [CrossRef]
26. Hu, J.; Sun, L.; Li, C.H.; Wang, X.; Jia, X.L.; Cai, Y.P. Water quality risk assessment for the Laoguanhe River of China using a stochastic simulation method. *J. Environ. Inform.* **2018**, *31*, 123–136. [CrossRef]
27. Bigu, J. Radon daughter and thoron daughter deposition velocity and unattached fraction under laboratory-controlled conditions and in underground uranium mines. *J. Aerosol Sci.* **1985**, *16*, 157–165. [CrossRef]

Publisher's Note: MDPI stays neutral with regard to jurisdictional claims in published maps and institutional affiliations.

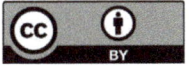

© 2020 by the authors. Licensee MDPI, Basel, Switzerland. This article is an open access article distributed under the terms and conditions of the Creative Commons Attribution (CC BY) license (http://creativecommons.org/licenses/by/4.0/).

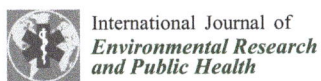

International Journal of
Environmental Research and Public Health

Article

Total Diet Study to Assess Radioactive Cs and ^{40}K Levels in the Japanese Population before and after the Fukushima Daiichi Nuclear Power Plant Accident

Hiroshi Terada [1,*], Ikuyo Iijima [2], Sadaaki Miyake [3], Kimio Isomura [4] and Hideo Sugiyama [1]

1. Department of Environmental Health, National Institute of Public Health, Saitama 351-0197, Japan; sugiyama.h.aa@niph.go.jp
2. Chemistry Division, Kanagawa Prefectural Institute of Public Health (Retired), Kanagawa 253-0087, Japan; ikijima@icloud.com
3. Biological Effect Research Group, Saitama Prefectural Institute of Public Health, Saitama 355-0133, Japan; miyake.sadaaki@pref.saitama.lg.jp
4. Hyogo Prefectural Institute of Public Health and Environmental Sciences (Retired), Kobe 652-0032, Japan; zaihuriboku@gmail.com
* Correspondence: terada.h.aa@niph.go.jp; Tel.: +81-48-458-6263

Received: 10 October 2020; Accepted: 31 October 2020; Published: 3 November 2020

Abstract: We conducted a total diet study (TDS) of ^{137}Cs, ^{134}Cs, and ^{40}K to assess their average dietary exposure levels in a Japanese adult population before and after the Fukushima Daiichi nuclear power plant (FDNPP) accident. Nineteen market baskets were evaluated in 2006–2011. In each basket, a TDS sample comprising tap water and 160–170 food items, which were combined into 13 groups, were collected for analysis by gamma-ray spectrometry. From 2006 to 2010, the ^{137}Cs activity concentration in the "fish and shellfish" group was 0.099 Bq/kg, representing the highest value obtained, whereas the total committed effective dose (CED) of radiocesium isotopes (^{137}Cs + ^{134}Cs) was 0.69 µSv. In 2011, "milk and dairy products" from Sendai City had a Cs activity concentration of 12 Bq/kg, representing the highest values among all food groups studied. However, the annual CED of radioactive Cs in Fukushima City was 17 µSv after the FDNPP accident, which is 60-fold lower than the maximum permissible dose of 1 mSv/year. The mean CED obtained for ^{40}K was 180 µSv, which is comparable to the global average. Our results reveal the average dietary exposure of ^{137}Cs, ^{134}Cs, and ^{40}K, which can aid in estimating the radiological safety of foods.

Keywords: total diet study; radioactive cesium; potassium-40; dietary intake; dose assessment; Fukushima accident

1. Introduction

To ensure food safety, it is essential to assess the exposure levels to toxic substances in food. Currently, there are three approaches for estimating the dietary intake of such substances: total diet study (TDS), duplicate portion study (DPS), and selective study of individual foodstuffs. A TDS, also referred to as a market basket study, has an advantage over the two alternatives in terms of its accuracy. Furthermore, TDS takes into account the effect of kitchen preparation on the levels of toxic substances in food, and provides information on which food groups are the main sources of contamination [1]. Therefore, TDSs have been supported and endorsed by the Food and Agriculture Organization of the United Nations (FAO) and the World Health Organization (WHO) since the 1970s. According to a survey carried out in 2015 by Health Canada, in cooperation with the WHO, approximately 53 countries around the world perform TDS analyses [2].

The first TDS was conducted in response to public concerns about a radioactive fallout from atmospheric nuclear testing [3,4]. Fallouts contain hundreds of different radionuclides. Among these,

^{137}Cs and ^{90}Sr are the most significant sources of internal exposure to radiation, owing to their long half-lives of 30.17 years and 28.8 years, respectively, as well as to their chemical similarities to essential elements (^{137}Cs resembles potassium and ^{90}Sr resembles calcium). Therefore, the U.S. Food and Drug Administration (FDA) has been carrying out TDSs focusing on these two radionuclides since 1961 [5].

In Japan, TDSs have been performed annually by the Ministry of Health, Labour and Welfare (MHLW) since 1977 [6,7]. Initially, pesticides and their metabolites, seven metals (Pb, Cd, total Hg, total As, Cu, Mn, and Zn), and total polychlorinated biphenyl (PCB) were analyzed in these studies [6,8]. Similarly, radioactivity monitoring has been conducted by the Nuclear Regulation Authority (NRA) since the 1950s. Radionuclide levels in airborne dust, rainwater, river water, seawater, soil, and food have been analyzed in this monitoring [9]. Until 2008, the NRA also conducted DPSs to evaluate the daily dietary intake of radionuclides [10–12]. Subsequently, TDSs of radionuclides began in 2003 by the MHLW to assess total exposure levels of radionuclides in the average Japanese diet, as well as the contribution of each food group to this total. Between 2003 and 2011, we carried out a TDS, which was supported by a Health and Labour Sciences Research Grant (HLSRG) from the MHLW [13–19]. From 2003 to 2005, the dietary exposure to man-made radionuclides (^{137}Cs, ^{134}Cs, and ^{90}Sr) and natural radionuclides (^{40}K, ^{214}Pb, ^{214}Bi, ^{228}Ac, ^{212}Pb, ^{208}Tl, and U) were determined. Sugiyama et al. [13] revealed that only trace amounts of ^{137}Cs were found in TDS samples, and that "fish and shellfish" contained 0.145 Bq/kg, representing the highest activity concentration measured. They also found that the daily dietary intake and the committed effective dose (CED) of ^{137}Cs were, at the very most, 0.080 Bq/person/day and 0.38 µSv, respectively, with the main sources of the exposure being from the "fish and shellfish", "meat and eggs", and "other vegetables, mushrooms and seaweeds" food groups.

The present study aimed to assess trends in dietary exposure levels to γ-emitting radionuclides, namely ^{137}Cs, ^{134}Cs, and ^{40}K, from typical Japanese diets via TDS. The concentrations, dietary intake, and CEDs of these radionuclides from 2006 to 2011 have been presented. The results from before and after the Fukushima Daiichi nuclear power plant (FDNPP) accident that occurred in March 2011 have been compared. We also attempted to summarize the results of the TDS performed between 2012 and 2019 by other institutions in Japan, because almost 10 years have passed since the FDNPP accident.

2. Materials and Methods

2.1. Sampling and Preparation

Each year, TDS samples have been collected from three or four cities in different regional blocks of Japan, except for the year 2010. Each sample collection is referred to as a market basket (MB). We collected as many locally produced food items as possible. The most preferred production areas in descending order were same prefecture, same regional block, and other regional blocks in Japan. As shown in Figure 1, 19 MBs were collected from all regional blocks of Japan, other than Minami-Kyushu, from 2006 to 2011. In each MB, 160 to 170 food items were purchased from local retailers. These items were classified into 13 food groups as follows: rice and rice products (Group I); cereals, seeds, nuts, and potatoes (Group II); sugars and confectionaries (Group III); fats and oils (Group IV); pulses and their products (Group V); fruits (Group VI); green and yellow vegetables (Group VII); other vegetables, mushrooms, and seaweeds (Group VIII); beverages (Group IX); fish and shellfish (Group X); meat and eggs (Group XI); milk and dairy products (Group XII); and seasonings (Group XIII). The relative proportion of each food item within a group was based on average regional food consumption data for individuals 20 years and over, which were obtained from the National Health and Nutrition Survey (NHNS) performed by the MHLW between 2002 and 2004. Individual food items were cooked, if necessary, and then combined for analysis into 13 food groups. In addition, tap water was collected in each MB for drinking water (Group XIV). Thus, in total 19 × 14 = 266 TDS samples were obtained. The sample weights of individual food groups were approximately 5 kg, with the exception of 12 kg for "rice and rice products" and 100 kg for "drinking water".

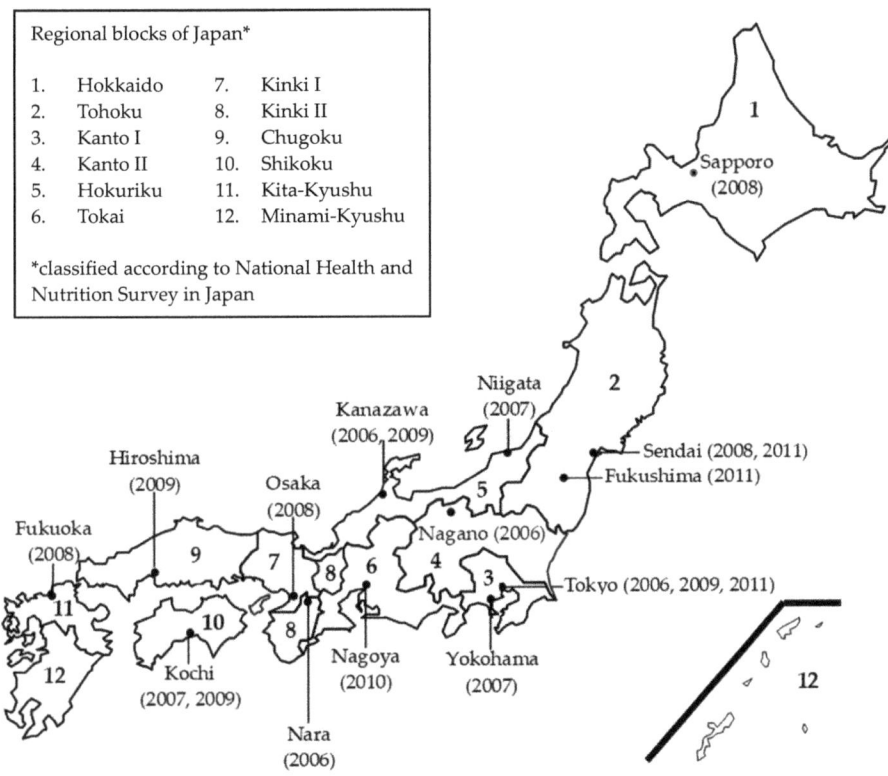

Figure 1. Sampling sites of included in the total diet study conducted from 2006 to 2011. Sampling year of each site is denoted in parenthesis.

TDS samples, other than "fats and oils" and "drinking water", were freeze-dried or heat-dried and then incinerated at 450 °C for 24 h into ash. The ash samples were placed in separate plastic containers with a capacity of 100 mL. The "drinking water" samples were condensed by heating and evaporated to dryness, and the residues were stored in the plastic containers, as described above. The "fats and oil" samples were stored in 1 L Marinelli beakers in their raw state.

2.2. Determination of ^{137}Cs, ^{134}Cs, and ^{40}K

Cs-137, Cs-134, and K-40 in the TDS samples were detected for a minimum of 80,000 s using high-purity Ge semiconductor detectors (2519 and GC2018 of CANBERRA Co., Meriden, CT, USA; EGPC 20-190-R of EURYSIS Co., Lingolsheim, Cedex-France; CNVD30-35195 of OXFORD Co., Oxon, Oxford, UK; and IGC40200 and IGC25190SD of PGT Co., Princeton, NJ, USA). Activity concentrations of the three radionuclides were corrected as of the end of the sampling period and expressed in Bq/kg of fresh weight. Energy and efficiency calibrations were performed using γ-ray volume sources (MX033U8PP and MX033MR, Japan Radioisotope Association, Tokyo, Japan). The limits of detection (LODs) for ^{137}Cs and ^{134}Cs were approximately 0.05 Bq/kg for all food groups, except for "fats and oils" and "seasonings".

2.3. Calculation of Dietary Intake and the Committed Effective Dose (CED) Values

The daily dietary intake of radioactive Cs and ^{40}K for adults was calculated from the activity concentrations of the three radionuclides in the samples, as described above. The radionuclide activity concentration was multiplied by the average food consumption value for the adult population, as determined by the NHNS, in each regional block to provide the radionuclide intake for each radionuclide and food group. Next, the calculated intake for each food group was summed to estimate the total dietary intake of a given radionuclide in each MB. The dietary intake of radioactive Cs was obtained by summation of ^{137}Cs and ^{134}Cs intake values. If a target radionuclide was not detected in a sample, the activity concentration of the non-detected (ND) radionuclide was assumed to be zero or the LOD value. The lower and upper limits of the total radionuclide intake values were estimated by assuming the ND value as zero and the LOD, respectively.

The CED values associated with Cs and ^{40}K for adults were estimated under the assumption of a one-year intake of the TDS samples, and were obtained by applying the dietary radionuclide intake values and dose coefficients for ingestion of each radionuclide, given by the International Commission on Radiological Protection (ICRP), to be 1.3×10^{-8} Sv/Bq for ^{137}Cs, 1.9×10^{-8} Sv/Bq for ^{134}Cs, and 4.6×10^{-9} Sv/Bq for ^{40}K [20]. The CED of radioactive Cs was calculated by summing those of ^{137}Cs and ^{134}Cs. The ND radionuclides were given a value of zero and the LOD for estimating the lower and upper limits of the CED values, respectively.

3. Results and Discussion

3.1. Levels of ^{137}Cs, ^{134}Cs, and ^{40}K

3.1.1. ^{137}Cs Levels before the FDNPP Accident

We collected 16 MBs from 13 cities between 2006 and 2010, resulting in a total of 224 TDS samples. Cesium-137 was the only anthropogenic radionuclide observed in these samples, as ^{134}Cs, which was released from the Chernobyl disaster, was not detected at all. Table 1 summarizes the ^{137}Cs activity concentrations in TDS samples from 2006 to 2010. The activity concentrations of ^{137}Cs in TDS samples were all below 0.1 Bq/kg during this period. The food group "fish and shellfish" had a ^{137}Cs activity concentration of 0.099 Bq/kg, representing the highest value measured, followed by "other vegetables, mushrooms and seaweeds" (0.092 Bq/kg), "meat and eggs" (0.083 Bq/kg), and "milk and dairy products" (0.057 Bq/kg). The highest mean ^{137}Cs activity concentrations were found in "fish and shellfish" (0.072 Bq/kg) followed by "other vegetables, mushrooms and seaweeds" (0.024 Bq/kg), "meat and eggs" (0.024 Bq/kg), and "milk and dairy products" (0.022 Bq/kg). These results are similar to the TDS carried out between 2003 and 2005 [13]. Cesium-137 was detected in all "fish and shellfish" samples, whereas it was not found in any samples of "fats and oils", "seasonings", and "drinking water". The detection rate of ^{137}Cs was about 30%, and was the highest in "fish and shellfish" (100%), followed by "milk and dairy products" (68.8%), "meat and eggs" (62.5%), and "other vegetables, mushrooms and seaweeds" (50.0%).

3.1.2. ^{137}Cs and ^{134}Cs Levels after the FDNPP Accident

We obtained 42 TDS samples from Sendai City, Fukushima City, and Tokyo in October and November of 2011, approximately six months after the FDNPP accident. According to the United Nations Scientific Committee on the Effects of Atomic Radiation (UNSCEAR) [21], the total release of ^{137}Cs, ^{134}Cs, and ^{131}I in the atmosphere resulting from the FDNPP incident was estimated to be 8.8 PBq, 9.0 PBq, and 124 PBq, respectively. Immediately after the FDNPP accident, some foodstuffs, such as spinach and milk, were highly contaminated with ^{131}I, which accumulates in the thyroid gland and may increase the risk of thyroid cancer [22–24]. However, ^{131}I levels decreased rapidly and became undetectable [25–27], owing to its short half-life of 8.02 days. Therefore, ^{131}I was not observed in the present study.

Table 1. Activity concentrations of ^{137}Cs in Japanese total diet study samples from 2006 to 2010.

	Food Group	Activity Concentrations of ^{137}Cs (Bq/kg)									Mean ± SD [*3]	Percentage of Detection (%) [*4]
		2006 (n = 4)		2007 (n = 3)		2008 (n = 4)		2009 (n = 4)		2010 (n = 1)		
		Min. [*1]	Max. [*2]	Min. [*1]	Max. [*2]	Min. [*1]	Max. [*2]	Min. [*1]	Max. [*2]			
I	Rice and rice products	<0.003	0.004	<0.005	0.0045	<0.004	0.0061	<0.008	0.013	0.020	0.0036 ± 0.0059	37.5
II	Cereals, nuts, and potatoes	<0.010	<0.025	<0.015	0.016	<0.014	0.034	<0.009	0.033	<0.010	0.0058 ± 0.012	25.0
III	Sugars and confectionaries	<0.018	0.035	<0.012	<0.052	<0.015	0.019	<0.022	<0.038	<0.150	0.0049 ± 0.011	18.8
IV	Fats and oils	<0.032	<0.056	<0.024	<0.049	<0.014	<0.065	<0.022	<0.078	<0.220	0	0
V	Pulses and their products	<0.040	<0.058	<0.024	0.016	<0.024	0.019	<0.014	0.032	<0.076	0.0042 ± 0.010	18.8
VI	Fruits	<0.010	<0.024	<0.010	0.027	<0.011	<0.037	<0.010	0.038	<0.026	0.0041 ± 0.011	12.5
VII	Green and yellow vegetables	<0.022	0.015	<0.016	0.018	<0.009	<0.039	<0.024	<0.029	<0.024	0.0021 ± 0.0057	12.5
VIII	Other vegetables, mushrooms, and seaweeds	<0.016	0.092	<0.029	0.069	<0.015	0.031	<0.022	0.024	<0.018	0.024 ± 0.031	50
IX [*5]	Beverages	<0.018	<0.024	<0.004	<0.015	<0.007	0.0073	<0.004	0.0049	<0.006	0.00077 ± 0.00210	12.5
X	Fish and shellfish	0.067	0.099	0.078	0.093	0.029	0.071	0.062	0.093	0.048	0.0720 ± 0.0205	100.0
XI	Meat and eggs	<0.023	0.041	<0.018	0.032	<0.020	0.083	<0.025	0.054	0.028	0.024 ± 0.024	62.5
XII	Milk and dairy products	<0.021	0.057	<0.025	0.018	<0.027	0.033	<0.042	0.051	0.035	0.022 ± 0.012	68.8
XIII [*6]	Seasonings	<0.012	<0.140	<0.075	<0.155	<0.054	<0.14	<0.028	<0.087	<0.089	0	0
XIV	Drinking water	<0.0002	<0.0004	<0.0001	<0.0004	<0.0001	<0.0005	<0.0001	<0.0003	<0.0002	0	0

n = number of the market basket(s) performed in each year. [*1] Minimum ^{137}Cs activity concentration in each year. [*2] Maximum ^{137}Cs activity concentration in each year. [*3] Mean and standard deviation values of ^{137}Cs activity concentrations, which were calculated under the assumption that the concentrations of the non-detected were zero. [*4] Detection rate of ^{137}Cs for each food group. [*5] This food group was categorized as "Seasonings and beverages" in 2006. [*6] This food group was categorized as "Others" in 2006.

Cesium-134 was not detected in any of the TDS samples between 2006 and 2010, but was observed in all food groups, with the exception of "fats and oils", in 2011 as a consequence of the FDNPP accident. Table 2 shows the ^{137}Cs and ^{134}Cs activity concentration of the TDS samples after the FDNPP accident. The detection rates of ^{137}Cs and ^{134}Cs were 88% and 69%, respectively. No sample exceeded the ^{137}Cs level of 0.1 Bq/kg during 2006 to 2010, whereas 19 samples exceeded this level in 2011. The activity concentrations of ^{137}Cs (Bq/kg) were in the range of <0.041–6.400 in Sendai City, <0.089–4.100 in Fukushima City, and <0.045–2.100 in Tokyo; while those of ^{134}Cs (Bq/kg) were <0.011–5.400 in Sendai City, <0.040–3.500 in Fukushima City, and <0.025–1.700 in Tokyo. The activity concentration ratios of ^{134}Cs to ^{137}Cs in the TDS samples were ranged from 0.38 to 0.94, and the mean and standard deviation values were calculated to be 0.73 and 0.14, respectively.

The highest activity concentration of radioactive Cs (^{137}Cs + ^{134}Cs) among the 42 TDS samples was 12 Bq/kg, and found in the "milk and dairy products" group from Sendai City. This food group also showed the highest Cs activity concentration in Tokyo (3.8 Bq/kg), while fruits carried the highest activity concentration in Fukushima City (7.6 Bq/kg). Cs activity concentrations in the fruits of Fukushima City were characteristically higher than those in Sendai City (0.093 Bq/kg) and Tokyo (0.17 Bq/kg). Although "green and yellow vegetables", such as spinach, showed extremely high Cs activity concentrations, with values exceeding 10,000 Bq/kg immediately following the FDNPP accident, their levels declined rapidly [26–28]. Thus, Cs activity concentrations in "green and yellow vegetables" were at most 0.58 Bq/kg in our TDS samples. The "meat and eggs" group was found to have higher Cs activity concentration before the FDNPP accident, while the relatively low activity concentration after the accident is due to the import of animal feed from foreign countries. Interestingly, ^{137}Cs and ^{134}Cs were not found in any "fats and oil" samples before or after the accident. This may be due to their poor solubility in lipids.

After the FDNPP accident, regulation of the levels of radionuclides in food was established by the MHLW. On 17 March 2011, the provisional regulation value (RPV) for radioactive Cs was established to be 200 Bq/kg for "drinking water" and "milk and dairy products", and 500 Bq/kg for vegetables, grain, meat, eggs, and fish [28,29]. Presently, the standard limits, which were put into place on 1 April 2012, are 100 Bq/kg for general foods, 50 Bq/kg for milk and infant foods, and 10 Bq/kg for drinking water [30,31]. In the present study, although Cs activity concentrations of the TDS samples increased significantly after the FDNPP accident, the concentrations were well below the regulatory levels. The highest radioactive Cs value of 12 Bq/kg in this TDS was 17 times lower than the RPV for "milk and dairy products", and four times lower than the standard limit for milk.

3.1.3. ^{40}K Levels

Potassium is an essential element in food products and humans. Potassium-40, whose natural abundance is 0.0117%, is the only naturally occurring radionuclide of potassium, and has a very long half-life of 1.248 billion years. Accordingly, ^{40}K in foods contributes considerably to internal exposure in the general public. The activity concentration values of ^{40}K in the TDS samples are listed in Table 3. In contrast to ^{137}Cs and ^{134}Cs, ^{40}K was detected in all food groups, and the levels were in the range of 10–100 Bq/kg in most of the TDS samples analyzed. The mean ^{40}K level values between 2006 and 2011 measured for individual food groups were the highest in "green and yellow vegetables", at 90 Bq/kg, followed by "pulses and their products" (84 Bq/kg), and "fish and shellfish" (83 Bq/kg). In contrast, mean ^{40}K values were relatively low in "fats and oils", "drinking water", "rice and rice products", and "beverages". The ^{40}K activity concentration was not significantly different before and after the FDNPP accident.

Table 2. Activity concentrations of ^{137}Cs and ^{134}Cs in Japanese total diet study samples in 2011.

	Food Group	Activity Concentrations of ^{137}Cs (Bq/kg)			Activity Concentrations of ^{134}Cs (Bq/kg)			Activity Concentrations of ^{137}Cs + ^{134}Cs (Bq/kg)		
		Sendai	Fukushima	Tokyo	Sendai	Fukushima	Tokyo	Sendai	Fukushima	Tokyo
I	Rice and rice products	0.270	1.500	0.079	0.210	1.200	0.057	0.480	2.600	0.140
II	Cereals, nuts, and potatoes	0.170	0.340	0.058	0.140	0.320	0.035	0.310	0.660	0.093
III	Sugars and confectionaries	0.120	0.180	0.053	0.054	0.130	<0.025	0.170	0.320	0.053
IV	Fats and oils	<0.087	<0.089	<0.045	<0.072	<0.100	<0.048	<0.160	<0.190	<0.093
V	Pulses and their products	<0.041	0.041	0.130	<0.025	<0.040	0.098	<0.066	0.041	0.230
VI	Fruits	0.0570	4.100	0.093	<0.036	3.500	0.074	<0.093	7.600	0.170
VII	Green and yellow vegetables	0.200	0.310	0.059	0.160	0.270	0.025	0.360	0.580	0.084
VIII	Other vegetables, mushrooms, and seaweeds	0.150	0.710	0.044	0.084	0.580	<0.028	0.230	1.300	0.044
IX [*1]	Beverages	0.017	0.015	0.018	<0.011	0.011	0.012	<0.028	0.026	0.030
X	Fish and shellfish	2.200	0.300	0.300	1.800	0.210	0.210	4.000	0.510	0.510
XI	Meat and eggs	0.074	0.063	0.056	0.047	<0.040	0.021	0.120	0.063	0.077
XII	Milk and dairy products	6.400	2.000	2.100	5.400	1.600	1.70	12.000	3.500	3.800
XIII [*2]	Seasonings	<0.230	0.052	0.140	<0.160	<0.088	<0.110	<0.390	0.052	0.140
XIV	Drinking water	0.0087	0.017	0.0048	0.0071	0.015	0.0038	0.016	0.032	0.0086

[*1] This food group was categorized as "Seasonings and beverages" in 2006. [*2] This food group was categorized as "Others" in 2006.

Table 3. Activity concentrations of ^{40}K in Japanese total diet study samples from 2006 to 2011.

	Food Group	Activity Concentrations of ^{40}K (Bq/kg) [1]									Mean ± SD [4] (Bq/kg)	Activity Concentrations of ^{40}K (Bq/kg) in 2011 [5]		
		2006 (n = 4)		2007 (n = 3)		2008 (n = 4)		2009 (n = 4)		2010 (n = 1)		Fukushima	Sendai	Tokyo
		Min. [2]	Max. [3]	Min. [2]	Max. [2]	Min. [2]	Max. [3]	Min. [2]	Max. [3]					
I	Rice and rice products	5.1	7.1	5.7	9.7	7.1	7.9	5.7	11.0	3.5	7.1 ± 1.7	31.0	8.3	5.4
II	Cereals, nuts, and potatoes	42.0	53.0	44.0	63.0	48.0	55.0	50.0	57.0	48.0	51.0 ± 5.1	52.0	62.0	54.0
III	Sugars and confectionaries	23.0	44.0	54.0	64.0	65.0	71.0	51.0	64.0	67.0	56.0 ± 14	65.0	67.0	49.0
IV	Fats and oils	<1.2	4.3	<0.81	0.9	<0.90	1.6	<0.22	1.2	<2.7	1.0 ± 1.3 [6]	<1.2	<1.2	<1.1
V	Pulses and their products	94.0	104.0	70.0	103.0	72.0	98.0	68.0	96.0	59.0	85.0 ± 15	78.0	80.0	76.0
VI	Fruits	41.0	54.0	46.0	57.0	48.0	55.0	44.0	61.0	61.0	52.0 ± 5.8	50.0	51.0	48.0
VII	Green and yellow vegetables	76.0	99.0	63.0	106.0	85.0	104.0	78.0	99.0	95.0	89.0 ± 11	95.0	79.0	103.0
VIII	Other vegetables, mushrooms, and seaweeds	47.0	106.0	93.0	136.0	47.0	105.0	39.0	103.0	55.0	81.0 ± 29	48.0	58.0	59.0
IX [7]	Beverages	23.0	28.0	7.9	9.0	7.4	11.0	3.2	9.3	8.1	12.0 ± 8.2	8.6	7.8	6.3
X	Fish and shellfish	74.0	95.0	81.0	88.0	70.0	87.0	75.0	99.0	77.0	82.0 ± 7.9	96.0	79.0	96.0
XI	Meat and eggs	64.0	89.0	68.0	85.0	61.0	80.0	60.0	82.0	77.0	73.0 ± 9.8	73.0	74.0	47.0
XII	Milk and dairy products	45.0	51.0	41.0	50.0	37.0	43.0	44.0	105.0	43.0	49.0 ± 15	48.0	46.0	51.0
XIII [8]	Seasonings	11.0	74.0	66.0	88.0	64.0	71.0	28.0	69.0	79.0	64.0 ± 19	76.0	82.0	81.0
XIV	Drinking water	0.019	0.061	0.015	0.05	0.017	0.087	0.021	0.040	0.039	0.041 ± 0.020	0.012	0.018	0.053

n = number of the market basket(s) performed in each year. [1] Before the Fukushima Daiichi nuclear power plant accident. [2] Minimum ^{40}K activity concentration in each year. [3] Maximum ^{40}K activity concentration in each year. [4] Mean and standard deviation values of ^{40}K activity concentration before the Fukushima Daiichi nuclear power plant accident. [5] After the Fukushima Daiichi nuclear power plant accident. [6] Calculated under the assumption that the ^{40}K activity concentrations of the non-detected were zero. [7] This food group was categorized as "Seasonings and beverages" in 2006. [8] This food group was categorized as "Others" in 2006.

3.2. Dietary Intake and CED Values of Radioactive Cs

3.2.1. Before the FDNPP Accident

Table 4 presents the total daily dietary intake values and CEDs of radioactive Cs and ^{40}K for adults in each MB. Between 2006 and 2010, the lower and upper limits of radioactive Cs intake varied from 0.0047 to 0.0320 Bq/person/day and from 0.060 to 0.122 Bq/person/day, respectively. The mean values obtained for the lower and upper limits during the same period were 0.020 Bq/person/day (SD = 0.0082) and 0.085 Bq/person/day (SD = 0.019), respectively. Similar results were obtained in a previous study [13]. The lower and upper limits in each MB were significantly different because of the low detection rates of ^{137}Cs and ^{134}Cs before the FDNPP accident (30% and 0%, respectively).

Table 4. Total daily dietary intake values and committed effective doses of radioactive Cs (^{137}Cs + ^{134}Cs) for adults in Japan, estimated via total diet studies from 2006 to 2011.

	Year	Region	City	Daily Intake (Bq/Person·Day)		Committed Effective Dose (μSv)	
				Lower Limit *1	Upper Limit *2	Lower Limit *1	Upper Limit *2
Before the FDNPP *3 accident	2006	Kanto I	Tokyo	0.0320	0.079	0.150	0.40
		Kanto II	Nagano	0.0270	0.081	0.150	0.40
		Hokuriku	Kanazawa	0.0190	0.061	0.130	0.45
		Kinki II	Nara	0.0210	0.065	0.089	0.34
	2007	Kanto I	Yokohama	0.0280	0.120	0.099	0.37
		Hokuriku	Niigata	0.0160	0.064	0.130	0.69
		Shikoku	Kochi	0.0100	0.100	0.074	0.37
	2008	Hokkaido	Sapporo	0.0220	0.087	0.049	0.58
		Tohoku	Sendai	0.0047	0.097	0.100	0.58
		Kinki I	Osaka	0.0310	0.060	0.022	0.55
		Kita-Kyushu	Fukuoka	0.0079	0.086	0.140	0.33
	2009	Kanto I	Tokyo	0.0290	0.071	0.037	0.51
		Hokuriku	Kanazawa	0.0230	0.100	0.140	0.40
		Chugoku	Hiroshima	0.0140	0.098	0.110	0.63
		Shikoku	Kochi	0.0160	0.072	0.064	0.55
	2010	Tokai	Nagoya	0.0220	0.120	0.077	0.41
	Mean ± SD *4			0.0200 ± 0.0083	0.085 ± 0.019	0.098 ± 0.041	0.47 ± 0.11
After the FDNPP *3 accident	2011	Tohoku	Sendai	2.20	2.20	12.0	13.0
		Tohoku	Fukushima	2.90	2.90	17.0	17.0
		Kanto I	Tokyo	0.67	0.69	3.8	3.9

*1 Assuming that the activity concentrations of the non-detected radionuclides were zero. *2 Assuming that the activity concentrations of non-detected radionuclides were equal to the limits of detection. *3 FDNPP: Fukushima Daiichi nuclear power plant. *4 Mean and standard deviation values before the Fukushima Daiichi nuclear power plant accident.

As previously described, the NRA conducted DPS studies of radionuclides until 2008, and compiled the results from 47 prefectures in Japan into a database [32]. According to the database, the daily intake of ^{137}Cs for adults between 2003 and 2008 ranged from below the detection limit to 0.56 Bq/person/day, and the mean was calculated to be 0.018 Bq/person/day (SD = 0.031), assuming that the activity concentration value of ND radionuclides was zero. Although a larger variation was observed, this finding is similar to the mean lower limit of radioactive Cs intake obtained in the present study.

The lower and upper limits of the CEDs of radioactive Cs were in the range of 0.022–0.150 μSv and 0.33–0.69 μSv, with mean values of 0.098 μSv (SD = 0.041) and 0.47 μSv (SD = 0.11), respectively. The current standard limits for radionuclides in food in Japan were established on the basis of an annual CED of 1 mSv, representing the maximum permissible dose due to food consumption [27,31].

Although the upper limit of the CEDs obtained were overestimated, due to the low detection rate of ^{137}Cs and ^{134}Cs, the highest CED of 0.69 µSv is approximately 1400 times lower than the maximum permissible dose, and thus would seem to pose no health risk.

3.2.2. After the FDNPP Accident

Since ^{137}Cs and ^{134}Cs were detected in most of the food groups after the FDNPP accident, the lower and upper limits of radioactive Cs intakes were calculated using actual activity concentrations of these radionuclides, rather than zero or LODs. Thus, the lower and upper limits were almost the same in each MB after the FDNPP accident, while they were significantly different before the accident. The lower limits of total radioactive Cs intake were estimated to be 2.9 Bq/person/day in Fukushima City, 2.2 Bq/person/day in Sendai City, and 0.67 Bq/person/day in Tokyo, after the FDNPP accident (Table 4).

The lower limits of the total CED of radioactive Cs in 2011 were 12 µSv in Sendai City, 17 µSv in Fukushima City, and 3.8 µSv in Tokyo. The high value obtained for Fukushima City is expected, as it is located the closest to the FDNPP incident. Figure 2 displays the lower limits of CED values of radioactive Cs from 2003 to 2011, and shows that values obtained after the FDNPP accident were about two orders of magnitude higher than before the accident. Nevertheless, the highest CED of radioactive Cs (17 µSv), which was the exposure level in half a year after the FDNPP accident, is approximately 60 times lower than the maximum permissible dose.

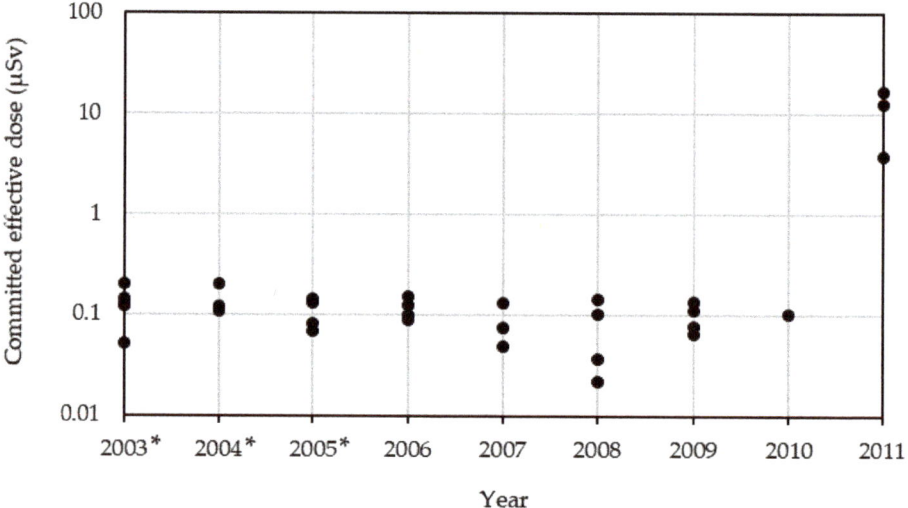

Figure 2. Committed effective doses of radioactive Cs (^{137}Cs + ^{134}Cs) obtained from each market basket (2003–2011). The closed circles show the results of each market basket. The doses were estimated with the assumptions of one-year intake values of the total diet samples, and the activity concentration values of non-detected radionuclides to be zero.

Figure 3 summarizes the CED values of radioactive Cs, organized by food group, in 2011. The three food groups with the highest contributions to the CEDs were "milk and dairy products" (66%), "fish and shellfish" (17%), and "rice and rice products" (8.2%) in Sendai City; "rice and rice products" (33%), fruits (32%), and "milk and dairy products" (15%) in Fukushima City; and "milk and dairy products" (69%), "rice and rice products" (7.6%), and "fish and shellfish" (7.0%) in Tokyo.

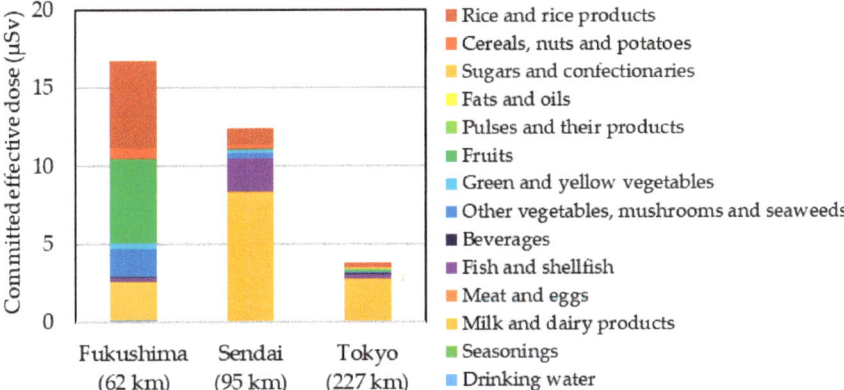

Figure 3. Committed effective doses of radioactive cesium (^{137}Cs + ^{134}Cs) by food groups in 2011. Distance from the Fukushima Daiichi nuclear power plant to each city is denoted in parentheses. This figure was modified from [19].

In 2011, TDSs of radioactive Cs and ^{40}K were also carried out by Tsutsumi et al. [33] and Miyazaki et al. [34]. Tsutsumi et al. analyzed MBs from Sendai City, Fukushima City, and Tokyo in September and November 2011, and revealed that the lower limits of total CED values of radioactive Cs were 17 µSv in Sendai City, 19 µSv in Fukushima City, and 2.1 µSv in Tokyo. They also found that "fish and shellfish", "fruits", "green and yellow vegetables", and "milk and dairy products" were the main contributors to the CED values obtained. Although the contributing food groups varied to some extent, their findings are similar to the total CED values of radioactive Cs obtained in the present study. Miyazaki et al. collected an MB from Nagoya City in August 2011, and measured CED values for radioactive Cs of 1.5 µSv, which was lower than that obtained in both our study and that of Tsutsumi et al. This might be because of the distance between the FDNPP accident site and Nagoya City, which at 446 km, is much larger than that to Sendai City (95 km), Fukushima City (62 km), or Tokyo (227 km).

After 2011, the TDSs have been performed by other institutions in Japan. The National Institute of Health Sciences have been conducting the TDS, which was targeting 15 areas, including Fukushima Prefecture, Miyagi Prefecture, and Tokyo, twice a year since 2011. Uekusa et al. [35] revealed that the maximum CEDs due to radioactive Cs decreased to 9.4 µSv (March 2012), 3.8 µSv (September 2012), and 7.1 µSv (March 2013) from 19 µSv in 2011 [33]. In the past two years, the results were as follows: 1.1 µSv (February–March 2018) [36], 1.1 µSv (September–October 2018) [37], 1.0 µSv (February–March 2019) [38], and 1.0 µSv (September–October 2019) [39]. The Tokyo Metropolitan Institute of Public Health also have been carrying out the TDS in Tokyo once a year. Their results between 2012 and 2019 showed that the CEDs due to radioactive Cs in Tokyo ranged from 0.20 µSv (2017) to 1.3 µSv (2012) [40]. All the results mentioned above indicated that the CEDs due to radioactive Cs clearly decreased from those in 2011, as expected. In 2019, the maximum CED of 1.0 µSv was 17 times lower than that from the present study, and was one-thousandth of the maximum permissible level. However, the maximum CED between 2012 and 2019 was still higher than the maximum upper limit of the CED, due to radioactive Cs before the FDNPP accident (0.69 µSv).

3.3. Dietary Intake and CED Values of ^{40}K

The minimum and maximum total dietary intake values of ^{40}K between 2006 and 2011 were 65 Bq/person/day and 94 Bq/person/day, respectively (Table 5), and the mean was calculated to be 79 Bq/person/day (SD = 7.0). Since ^{40}K was found in almost all TDS samples, the upper limit was in accordance with the lower limit in each MB. The intake values of ^{40}K showed smaller variation than those obtained for Cs, and no significant difference was observed before or after the FDNPP accident.

Table 5. Total daily dietary intake values and committed effective doses of ^{40}K for adults in Japan, estimated via total diet studies from 2006 to 2011.

Year		Region	City	Daily Intake (Bq/Person·Day)	Committed Effective Dose (µSv)
Before the FDNPP *1 accident	2006	Kanto I	Tokyo	76	170
		Kanto II	Nagano	78	180
		Hokuriku	Kanazawa	77	180
		Kinki II	Nara	65	150
	2007	Kanto I	Yokohama	91	210
		Hokuriku	Niigata	94	210
		Shikoku	Kochi	79	180
	2008	Hokkaido	Sapporo	81	180
		Tohoku	Sendai	78	180
		Kinki I	Osaka	80	180
		Kita-Kyushu	Fukuoka	69	160
	2009	Kanto I	Tokyo	76	170
		Hokuriku	Kanazawa	72	160
		Chugoku	Hiroshima	85	190
		Shikoku	Kochi	79	180
	2010	Tokai	Nagoya	75	170
	Mean ± SD *2			78.0 ± 7.3	178 ± 16
After the FDNPP *1 accident	2011	Tohoku	Sendai	88	200
		Tohoku	Fukushima	81	180
		Kanto I	Tokyo	78	180

*1 FDNPP: Fukushima Daiichi nuclear power plant. *2 Mean and standard deviation value before the Fukushima Daiichi nuclear power plant accident.

The present study was based on food consumption data derived from the NHNS between 2002 and 2004, as previously described. According to the NHNS, the daily K intake for adults was 2.452 g/person/day in 2002 [41], 2.426 g/person/day in 2003 [42], and 2.372 g/person/day in 2004 [43]. Since 1 g of K corresponds to 30.3 Bq of ^{40}K, the intake of this radionuclide can be estimated to be 74 Bq/person/day in 2002, 74 Bq/person/day in 2003, and 72 Bq/person/day in 2004; this is in close agreement with the mean ^{40}K intake value obtained in the present study. On the other hand, ^{40}K intake between 2003 and 2008 varied from 5 to 150 Bq/person/day, according to a DPS conducted by the NRA [32]. The mean ^{40}K intake was calculated to be 57 Bq/person/day (SD = 16), and was clearly different from our finding. The DPS was performed on five consecutive days from June to January, whereas the NHNS was conducted for only a single day in November, to ensure the participation of a sufficient number of households. Thus, it should be noted that seasonal changes in food item availability and individual daily variations in food intake cannot be assessed using the NHNS and this TDS [7,44].

The minimum, maximum, and mean total CED values of natural occurring radionuclide ^{40}K between 2006 and 2011 were 150 µSv, 210 µSv, and 180 µSv (SD = 16), respectively, which are in close agreement with a previous TDS [13]. The mean value obtained was approximately ten times higher than the maximum CED obtained for artificial radioactive Cs in the present study, and was comparable to the worldwide average of 170 µSv [45]. Figure 4 shows the percent contributions of the contributing food groups to the CED values of ^{40}K in 2011. The food group "other vegetables, mushrooms, and seaweeds" had the greatest contribution to the CED values in Sendai City (31%), Fukushima City (26%), and Tokyo (32%). These results were similar to those of Tsutsumi et al. [33] and Miyazaki et al. [34].

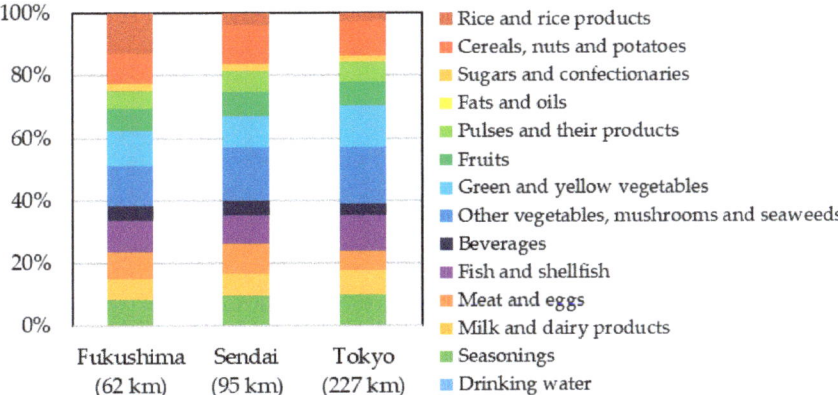

Figure 4. Percentage contributions of food groups to the committed effective doses of ^{40}K in 2011. Distance from the Fukushima Daiichi nuclear power plant to each city is denoted in parentheses. This figure was modified from [19].

3.4. TDS of Radionuclides Conducted by Other Countries

The second International Workshop on Total Diet Studies compiled a list of core (screening), intermediate, and comprehensive (refined assessment) priority chemicals that should be considered for inclusion in a TDS [46]. Radionuclides are categorized into the intermediate list, and there are three countries that routinely conduct TDSs, including Japan [2].

The United States has been performing TDSs continuously since 1961, as mentioned previously. The FDA routinely analyzes the following radionuclides in their TDS analysis: ^{137}Cs, ^{90}Sr, ^{106}Ru, ^{131}I, and ^{40}K. According to the FDA's report [47], the following three of 2984 samples were above the reporting limit of 5 Bq/kg for ^{137}Cs between 2006 and 2014: "baby foods, squash" in 2007 (93.3 Bq/kg), "raisin bran cereal" in 2009 (10.8 Bq/kg), and "salad dressing, creamy/buttermilk type, low calorie" in 2014 (40.5 Bq/kg).

Canada also continuously carries out TDSs of radionuclides. Health Canada has been monitoring natural (^{40}K and ^{210}Pb) and artificial (^{137}Cs, ^{134}Cs, ^{131}I, ^{241}Am, ^{57}Co, and ^{60}Co) radionuclides in foods since 2000. Their results between 2015 and 2017 showed that all 480 samples tested contained ^{137}Cs and ^{134}Cs levels below the minimum detection limit, showing a value of approximately 1.3 Bq/kg [48].

The result obtained from the American study was comparable to our finding, in that only one of the 266 TDS samples exceeded ^{137}Cs levels of 5 Bq/kg. Similarly, the Canadian study was consistent with respect to ^{137}Cs levels, specifically for those observed before the FDNPP accident in the present study. However, such a comparison should be interpreted with caution, since the number of composite samples analyzed in each MB differed between the three countries (approximately 280 for the United States, approximately 160 for Canada, and 14 for the present study) [5,49]. In the present study, individual food items with high levels of ^{137}Cs may be underrepresented, due to the grouping of a greater number of food items within each category, which could have lower levels of the radionuclide [1,50]. This dilution effect might have caused the ^{137}Cs levels after the FDNPP accident in the present study to be lower than those of "baby foods, squash", etc., as mentioned above. Meanwhile, the detection rate of ^{137}Cs in the present study was much higher than that in the United States and Canada, owing to the lower LOD values of ^{137}Cs. The present study evaluated the exposure level to ^{137}Cs as previously described, whereas the United States and Canada did not, because ^{137}Cs was not detected in nearly any samples.

China [51] and Lebanon [52] also conducted TDSs of radionuclides in 1990 and 2004, respectively. For each MB, both countries collected 12 composite samples, similar to the approach used in the present study. Cs-137 activity concentration in their TDS was found to be below 0.1 Bq/kg for most of the food groups, with the exception of potatoes, which had a value of 10.21 Bq/kg in China; that is consistent with our findings prior to the FDNPP accident.

4. Conclusions

The present study provides an estimate of the average dietary exposure of ^{137}Cs, ^{134}Cs, and ^{40}K for adults in Japan. Before the FDNPP accident, activity concentrations of ^{137}Cs were in the range of those reported in other countries, and dietary intake values and CEDs were consistent with our previous TDS. Similarly, after the FDNPP accident, the activity concentration and exposure levels of radioactive Cs were well below the regulatory levels, despite an increase in two orders of magnitude being measured. The exposure levels of ^{40}K did not differ before and after the FDNPP accident. The mean CED of ^{40}K was comparable to the international average, and was 10 times higher than the highest CED of radioactive Cs obtained in the present study.

On an international level, TDSs of radionuclides are scarce, and currently, only Japan evaluates trends in exposure levels to these contaminants. Thus, our findings provide invaluable information with regard to the radiological safety of foods. However, the present study has some limitations. First, the exposure levels immediately after the FDNPP accident could not be estimated, because the TDS in 2011 was performed approximately six months after the accident. Second, seasonal variation cannot be assessed, as the NHNS and this TDS were performed in only one season each year. Finally, the present study did not examine the exposure of children, or exposure to other radionuclides, such as ^{90}Sr, Pu, and ^{106}Ru, which are targets of standard limit regulations in foods. Therefore, further studies are required to determine the dietary exposure levels of these radionuclides for both adults and children.

Author Contributions: Conceptualization, H.T., I.I., S.M., K.I. and H.S.; methodology, H.T., I.I., S.M., K.I. and H.S.; formal analysis, H.T. and H.S.; investigation, H.T., I.I., S.M., K.I. and H.S.; resources, I.I., S.M., K.I. and H.S.; data curation, H.T. and H.S.; writing—original draft preparation, H.T.; writing—review and editing, H.T., H.S.; visualization, H.T.; supervision, H.S.; project administration, H.S.; funding acquisition, H.S. All authors have read and agreed to the published version of the manuscript.

Funding: This research was funded by the MHLW HLSRG (Research on Food Safety) (grant nos. H16-Shokuhin-Ippan-015, H19-Shokuhin-Ippan-003, and H22-Shokuhin-Ippan-017).

Acknowledgments: The authors would like to thank Michiko Koyano for her technical support in sample preparation.

Conflicts of Interest: The authors declare no conflict of interest.

References

1. Joint FAO/WHO Food Contamination Monitoring Programme, Global Environment Monitoring System and WHO. *Guidelines for the Study of Dietary Intakes of Chemical Contaminants*; WHO: Geneva, Switzerland, 1985; ISBN 978-92-4170-087-0.
2. WHO Regional Office for the Western Pacific. 5th International Workshop on Total Diet Studies, Seoul, Republic of Korea, 13–14 May 2015: Meeting Report. Available online: https://iris.wpro.who.int/bitstream/handle/10665.1/11686/20150514_KOR_eng.pdf (accessed on 28 October 2020).
3. Laug, E.P.; Mikalis, A.; Bollinger, H.M.; Dimitroff, J.M.; Deutsch, M.J.; Duffy, D.; Pillsbury, H.C.; Mills, P.A. Total Diet Study: A. Strontium-90 and Cesium-137 Content; B. Nutrient Content; C. Pesticide Content. *J. Assoc. Off. Agric. Chem.* **1963**, *46*, 749–752.
4. Egan, K. The Origin of Total Diet Studies. In *Total Diet Studies*; Moy, G.G., Vannoort, R.W., Eds.; Springer: New York, NY, USA, 2013; pp. 11–18. ISBN 978-1-4419-7688-8.
5. FDA. Total Diet Study. Available online: https://www.fda.gov/food/science-research-food/total-diet-study (accessed on 28 October 2020).
6. Maitani, T. Evaluation of Exposure to Chemical Substances through Foods—Exposure to Pesticides, Heavy Metals, Dioxins, Acrylamide and Food Additives in Japan—. *J. Health Sci.* **2004**, *50*, 205–209. [CrossRef]
7. Kayama, F.; Nitta, H.; Nakai, S.; Sasaki, S.; Horiguchi, H. Total Diet Studies in Japan. In *Total Diet Studies*; Moy, G.G., Vannoort, R.W., Eds.; Springer: New York, NY, USA, 2013; pp. 317–326. ISBN 978-1-4419-7688-8.

8. Gorchev, H.G.; Jelinek, C.F. A review of the dietary intakes of chemical contaminants. *Bull. World Health Organ.* **1985**, *63*, 945–962. [PubMed]
9. Ota, Y. Present Status and Prospect of Ultralow Level Radioactivity Measurements (3). Environmental Radioactivity in Japan. *Radioisotopes* **2006**, *55*, 351–359. (In Japanese) [CrossRef]
10. Akaishi, J.; Kasai, A.; Fujita, M. Trends with Time of Fallout ^{90}Sr, ^{137}Cs and ^{95}Zr-^{95}Nb in Total Diet and the Concentration in the Air. *J. Radiat. Res.* **1966**, *7*, 8–17. [CrossRef]
11. Suzuki, Y.; Nakamura, R.; Kawachi, E.; Ueda, T. Cesium-137 Contents in Japanese Diet from 1963 to 1971. *J. Radiat. Res.* **1974**, *15*, 181–188. [CrossRef]
12. Iijima, I.; Takagi, H.; Tomura, K.; Watanuki, T.; Sugiyama, H. Evaluation of Cesium-137 (^{137}Cs) and Elements Intake from Daily Diets in Residents of Kanagawa Prefecture, Japan. *J. Health Sci.* **2009**, *55*, 192–205. [CrossRef]
13. Sugiyama, H.; Terada, H.; Takahashi, M.; Iijima, I.; Isomura, K. Contents and Daily Intakes of Gamma-Ray Emitting Nuclides, ^{90}Sr, and ^{238}U using Market-Basket Studies in Japan. *J. Health Sci.* **2007**, *53*, 107–118. [CrossRef]
14. Sugiyama, H.; Terada, H.; Takahashi, M.; Iijima, I.; Isomura, K. Research on investigation and evaluation of the intake of radionuclides in the food. In *Summary and Sharing Report of Research on Investigation and Evaluation of the Intake of Toxic Substances and Others in the Food (FY2006)*; MHLW HLSRG (Research on Food Safety): Tokyo, Japan, 2007; pp. 55–81. (In Japanese)
15. Sugiyama, H.; Terada, H.; Iijima, I.; Isomura, K. Research on investigation and evaluation of the intake of radionuclides in the food. In *Summary and Sharing Report of Research on Investigation and Evaluation of the Intake of Toxic Substances and Others in the Food (FY2007)*; MHLW HLSRG (Research on Food Safety): Tokyo, Japan, 2008; pp. 67–92. (In Japanese)
16. Sugiyama, H.; Terada, H.; Koyano, M.; Iijima, I.; Isomura, K. Research on investigation and evaluation of the intake of radionuclides in the food. In *Summary and Sharing Report of Research on Investigation and Evaluation of the Intake of Toxic Substances and Others in the Food (FY2008)*; MHLW HLSRG (Research on Food Safety): Tokyo, Japan, 2009; pp. 53–87. (In Japanese)
17. Sugiyama, H.; Terada, H.; Koyano, M.; Iijima, I.; Miyake, S. Research on investigation and evaluation of the intake of radionuclides in the food. In *Summary and Sharing Report of Research on Investigation and Evaluation of the Intake of Toxic Substances and Others in the Food (FY2009)*; MHLW HLSRG (Research on Food Safety): Tokyo, Japan, 2010; pp. 65–95. (In Japanese)
18. Sugiyama, H.; Terada, H.; Koyano, M.; Iijima, I.; Miyake, S. Research on investigation and evaluation of the intake of radionuclides in the food. In *Sharing Report of Research on Evaluation of the Intake of Toxic Substances such as Dioxins via Food and its Methodological Development (FY2010) (Tentative Translation)*; MHLW HLSRG (Research on Food Safety): Tokyo, Japan, 2011. (In Japanese)
19. Sugiyama, H.; Terada, H.; Koyano, M.; Iijima, I.; Miyake, S. Research on evaluation of exposure to radionuclides via food. In *Summary and Sharing Report of Research on Evaluation of the Intake of Toxic Substances such as Dioxins via Food and Its Methodological Development (FY2011) (Tentative Translation)*; MHLW HLSRG (Research on Food Safety): Tokyo, Japan, 2012; pp. 69–108. (In Japanese)
20. ICRP. Age-dependent Doses to Members of the Public from Intake of Radionuclides: Part 5. Compilation of Ingestion and Inhalation Dose Coefficients. *Ann. ICRP* **1996**, *26*, 1–91. [CrossRef]
21. UNSCEAR. *UNSCEAR 2013 Report Annex A: Levels and Effects of Radiation Exposure Due to the Nuclear Accident after 2011 Great East-Japan Earthquake and Tsunami*; United Nations: New York, NY, USA, 2014; ISBN 978-92-1-142291-7.
22. Likhtarov, I.; Kovgan, L.; Vavilov, S.; Chepurny, M.; Bouville, A.; Luckyanov, N.; Jacob, P.; Voillequé, P.; Voigt, G. Post-Chornobyl thyroid cancers in Ukraine. Report 1: Estimation of thyroid doses. *Radiat. Res.* **2005**, *163*, 125–136. [CrossRef]
23. WHO. *Health Effects of the Chernobyl Accident and Special Health Care Programmes. Report of the UN Chernobyl Forum Expert Group "Health"*; Bennett, B., Repacholi, M., Carr, Z., Eds.; WHO: Geneva, Switzerland, 2006; ISBN 978-92-4-159417-2.
24. Bouville, A.; Likhtarev, I.A.; Kovgan, L.N.; Minenko, V.F.; Shinkarev, S.M.; Drozdovitch, V.V. Radiation dosimetry for highly contaminated Belarusian, Russian and Ukrainian populations, and for less contaminated populations in Europe. *Health Phys.* **2007**, *93*, 487–501. [CrossRef] [PubMed]

25. Unno, N.; Minakami, H.; Kubo, T.; Fujimori, K.; Ishiwata, I.; Terada, H.; Saito, S.; Yamaguchi, I.; Kunugita, N.; Nakai, A.; et al. Effect of the Fukushima Nuclear Power Plant Accident on Radioiodine (131I) Content in Human Breast Milk. *J. Obstet. Gynaecol. Res.* **2012**, *38*, 772–779. [CrossRef] [PubMed]
26. Ohse, K.; Kihou, N.; Kurishima, K.; Inoue, T.; Taniyama, I. Changes in concentrations of ^{131}I, ^{134}Cs and ^{137}Cs in leafy vegetables, soil and precipitation in Tsukuba city, Ibaraki, Japan, in the first 4 months after the Fukushima Daiichi nuclear power plant accident. *Soil Sci. Plant Nutr.* **2015**, *61*, 225–229. [CrossRef]
27. Terada, H.; Yamaguchi, I.; Shimura, T.; Svendsen, E.R.; Kunugita, N. Regulation values and current situation of radioactive materials in food. *J. Natl. Inst. Public Health* **2018**, *67*, 21–33.
28. Hamada, N.; Ogino, H. Food safety regulations: What we learned from the Fukushima nuclear accident. *J. Environ. Radioact.* **2012**, *111*, 83–99. [CrossRef]
29. MHLW. Handling of Food Contaminated by Radioactivity. Available online: https://www.mhlw.go.jp/stf/houdou/2r9852000001558e-img/2r98520000015av4.pdf (accessed on 28 October 2020).
30. MHLW. The Ministerial Ordinance Partially Revising the Ministerial Ordinance on Milk and Milk Products Concerning Compositional Standards, etc.; the Notification on Designating the Radioactive Substances Designated by the Minister of Health, Labour and Welfare under the Provisions of Item(I)(1) of the Attached Table 2 of the Ministerial Ordinance on Milk and Milk Products Concerning Compositional Standards, etc.; and the Notification on Partial Revision of Specification and Standards for Food, Food Additives etc. Available online: https://www.mhlw.go.jp/english/topics/2011eq/dl/food-120821_1.pdf (accessed on 28 October 2020).
31. Iwaoka, K. The Current Limits for Radionuclides in Food in Japan. *Health Phys.* **2016**, *111*, 471–478. [CrossRef]
32. NRA. Environmental Radiation Database. Available online: https://search.kankyo-hoshano.go.jp/servlet/search.top (accessed on 28 October 2020).
33. Tsutsumi, T.; Nabeshi, H.; Ikarashi, A.; Hachisuka, A.; Matsuda, R. Estimation of the Committed Effective Dose of Radioactive Cesium and Potassium by the Market Basket Method. *J. Food Hyg. Soc. Jpn.* **2013**, *54*, 7–13. (In Japanese) [CrossRef]
34. Miyazaki, H.; Kato, H.; Kato, Y.; Tsuchiyama, T.; Terada, H. Estimation of the Intake of Radioactive Cesium Based on Analysis of Total Diet Samples in Nagoya. *J. Food Hyg. Soc. Jpn.* **2013**, *54*, 151–155. (In Japanese) [CrossRef]
35. Uekusa, Y.; Nabeshi, H.; Tsutsumi, T.; Hachisuka, A.; Matsuda, R.; Teshima, R. Estimation of Dietary Intake of Radioactive Materials by Total Diet Methods. *J. Food Hyg. Soc. Jpn.* **2014**, *55*, 177–182. (In Japanese) [CrossRef]
36. MHLW. Survey Results of Dose from Radioactive Cs in Foods (February–March 2018). (Tentative Translation). Available online: https://www.mhlw.go.jp/content/11134000/000462888.pdf (accessed on 28 October 2020). (In Japanese)
37. MHLW. Survey Results of Dose from Radioactive Cs in Foods (September–October 2018). (Tentative Translation). Available online: https://www.mhlw.go.jp/content/11134000/000520599.pdf (accessed on 28 October 2020). (In Japanese)
38. MHLW. Survey Results of Dose from Radioactive Cs in Foods (February–March 2019). (Tentative Translation). Available online: https://www.mhlw.go.jp/content/11134000/000630323.pdf (accessed on 28 October 2020). (In Japanese)
39. MHLW. Survey Results of Dose from Radioactive Cs in Foods (September–October 2019). (Tentative Translation). Available online: https://www.mhlw.go.jp/content/11134000/000643447.pdf (accessed on 28 October 2020). (In Japanese)
40. Tokyo Metropolitan Government. Survey Results of Chemical Substances Intake via Foods. (Tentative Translation). Available online: https://www.fukushihoken.metro.tokyo.lg.jp/smph/kankyo/kankyo_eisei/kagakutaisaku/shokuhin/kekka.html (accessed on 28 October 2020). (In Japanese).
41. MHLW. *The National Nutrition Survey in Japan, 2002*; Daiichi Shuppan: Tokyo, Japan, 2004; ISBN 978-4-8041-1082-0. (In Japanese)
42. MHLW. *The National Health and Nutrition Survey in Japan, 2003*; Daiichi Shuppan: Tokyo, Japan, 2006; ISBN 978-4-8041-1122-3. (In Japanese)
43. MHLW. *The National Health and Nutrition Survey in Japan, 2004*; Daiichi Shuppan: Tokyo, Japan, 2006; ISBN 978-4-8041-1151-4. (In Japanese)

44. Ikeda, N.; Takimoto, H.; Imai, S.; Miyachi, M.; Nishi, N. Data Resource Profile: The Japan National Health and Nutrition Survey (NHNS). *Int. J. Epidemiol.* **2015**, *44*, 1842–1849. [CrossRef]
45. UNSCEAR. *Sources and Effects of Ionizing Radiation, UNSCEAR 2000 Report to the General Assembly, with Scientific Annexes*; United Nations: New York, NY, USA, 2000; ISBN 978-9211422382.
46. International Workshop on Total Diet Studies (2nd. 2002: Brisbane, Australia); WHO Food Safety Programme. *GEMS/Food Total Diet Studies: Report of the 2nd International Workshop on Total Diet Studies, Brisbane, Australia, 4–15 February 2002*; WHO: Geneva, Switzerland, 2002; ISBN 92-4-156219-6.
47. FDA. Total Diet Study. In *Radionuclide Results Summary Statistics. Market Baskets 2006 through 2014*. Available online: https://www.fda.gov/media/94785/download (accessed on 28 October 2020).
48. Health Canada. Canadian Total Diet Study—Radionuclides. Available online: https://open.canada.ca/data/en/dataset/062c769f-57d7-432e-9d33-1e333a87d6d0 (accessed on 28 October 2020).
49. Health Canada. Canadian Total Diet Study. Available online: https://www.canada.ca/en/health-canada/services/food-nutrition/food-nutrition-surveillance/canadian-total-diet-study.html (accessed on 28 October 2020).
50. European Food Safety Authority; FAO; WHO. Towards a harmonised total diet study approach: A guidance document. *EFSA J.* **2011**, *9*, 2450. [CrossRef]
51. Chen, J.; Gao, J. The Chinese Total Diet Study in 1990. Part I. Chemical Contaminants. *J. AOAC Int.* **1993**, *76*, 1193–1205. [CrossRef] [PubMed]
52. Nasreddine, L.; Hwalla, N.; El Samad, O.; LeBlanc, J.C.; Hamzé, M.; Sibiril, Y.; Parent-Massin, D. Dietary Exposure to Lead, Cadmium, Mercury and Radionuclides of an Adult Urban Population in Lebanon: A Total Diet Study Approach. *Food Addit. Contam.* **2006**, *23*, 579–590. [CrossRef]

Publisher's Note: MDPI stays neutral with regard to jurisdictional claims in published maps and institutional affiliations.

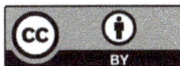

© 2020 by the authors. Licensee MDPI, Basel, Switzerland. This article is an open access article distributed under the terms and conditions of the Creative Commons Attribution (CC BY) license (http://creativecommons.org/licenses/by/4.0/).

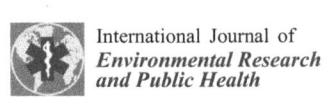

Article

Passive-Type Radon Monitor Constructed Using a Small Container for Personal Dosimetry

Yuki Tamakuma [1,2], Chutima Kranrod [1], Takahito Suzuki [2,†], Yuki Watanabe [3,‡], Thamaborn Ploykrathok [1,§], Ryoju Negami [2], Eka Djatnika Nugraha [2], Kazuki Iwaoka [4], Mirosław Janik [4], Masahiro Hosoda [1,2] and Shinji Tokonami [1,*]

1. Institute of Radiation Emergency Medicine, Hirosaki University, 66-1 Honcho, Hirosaki, Aomori 036-8564, Japan; tamakuma@hirosaki-u.ac.jp (Y.T.); kranrodc@hirosaki-u.ac.jp (C.K.); thamaborn.p@outlook.com (T.P.); m_hosoda@hirosaki-u.ac.jp (M.H.)
2. Graduate School of Health Sciences, Hirosaki University, 66-1 Honcho, Hirosaki, Aomori 036-8564, Japan; suzuki-takahito@fujielectric.com (T.S.); h20gg204@hirosaki-u.ac.jp (R.N.); h20gg701@hirosaki-u.ac.jp (E.D.N.)
3. School of Health Sciences, Hirosaki University, 66-1 Honcho, Hirosaki, Aomori 036-8564, Japan; watanabe.yuki@jaea.go.jp
4. National Institutes for Quantum and Radiological Science and Technology, 4-9-1 Anagawa, Inage, Chiba 263-0024, Japan; iwaoka.kazuki@qst.go.jp (K.I.); janik.miroslaw@qst.go.jp (M.J.)
* Correspondence: tokonami@hirosaki-u.ac.jp; Tel.: +81-172-39-5404
† Present address: Fuji Electric Co., Ltd., 1 Fujimachi, Hino, Tokyo 191-8502, Japan.
‡ Present address: Radiation Protection Department, Nuclear Fuel Cycle Engineering Laboratories, Japan Atomic Energy Agency, 4-33 Muramatsu, Tokai, Ibaraki 319-1194, Japan.
§ Present address: Department of Nuclear Engineering, Faculty of Engineering, Chulalongkorn University, Bangkok 10330, Thailand.

Received: 14 July 2020; Accepted: 2 August 2020; Published: 5 August 2020

Abstract: The International Commission on Radiological Protection (ICRP) recently recommended a new dose conversion factor for radon based on the latest epidemiological studies and dosimetric model. It is important to evaluate an inhalation dose from radon and its progeny. In the present study, a passive radon personal monitor was designed using a small container for storing contact lenses and its performance was evaluated. The conversion factor for radon (^{222}Rn), the effect of thoron (^{220}Rn) concentration and the air exchange rate were evaluated using the calibration chamber at Hirosaki University. The minimum and maximum detectable radon concentrations were calculated. The conversion factor was evaluated as 2.0 ± 0.3 tracks cm^{-2} per kBq h m^{-3}; statistical analyses of results showed no significant effect from thoron concentration. The minimum and maximum detectable radon concentrations were 92 Bq m^{-3} and 231 kBq m^{-3} for a measurement period of three months, respectively. The air exchange rate was estimated to be 0.26 ± 0.16 h^{-1}, whose effect on the measured time-integrated radon concentration was small. These results indicate that the monitor could be used as a wearable monitor for radon measurements, especially in places where radon concentrations may be relatively high, such as mines and caves.

Keywords: passive radon monitor; development; sensitivity; detection limit; air-exchange rate

1. Introduction

Radon is one of the naturally occurring radionuclides, which is well known as the second leading risk factor for lung cancer after tobacco smoking [1]. According to the United Nations Scientific Committee on the Effects of Atomic Radiation (UNSCEAR) 2008 report on the sources and effects of ionizing radiation [2], the world mean value of annual effective dose by natural radiation sources is 2.4 mSv, and half of this dose is attributed to radon (^{222}Rn), thoron (^{220}Rn), and their progenies.

Radon and thoron, which are radioactive noble gases, are normally generated by radioactive decay from radium (^{226}Ra and ^{224}Ra) in soil, rocks, and building materials. Indoor radon concentrations tend to be higher than outdoor concentrations due to the ventilation rate. Many indoor radon concentration surveys have been carried out in various countries [3–7]. The world mean indoor radon concentration was reported to be 40 Bq m^{-3} [8]. However, radon concentrations in mines and caves are higher than indoor concentrations because radon generated from surrounding rocks and soil can be easily accumulated due to the low ventilation. Recently, it has been reported that mean radon concentrations at several mines and caves were over ~1000 Bq m^{-3} [9–12].

In 2017, the International Commission on Radiological Protection (ICRP) recommended a new dose conversion factor of 3 mSv per mJ h m^{-3} for radon in buildings and underground mines based on current epidemiological studies and dosimetric model [13,14]. This value corresponds to 17 nSv per Bq h m^{-3}, which is almost twice the dose conversion factor of 9 nSv per Bq h m^{-3} given by the UNSCEAR 2006 report on the sources and effects of ionizing radiation [15]. Many countries will approve the new dose conversion factor of ICRP for the occupational environment under the existing situation [16]. Therefore, it is important to evaluate an inhalation dose from radon and its progeny, especially for workers in mines and caves.

Generally, radon concentration is measured using passive-type monitors recording long-term measurements [17]. However, passive-type monitors have an upper limit of detection. The overlaps of tracks made by alpha particles in the measurement at a high radon concentration area lead to the underestimation of radon concentration. Thus, the sensitivity to radon should be lower than that of previous monitors to measure radon concentrations in the prone area. These monitors are large and inconvenient to carry and they are not designed to be carried by workers. Therefore, a passive radon monitor with low sensitivity to radon for measurement in radon-prone areas that is small enough to be carried during the work period is needed for evaluation of inhalation dose. In the present study, such a passive radon personal monitor was designed and its performance was evaluated.

2. Materials and Methods

2.1. Overview of the Passive Radon Rersonal Monitor

A passive radon personal monitor is shown in Figure 1a. A small container for storing contact lenses was adapted because it is cheap, and easy to obtain and handle. Each container volume was ~3.2 cm^3. A solid-state track detector (CR-39; BARYOTRAK, Nagase Landauer, Ltd., Tsukuba, Japan), 1.0 × 1.0 cm, was used as the detecting material and one piece of CR-39 was held in place at the top of each container with sticky clay (Figure 1b). Electroconductive materials have been used for the container of previous passive radon monitors to avoid electrostatic phenomena, which may cause a non-uniform deposition of radon progeny [18,19]. Thus, an electroconductive coating material (D-362, Fujikura Kasei Co., Ltd., Tokyo, Japan) was used on the container's inner wall. Each container was closed by an attached lid; this makes an invisible air gap that prevents thoron from passing into the monitor. The radon concentration (X_{Rn}) was calculated using the following Equation (1):

$$X_{Rn} = \frac{N - N_0}{CF_{Rn} \cdot T} \quad (1)$$

where X_{Rn} is the mean concentration of radon during the exposure period in kBq m^{-3}; N and N_0 (tracks cm^{-2}) are the track density in the measurement and the background, respectively; CF_{Rn} (tracks cm^{-2} per kBq h m^{-3}) is the conversion factor to radon concentration, which is obtained by a calibration experiment; and T is the exposure time in hours.

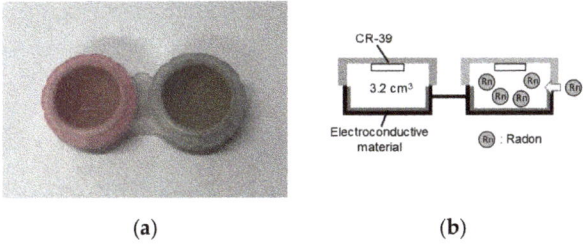

(a) (b)

Figure 1. External view of the passive radon personal monitor constructed using a small container for storing contact lenses (**a**) and a schematic representation of the monitor (**b**).

2.2. Conversion Factor to Radon Concentration

To obtain the conversion factor (CF) to radon concentration, this monitor was placed in the radon calibration chamber [20] at the Institute of Radiation Emergency Medicine (IREM) at Hirosaki University. The radon concentrations in the chamber were continuously monitored by a scintillation cell (300A, Pylon Electronics Inc., Ottawa, ON, Canada) with a portable radon monitor (AB-5, Pylon Electronics Inc., Ottawa, ON, Canada). Three different exposure tests were carried out. Five monitors, totaling 10 CR-39 pieces, were exposed for each exposure condition. After exposure tests, CR-39 pieces were taken from the containers and were chemically etched with a 6.0 M NaOH solution at 60 °C for 24 h. The alpha tracks were counted using ImageJ software (National Institutes of Health, Bethesda, MD, USA) with photos of etched CR-39 pieces. Ten reading areas of 0.01 cm^2, which corresponds to 0.1 cm^2, were randomly selected to count the number of the tracks. The CFs for each CR-39 were calculated using Equation (1), and then the arithmetic mean of the CF value was evaluated.

2.3. Effect of Thoron Interference

To evaluate the effect of thoron concentration, this monitor was placed in the thoron chamber at IREM. Thoron concentrations were continuously monitored with an electrostatic collection radon-thoron monitor (RAD7, Durridge. Co. Inc., Billerica, MA, USA). A grab sampling technique using a scintillation cell with a portable radiation monitor was used for the correction of values measured by the RAD7 [21]. Temperature and relative humidity in the thoron chamber were simultaneously monitored with an environmental monitor (TR-73U, T&D Co., Matsumoto, Japan). After exposure, the alpha tracks were counted in the same way as for radon exposure. The tracks of the exposed group and background were compared using two-sided Student's t-tests. The difference was considered significant for $p < 0.05$. Excel 2016 software (Microsoft, Washington WA, USA) and R version 3.5.2 were used to perform the statistical analyses.

2.4. Minimum and Maximum Detectable Radon Concentrations

The minimum detectable radon concentration was evaluated using the method of the International Organization for Standardization (ISO 11929) [22]. The following equation was used for the calculation of the minimum detectable radon concentration:

$$y^* = \frac{k\sqrt{2n_0}}{S \cdot CF \cdot T} \qquad (2)$$

$$y^{\#} = \frac{2y^* + \frac{k^2}{S \cdot CF \cdot T}}{1 - k^2\{u_{rel}^2(S) + u_{rel}^2(CF)\}} \qquad (3)$$

where y^* and $y^\#$ are the decision threshold and the minimum detectable radon concentration (kBq m^{-3}), respectively; k is the quantile of the standardized normal distribution for probabilities of 0.95 (i.e., $k = 1.65$); n_0 is the number of background tracks (tracks); S is the total reading area (cm^2); CF is the conversion factor for radon concentration (tracks cm^{-2} per kBq h m^{-3}); T is the exposure time (h); and $u_{rel}(x)$ is the standard relative uncertainty for the parameter x. The standard relative uncertainty for the total reading area $u_{rel}(S)$ was assumed to be zero.

In addition, the maximum detectable radon concentration can be calculated using Equation (1) and the maximum track density estimated by an average track diameter measured using an optical microscopy (Model LVS, Kenis Ltd., Japan). The maximum alpha track density N_{max} (tracks cm^{-2}) can be calculated by:

$$N_{max} = \frac{1}{d_t^2} \tag{4}$$

where d_t is the average alpha track diameter (cm). Then, the maximum detectable concentration $X_{Rn,\,max}$ in kBq m^{-3} is expressed as:

$$X_{Rn,\,max} = \frac{N_{max} - N_0}{CF_{Rn} \cdot T}. \tag{5}$$

2.5. Air Exchange Rate

The air exchange rate was evaluated using an exposure–degassing–enclosure method reported by Omori et al. [23]. The 20 monitors with CR-39s were exposed in the radon chamber at IREM, where the radon concentration was stabilized. The radon concentrations were monitored every hour by the pulse-type ionizing chamber (AlphaGUARD, PQ2000PRO, Genitron Instruments GmbH, Frankfurt, Germany), which was calibrated by Physilalish Technische Bundesanstalt (Braunschweig, Germany). After the 48 h exposure, the monitors were taken out of the radon chamber and degassed by leaving them in an experimental room where the radon concentration was low. The degassing time was set to be 0, 1, 2, 3, 4, 6, 8, 10, 12 and 16 h, and the radon gas in the monitor rapidly goes out through the invisible air gap to the experimental room in this period. The monitors were enclosed in a radon-proof bag made from polyethylene for 288 h when each degassing time passed. Table 1 shows the average radon concentration, the environmental parameters in the radon chamber, and the experimental room during the experiment. The average radon concentration observed in the environmental room was quite low compared to that measured in the radon chamber, which indicated the existence of radon in the experimental room during the degassing time would be negligible. After the enclosure, the CR-39s were etched in the same way. For the analysis, 40 reading areas in each CR-39 were taken to avoid increasing the deviation of the track density in this study because the expected difference in the track density for each degassing condition was small.

Table 1. Radon concentration and environmental parameters in the radon chamber and an experimental room.

Parameter	Radon Chamber		Experimental Room	
	Average	Standard Deviation	Average	Standard Deviation
Radon concentration (Bq m^{-3})	13,300	1603	7.7	3.0
Temperature (°C)	27.7	0.4	26.3	1.5
Relative humidity (%)	50.1	2.5	34.7	6.1
Air pressure (hPa)	1002	2	1003	7

3. Results

3.1. Conversion Factor to Radon Concentration

Three different exposures were controlled as 132 ± 1, 309 ± 3, and 564 ± 5 kBq h m^{-3}. Using these data, Figure 2 shows the relationship between the time-integrated radon concentration and the alpha track density. The CF to radon concentration was found to be 2.0 ± 0.3 tracks cm^{-2} per kBq h m^{-3}.

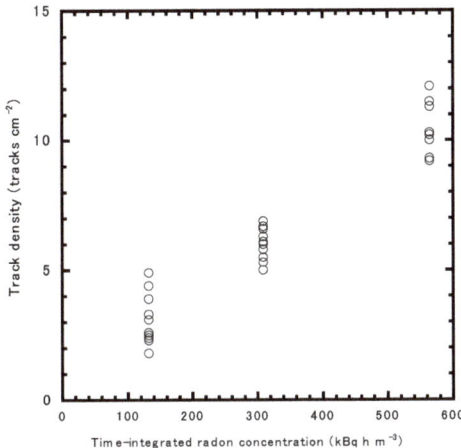

Figure 2. The relationship between the time-integrated radon concentration and alpha track density. Ten CR-39 pieces were exposed for each condition.

3.2. Effect of Thoron Interference

The mean thoron concentration, temperature, and relative humidity were 6785 ± 2122 Bq m^{-3}, 25.5 ± 0.2 °C, and 9 ± 4%, respectively. Time-integrated thoron concentration was controlled as 329 ± 6 kBq h m^{-3}. As shown in Figure 3, the track densities for background and exposed CR-39 were 43 ± 17 and 47 ± 27 tracks cm^{-2}, respectively. As a result of the statistical analysis, no significant difference in the track density was observed between the background and exposed group ($p = 0.76$).

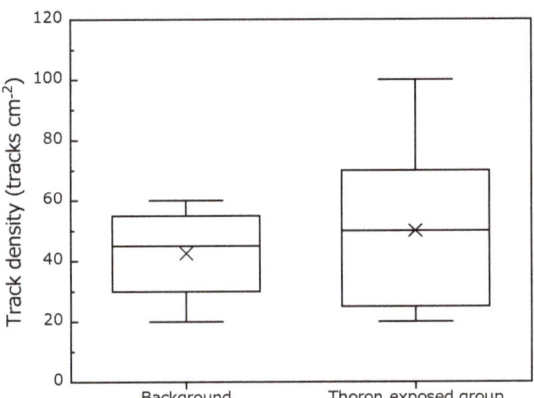

Figure 3. Track densities for the background and thoron-exposed group in unit of tracks cm^{-2}. Bottom and top whiskers are the 25th and 75th percentiles, respectively. The lines across the boxes and the cross marks represent the median and the arithmetic mean value, respectively.

3.3. Minimum and Maximum Detectable Radon Concentrations

Parameters used for the calculation of the minimum detectable radon concentration are summarized in Table 2. Notably, the working time of 8 h per day was considered for the calculation; thus, the measurement times were set to be 720 and 1440 h for three and six months, respectively. The minimum detectable concentrations with a measurement interval of three and six months were evaluated as 92 and 46 Bq m^{-3}, respectively.

Table 2. Parameters used for the calculation of the minimum detectable radon concentration.

Item	Symbol	Value	Remarks
Quantiles of the standardized normal distribution	k	1.65	For probabilities of 0.95
Number of background track	n_0	4.3 tracks	Derived from the background track density of 43 tracks cm^{-2}
Total reading area	S	0.1 cm^2	Ten reading areas of 0.01 cm^2
Conversion factor for radon concentration	CF	2.0 tracks cm^{-2} per kBq h m^{-3}	
Measurement time	T	720 h 1440 h	3 months 6 months
Relative standard uncertainty for the total reading area	$u_{rel}(S)$	0	
Relative standard uncertainty For the conversion factor	$u_{rel}(CF)$	0.15	

The average alpha track diameter was estimated as 10 μm. Thus, the maximum detectable radon concentrations with three- and six-month measurements were evaluated as 231 and 116 kBq m^{-3}, respectively.

3.4. Air Exchange Rate

Figure 4 illustrates the alpha track density with a standard deviation against the degassing time. The track density slowly decreased with a degassing time of 0–8 h. Theoretically, the decreasing trend can be fitted by a single exponential function. As a result, the air exchange rate was estimated to be 0.26 ± 0.16 h^{-1}. The result indicates that the air in the monitor is almost exchanged after 8 h from the end of exposure.

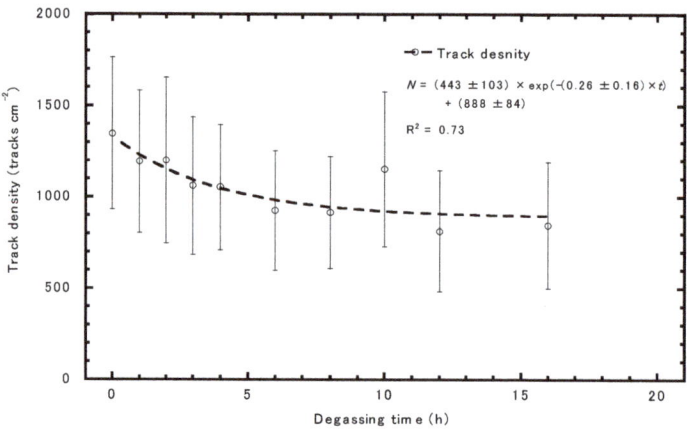

Figure 4. The alpha track density against the degassing time.

4. Discussion

4.1. Conversion Factor to Radon Concentration

The CFs of various passive integrated radon monitors are summarized in Table 3. Many kinds of passive integrated radon monitors have been developed by different groups, and the CFs are different for each one [18,24–27]. The CF for the present monitor was almost same or lower compared with the factors for other monitors. This might be due to the difference in the type of solid-state nuclear track detector (SSNTD) used in the monitors. The CFs shown in previous papers might have been evaluated using a different type of SSNTD that has a lower sensitivity than the CR-39 used in the present study. Thus, the CF for RADUET, widely used for a large-scale radon survey, was also evaluated by the same method using two types of CR-39s at the same time to check the difference in sensitivity attributed to the SSNTD. One was provided by Nagase Landauer Ltd., which was used in the present study, and the other was provided by RadoSys Ltd., which was used by Tokonami et al. [18]. The CFs for RADUET evaluated in the present study and the previous paper are summarized in Table 4. The CFs of the CR-39 by Nagase Landauer Ltd. and RadoSys Ltd. were estimated to be 4.4 ± 0.1 and 2.8 ± 0.1 tracks cm^{-2} per kBq h m^{-3}, respectively. This result suggested that the sensitivity of SSNTD significantly affects the CF of a passive radon monitor. Notably, the image analysis system and the chemical etching condition might also be significant factors affecting the CF.

Table 3. Conversion factors of various passive radon monitors.

Measuring Device	Conversion Factor (Tracks cm^{-2} per kBq h m^{-3})	Reference
Present radon monitor	2.0	
RADUET [1]	2.3	[18]
KfK monitor [2]	0.9	[24]
Radtrak	2.8	[25]
NRPB/SSI [3]	2.2	[26]
Radon-thoron discriminative dosimeter [1]	1.2	[27]

[1] The CFs of these monitors were evaluated for those with a low air ventilation rate. [2] KfK: Kernforschungszentrum Karlsruhe [3] NRPB/SSI: National Radiological Protection Board/Statens strålskyddsinstitut.

Table 4. The conversion factors of RADUET evaluated by two types of CR-39s in the present study and in a previous study. RADUETs, which contain both CR-39s, were simultaneously exposed to radon atmosphere for evaluation of the difference in CFs.

Item	Conversion Factor (Tracks cm^{-2} per kBq h m^{-3})	
	Nagase Landauer	RadoSys [1]
Present study	4.4	2.8
Previous report [2]	-	2.3

[1] CR-39s were chemically etched using a 6.25M NaOH solution at 90 °C for 6 h. [2] The data were cited from Tokonami et al. [18].

McLaughlin and Fitzgerald developed a model to calculate a CF for a cylindrically-shaped passive radon monitor [28]. According to the model, the CFs of the monitors, which have radii of 1.0 and 2.0 cm, corresponding to the present monitor and RADUET, respectively, were estimated to be 1.8 and 3.7 tracks cm^{-2} per kBq h m^{-3}, respectively. Compared with the empirical values, the differences in the present monitor and RADUET were 12% and 16%, respectively. Notably, these values calculated by the model include an uncertainty because the model made assumptions that do not reflect the exact geometry and shape of a detector for simplification. The ratio of the two values by the model was calculated as 2.1, whereas that of experimentally evaluated in this study was 2.2. We found a reasonably good agreement between the ratios regardless of the simplified model, indicating that the sensitivity was lower compared with the previous monitor, and the difference in the CFs between the present monitor and RADUET was attributed to the shape of the monitor.

We found that the air gap between the lid and the container prevented thoron from entering the monitor. This result suggested that the effect of thoron concentration is small enough for radon measurements that it could be ignored.

4.2. Minimum and Maximum Detectable Radon Concentrations

The results suggested that the present monitor would be useful for radon measurements in places where radon concentrations might be relatively high, such as mines and caves. According to a previous report, radon concentrations in mines and tourist caves have daily and seasonal variations, and its mean annual concentration was around 3500 Bq m^{-3} with a standard deviation of 1833 Bq m^{-3} [12]. There are very few underground mines in Japan so far, but there are some tourist caves; a wearable monitor may be useful as a simple radiation protection instrument for workers.

The long-term indoor radon concentrations are measured using a passive radon monitor, which is put on a shelf or hung on a wall and roof for three or six months. In this case, the minimum detectable radon concentrations are evaluated to be 31 and 15 Bq m^{-3} for three- and six-month measurements, respectively. It has been reported in several foreign countries that their mean indoor radon concentrations are relatively higher than these values [29–34]. Therefore, the passive radon monitor developed in this study will be useful not only as a wearable monitor for personal dosimetry due to radon inhalation but also for indoor radon measurements in many countries.

4.3. Air Exchange Rate

The trend in the alpha track density against the degassing time in Figure 4 was found to be similar to that reported by Omori et al. [23]. Omori et al. [23] reported that the experimental value was in good agreement with the theoretically calculated value. The air exchange rate of RADUET was previously reported as 0.71 h^{-1}, which is higher than that of the present monitor of 0.26 h^{-1} [23]. This indicated that the present monitor has a higher diffusion barrier than RADUET. The monitor is closed by the container's lid with a screw, which could make the high diffusion barrier, whereas RADUET was designed to be easy to dismantle. As shown in Figure 4, it takes approximately 8 h to completely exchange the air in the monitor, which is why the effect of thoron could be neglected.

To evaluate the effect of air exchange rate on the measurement result when being used as a wearable monitor, the theoretical time-integrated radon concentration in the monitor was calculated considering the working period. It was assumed that workers wear the monitor for a working period of eight hours, and do not wear it at other times. If the radon concentration is 1000 Bq m^{-3}, the theoretical time-integrated radon concentration in the monitor is estimated to be 7.6 kBq h m^{-3}, whereas the actual value is 8.0 kBq h m^{-3}. We found that the difference was estimated to be 5%, which is low compared with other uncertainties such as a counting error. Therefore, the present monitor can be useful as a wearable monitor to evaluate occupational exposure to radon.

5. Conclusions

A passive radon personal monitor was designed using a small container for storing contact lenses and its performance was tested. The conversion factor to radon concentration and the effect of thoron concentration on the measurement result were evaluated using the calibration chamber at Hirosaki University. The conversion factor for radon was evaluated as 2.0 ± 0.3 tracks cm^{-2} per kBq h m^{-3} and could be smaller than those with the previous monitors. No significant effect of thoron was observed in the two-sided Student's t-test. The minimum and maximum detectable radon concentrations were estimated as 92 Bq m^{-3} and 231 kBq m^{-3} for a measurement period of three months, respectively. The air exchange rate was evaluated to be 0.26 h^{-1}, and the effect could be ignored even if it is used only during the working period. These results indicated that this monitor would be useful as a wearable monitor for radon measurements, especially in caves and mines, and for indoor radon measurements where relatively high radon concentrations are present.

Author Contributions: Conceptualization, Y.T., M.H., and S.T.; methodology, Y.T., C.K., M.H., and S.T.; validation, Y.T., M.H., and S.T.; formal analysis, T.S., Y.W., T.P., R.N., and E.D.N.; investigation, T.S., Y.W., T.P., R.N., E.D.N., K.I., and M.J.; resources, K.I., M.J., M.H., and S.T.; data curation, Y.T.; writing—original draft preparation, Y.T.; writing—review and editing, Y.T., C.K., E.D.N., M.J., M.H., and S.T.; visualization, Y.T.; supervision, M.H. and S.T.; project administration, Y.T., M.H., and S.T.; funding acquisition, M.H. and S.T. All authors have read and agreed to the published version of the manuscript.

Funding: This research was partially funded by the Japan Society for the Promotion of Science KAKENHI (18K10023, 18KK0261, and 20H00556), the Environmental Radioactivity Research Network Center (E-20-10) and Hirosaki University Institutional Research Grant.

Conflicts of Interest: The authors declare no conflict of interest.

References

1. World Health Organization. *WHO Handbook on Indoor Radon: A Public Health Perspective*; WHO: Geneva, Switzerland, 2009.
2. United Nations Scientific Committee on the Effects of Atomic Radiation. *UNSCEAR 2008 Report, Sources and Effects of Ionizing Radiation*; Volume I: Annex B Exposures of the Public and Workers from Various Sources of Radiation; UNSCEAR: New York, NY, USA, 2010.
3. Bochicchio, F.; Venuti, C.G.; Nuccetelli, C.; Piermattei, S.; Risica, S.; Tommasino, L.; Torri, G. Results of the representative Italian national survey on radon indoors. *Health Phys.* **1996**, *71*, 741–748. [CrossRef] [PubMed]
4. Letourneau, G.E.; McGregor, G.R.; Walker, B.W. Design and interpretation of large surveys for indoor exposure to radon daughters. *Radiat. Prot. Dosim.* **1984**, *7*, 303–308. [CrossRef]
5. Marcinowski, F. Nationwide survey of residential radon levels in the US. *Radiat. Prot. Dosim.* **1992**, *45*, 419–424. [CrossRef]
6. Sanada, T.; Fujimoto, K.; Miyamoto, K.; Doi, M.; Tokonami, S.; Uesugi, M.; Takata, Y. Measurement of nationwide indoor Rn concentration in Japan. *J. Environ. Radioact.* **1999**, *45*, 129–137. [CrossRef]
7. Omori, Y.; Hosoda, M.; Takashi, F.; Sanada, T.; Hirao, S.; Ono, K.; Furukawa, M. Japanese population dose from natural radiation. *J. Radiol. Prot.* **2020**, in press. [CrossRef] [PubMed]
8. United Nations Scientific Committee on the Effects of Atomic Radiation. *UNSCEAR 2000 Report, Sources and Effects of Ionizing Radiation*; Volume I: Annex B Exposures from Natural Radiation Sources; UNSCEAR: New York, NY, USA, 2000.
9. Thinová, L.; Froňka, A.; Rovenská, K. The overview of the radon and environmental characteristics measurements in the Czech show caves. *Radiat. Prot. Dosim.* **2015**, *164*, 502–509. [CrossRef]
10. Dinu, A.C.; Călugăr, M.I.; Burghele, B.D.; Dumitru, O.A.; Cosma, C.; Onac, B.P. Radon levels in Romanian caves: An occupational exposure survey. *Environ. Geochem. Health* **2017**, *39*, 1085–1099. [CrossRef]
11. Shahrokhi, A.; Vigh, T.; Németh, C.; Csordás, A.; Kovács, T. Radon measurements and dose estimate of workers in a manganese ore mine. *Appl. Radiat. Isot.* **2017**, *124*, 32–37. [CrossRef]
12. Sainz, C.; Rábago, D.; Fernández, E.; Quindós, J.; Quindós, L.; Fernández, A.; Fuente, I.; Arteche, J.L.; Quindós, L.S.; Celaya, S. Variations in radon dosimetry under different assessment approaches in the Altamira Cave. *J. Radiol. Prot.* **2020**, *40*, 367–380. [CrossRef]
13. International Commission on Radiological Protection. *Occupational Intakes of Radionuclides: Part 3*; Annals of the ICRP: New York, NY, USA, 2017.
14. Tokonami, S. Some thought on new dose conversion factors for radon progeny inhalation. *Jpn. J. Health Phys.* **2018**, *53*, 282–293. [CrossRef]
15. United Nations Scientific Committee on the Effects of Atomic Radiation. *UNSCEAR 2006 Report, Effects of Ionizing Radiation*; Volume II: Annex E Sources-to-Effects Assessment for Radon in Homes and Workplaces; UNSCEAR: New York, NY, USA, 2009.
16. Hosoda, M. Report on a technical meeting on the implications of the new dose conversion factors for radon. *Jpn. J. Health Phys.* **2019**, *54*, 226–230. [CrossRef]

17. Kudo, H.; Tokonami, S.; Omori, Y.; Ishikawa, T.; Sahoo, S.K.; Akata, N.; Hosoda, M. Comparative dosimetry for radon and thoron in high background radiation areas in China. *Radiat. Prot. Dosim.* **2015**, *167*, 155–159. [CrossRef] [PubMed]
18. Tokonami, S.; Takahashi, H.; Kobayashi, Y.; Zhuo, W. Up-to-date radon-thoron discriminative detector for a large-scale survey. *Rev. Sci. Instrum.* **2005**, *76*, 113505. [CrossRef]
19. Szeiler, G.; Somlai, J.; Ishikawa, T.; Omori, Y.; Mishra, R.; Sapra, B.K.; Mayya, Y.S.; Tokonami, S.; Csordás, A.; Kovács, T. Preliminary results from an indoor radon thoron survey in Hungry. *Radiat. Prot. Dosim.* **2012**, *152*, 243–246. [CrossRef] [PubMed]
20. Pornnumpa, C.; Oyama, Y.; Iwaoka, K.; Hosoda, M.; Tokonami, S. Development of radon and thoron exposure system at Hirosaki University. *Radiat. Environ. Med.* **2018**, *7*, 13–20.
21. Tokonami, S.; Yang, M.; Yonehara, H.; Yamada, Y. Simple, discriminative measurement technique for radon and thoron concentrations with a single scintillation cell. *Rev. Sci. Instrum.* **2002**, *73*, 69–72. [CrossRef]
22. International Organization for Standardization. *Determination of the Characteristic Limits (Decision Threshold, Detection Limit and Limits of the Confidence Interval) for Measurements of Ionizing Radiation—Fundamentals and Application ISO11929*; ISO: Geneva, Switzerland, 2010.
23. Omori, Y.; Janik, M.; Sorimachi, A.; Ishikawa, T.; Tokonami, S. Effects of air exchange property of passive-type radon-thoron discriminative detectors on performance of radon and thoron measurements. *Radiat. Prot. Dosim.* **2012**, *152*, 140–145. [CrossRef]
24. Urban, M.; Piesch, E. Low level environmental radon dosimetry with a passive track etch detector device. *Radiat. Prot. Dosim.* **1981**, *1*, 97–109.
25. Pearson, M.D.; Spangler, R.R. Calibration of alpha-track monitors for measurement of thoron (220Rn). *Health Phys.* **1991**, *60*, 697–701.
26. Tokonami, S. Summary of dosimetry (radon and thoron) studies. In Proceedings of the Sixth International Conference on High Levels of Natural Radiation Areas, Osaka, Japan, 6–10 September 2004; Volume 1276, pp. 151–154.
27. Doi, M.; Kobayashi, S. The passive radon-thoron discriminative dosimeter for practical use. *Jpn. J. Health Phys.* **1994**, *29*, 155–166. [CrossRef]
28. McLaughlin, J.P.; Fitzgerald, B. Model for determining the response of passive alpha particle detectors to radon and its progeny in cylindrical detecting volumes. *Radiat. Prot. Dosim.* **1994**, *56*, 241–246. [CrossRef]
29. Quindos, L.S.; Fernandez, P.L.; Soto, J. National survey on indoor radon in Spain. *Environ. Int.* **1991**, *17*, 449–453. [CrossRef]
30. Espinosa, G.; Golzarri, J.I.; Rickards, J.; Gammage, R.B. Distribution of indoor radon levels in Mexico. *Radiat. Meas.* **1991**, *31*, 355–358. [CrossRef]
31. Khan, A.J. A study of indoor radon levels in Indian dwellings, influencing factors and lung cancer risks. *Radiat. Meas.* **2000**, *32*, 92–97. [CrossRef]
32. Kim, C.K.; Lee, S.C.; Lee, D.M.; Chang, B.U.; Rho, B.H.; Kang, H.D. Nationwide survey of radon levels in Korea. *Health Phys.* **2003**, *84*, 354–360. [CrossRef]
33. Radolić, V.; Vuković, B.; Stanić, D.; Katić, M. National survey of indoor radon levels in Croatia. *J. Radioanal. Chem.* **2006**, *269*, 87–90. [CrossRef]
34. Dowdal, A.; Murphy, P.; Pollard, D.; Fenton, D. Update of Ireland's national average indoor radon concentration—Application of a new survey protocol. *J. Environ. Radioact.* **2017**, *169–170*, 1–8. [CrossRef]

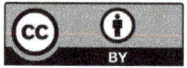

© 2020 by the authors. Licensee MDPI, Basel, Switzerland. This article is an open access article distributed under the terms and conditions of the Creative Commons Attribution (CC BY) license (http://creativecommons.org/licenses/by/4.0/).

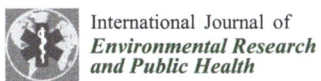

Article

Assessment of Radiation Dose from the Consumption of Bottled Drinking Water in Japan

Aoife Kinahan [1,*], Masahiro Hosoda [2], Kevin Kelleher [1], Takakiyo Tsujiguchi [2], Naofumi Akata [3], Shinji Tokonami [3], Lorraine Currivan [1] and Luis León Vintró [4]

1. Environmental Protection Agency, Clonskeagh Square, Clonskeagh, D14 H424 Dublin 14, Ireland; K.Kelleher@epa.ie (K.K.); L.Currivan@epa.ie (L.C.)
2. Graduate School of Health Science, Hirosaki University, 66-1 Hon-cho, Hirosaki, Aomori 036-8564, Japan; m_hosoda@hirosaki-u.ac.jp (M.H.); r.tsuji@hirosaki-u.ac.jp (T.T.)
3. Institute of Radiation Emergency Medicine, Hirosaki University, 66-1 Hon-cho, Hirosaki, Aomori 036-8564, Japan; akata@hirosaki-u.ac.jp (N.A.); tokonami@hirosaki-u.ac.jp (S.T.)
4. School of Physics, University College Dublin, Dublin 4, Ireland; luis.leon@ucd.ie
* Correspondence: A.Kinahan@epa.ie; Tel.: +353-01-268-0100

Received: 23 June 2020; Accepted: 8 July 2020; Published: 11 July 2020

Abstract: Activity concentrations of ^{234}U, ^{235}U, ^{238}U, ^{226}Ra, ^{228}Ra, ^{222}Rn, ^{210}Po, ^{210}Pb, ^{40}K, ^{3}H, ^{14}C, ^{134}Cs and ^{137}Cs were determined in 20 different Japanese bottled drinking water commercially available in Japan. The origins of the mineral water samples were geographically distributed across different regions of Japan. Activity concentrations above detection limits were measured for the radionuclides ^{234}U, ^{235}U, ^{238}U, ^{226}Ra, ^{228}Ra and ^{210}Po. An average total annual effective dose due to ingestion was estimated for adults, based on the average annual volume of bottled water consumed in Japan in 2019, reported to be 31.7 L/y per capita. The estimated dose was found to be below the recommended World Health Organisation (WHO) guidance level of 0.1 mSv/y for drinking water quality. The most significant contributor to the estimated dose was ^{228}Ra.

Keywords: dose assessment; Japan; bottled water; guidance level; WHO; natural radionuclides; artificial radionuclides; effective dose; ingestion

1. Introduction

People are continuously exposed, both externally and internally, to ionising radiation from naturally occurring sources, such as cosmic rays and terrestrial radioactivity, as well as artificial sources, such as weapons fallout and authorized and accidental releases from the nuclear industry. The main pathways for internal exposure to radiation are inhalation and the ingestion of food and water. On average, people typically receive an estimated dose of 0.3 mSv/y due to the ingestion of naturally occurring radionuclides such as ^{238}U, ^{232}Th, their daughter products and ^{40}K in their diet [1]. Drinking water contributes to approximately 0.01 mSv of this dose [2]. While this is a small fraction of the overall ingested dose, drinking water needs to be monitored, as there can be large variations in the radioactivity content in water as a result of the underlying geology of the water source. Higher radioactivity concentrations in drinking water can result in a higher contribution to the overall ingested dose. The World Health Organisation (WHO) has issued guidelines for drinking water quality. If the radioactivity dose from drinking water is below the WHO recommended guidance level of 0.1 mSv/y, water is deemed safe for human consumption from a radiological perspective [3].

The volume of bottled water being consumed has increased steadily worldwide for the past 14 years, and this trend is also reflected in the consumption of bottled water in Japan. According to the report by the Mineral Water Association of Japan, the annual intake of bottled water consumed in Japan in 2019 was reported to be 31.7 L/y per capita [4]. As shown in Figure 1, this is still significantly lower than bottled water consumption in many EU countries and the USA. However, a significant increase in the consumption of bottled water has occurred in Japan since 2011 [4], which has been attributed to consumer behavior after the Fukushima Dai-ichi Nuclear Power Plant (FDNPP) accident.

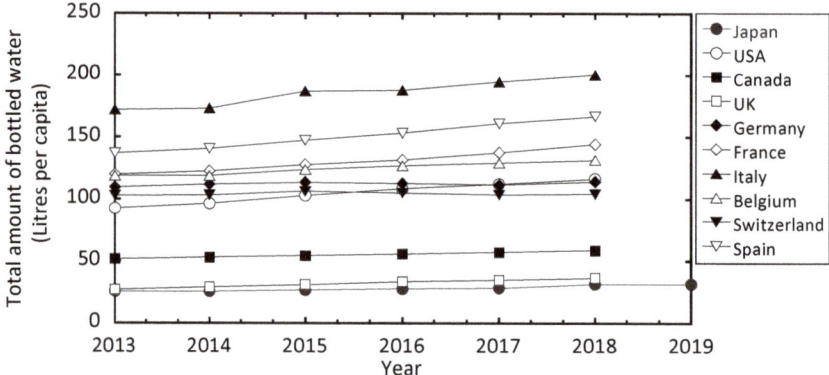

Figure 1. Trend graph for the consumption of bottled water in 10 different countries, including Japan [4].

In this study, an estimation is made of the radioactivity dose ingested from the consumption of bottled water in Japan, based on the measurement of activity concentrations for a range of radiologically significant natural and artificial radionuclides in a selection of 20 different bottled waters collected throughout the country. The inclusion of artificial radionuclides such as ^{3}H, ^{14}C (also naturally occurring), ^{134}Cs and ^{137}Cs is considered particularly important from a radiation risk communication perspective, particularly after the FDNPP accident in 2011. Currently, 33 nuclear reactors remain operable in Japan, of which 9, located in 5 separate power plants, are in operation [5].

A review of the scientific literature shows that a number of previous studies were carried out to determine the radioactivity levels in bottled water consumed in Japan. For example, Shiraishi et al. investigated the effective dose due to ^{232}Th and ^{238}U in imported mineral waters [6], and Shozugawa analysed four Japanese bottled waters for ^{134}Cs and ^{137}Cs following the FDNPP accident in 2011 [7]. However, no single study has attempted to analyse Japanese bottled waters for a comprehensive suite of radionuclides, although similar studies have been conducted in other countries for estimating the activity concentration and ingestion doses arising from the consumption of natural radionuclides in bottled water [8–22].

The annual effective dose arising from the consumption of bottled water is estimated in this study, which represents the first comprehensive study of this kind to be undertaken in relation to Japanese bottled water. The results presented are based on the analysis of 20 Japanese bottled water samples for natural and artificial radionuclides.

2. Materials and Methods

2.1. Sampling and Chemical Characteristics of Bottled Water

Drinking water samples from 20 different bottled water companies were purchased from Japanese supermarkets. The water sources were distributed across the country of Japan (Figure 2), which gives a wider geographical distribution to capture any potential effects of variability of the underlying geology of the regions. To increase representativeness, multiple bottles were purchased for each bottled water company and combined into a single sample. All water samples originated from natural mineral water sources.

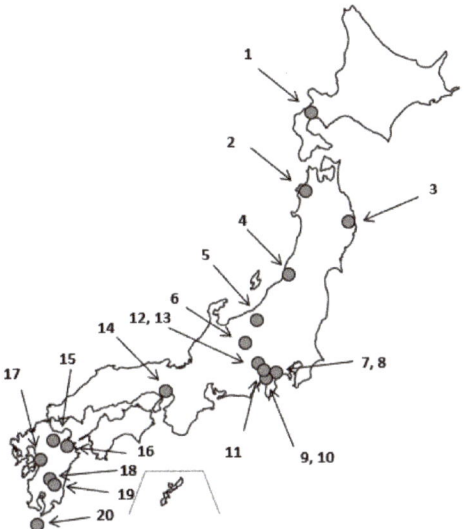

Figure 2. Locations of 20 bottle water samples.

To determine the chemical characteristics of the bottled water, pH and water hardness were evaluated using a pH meter (Eutech pH 700, Thermo Fisher Scientific, Waltham, MA, USA) and by determining the contents of magnesium (Mg) and calcium (Ca) by ICP–MS (ELAN 9000, Perkin Elmer, Germany), respectively. The water hardness ($CaCO_3$ content) was calculated using Equation (1).

$$\text{Total Hardness (mg/L as } CaCO_3) = 2.5Ca + 4.1Mg \tag{1}$$

According to WHO guidelines [23], waters are classified on the basis of their hardness into soft ($CaCO_3$ < 60), moderately hard (60 < $CaCO_3$ < 120), hard (120 < $CaCO_3$ < 180) and very hard ($CaCO_3$ > 180).

2.2. Radionuclide Determination

All samples were analysed for radioactivity in the Environmental Protection Agency, Ireland's radiation monitoring laboratory, which is accredited to ISO 17025 [24]. Table 1 gives a summary of the radionuclides analysed and the analytical techniques used for their determination. The methods and associated references are discussed in more detail below.

Table 1. Summary of the methods used for the analysis. HPGe, high-purity germanium.

Radionuclide	Preparation	Analytical Techniques
^3H, ^{14}C	8:12 mL water:/Ultima Gold ™ LLT 7:1:12 mL water/spike/Ultima Gold ™ LLT	Liquid scintillation counting
^{222}Rn	8:12 mL water/organic scintillation cocktail	Liquid scintillation counting
^{40}K, ^{134}Cs, ^{137}Cs	500 mL Marinelli	Direct counting on HPGe
^{40}K	Acidified	ICP–MS (evaluated from stable potassium to ^{40}K)
^{210}Po	500 mL water, acidified, spontaneous deposition	Alpha spectrometry
^{210}Pb	500 mL water, acidified, spontaneous deposition (after 6 months)	Alpha spectrometry
^{226}Ra, ^{228}Ra	1 to 4 L water, barium co-precipitation method, stored for one month prior to measurement	Gamma spectrometry (HPGe)
^{234}U, ^{235}U, ^{238}U	Acidified	ICP–MS (evaluated from total uranium)

2.2.1. Tritium and Carbon-14 Determination

For the determination of ^3H and ^{14}C, the spiked duplicate method was employed. Eight (8) mL of each water sample was taken for each radionuclide and mixed with 12 mL of Ultima Gold™ LLT

(Perkin Elmer, Groningen, The Netherlands) liquid scintillation cocktail. A duplicate sample was made with 7 mL of water sample and 1 mL of a calibrated ^{3}H or ^{14}C standard and mixed with 12 mL of Ultima Gold™ LLT. These samples were analysed for 720 min using a Tri-Carb® 3170TR/SL (Perkin Elmer, Waltham, MA, USA) low-level liquid scintillation counter. Analysis of the sample and the spiked duplicate sample was used to account for chemical and colour quenching in each sample. Optimised counting parameters were used with energy windows of 0.0–18.6 keV for ^{3}H and 0.0–156.0 keV for ^{14}C.

2.2.2. Radon Determination

For the determination of ^{222}Rn, 8 mL of sample was poured into a 20 mL scintillation vial containing Perkin Elmer, Ultima Gold™ F liquid scintillation cocktail. The vial was shaken for 60 s and counted on a Perkin Elmer Tri-Carb® 3170TR/SL low-level liquid scintillation counter for 60 min, after 4 h of dark equilibration and to allow for the short-lived daughter products to reach secular equilibrium. These short-lived daughter products were measured to assess radon activity. The alpha energy window was optimised to 300–1000 keV. The principle of this method is based on the ISO standard, ISO 13164–Part 4 [25].

2.2.3. Potassium and Caesium Determination

^{40}K and ^{134,137}Cs were analysed by direct counting on a gamma spectrometry system using in-house analytical methods accredited to the ISO 17025 standard [24]. The samples were measured with a high-purity germanium (HPGe) p-type co-axial detector (GC7520/S Mirion Technologies Inc., San Ramon, CA, USA). Radiocaesium concentrations in the water samples were determined by counting photons in the full-energy peak channels of 605 keV for ^{134}Cs, 662 keV for ^{137}Cs and 1461 keV for ^{40}K. The measurement time was 86,400 s. The uncertainty for the activity concentration was evaluated taking into account the uncertainties of the counts for the sample and background. Coincidence summing, self-attenuation and decay corrections were applied using Canberra ApexGamma software (Mirion Technologies Inc., San Ramon, CA, USA) in conjunction with GESPECOR Monte-Carlo software (CID Media GmbH, Hasselroth, Germany).

The stable potassium content was also determined by ICP–MS (ELAN 9000, Perkin Elmer, Waltham, MA, USA). Fifty (50) mL of water sample was preserved in 0.5%v/v nitric acid. The principle of this method is based on the ISO standard, ISO 17294-2:2016 [26]. The isotopic abundance of ^{40}K in natural potassium is 0.0117%, where ^{40}K has a specific activity concentration of 3.1×10^{-2} Bq/kg. The amount of K-40 present in the sample was calculated by multiplying the amount of potassium measured (mg/L) by the activity concentration (Bq/kg) and isotopic abundance.

2.2.4. Uranium Determination

The activity concentrations of ^{234,235,238}U were determined by ICP–MS (ELAN 9000, Perkin Elmer, Waltham, MA, USA). Fifty (50) mL of water sample was preserved in 0.5% v/v nitric acid. The total uranium content was assessed. The principle of this method is based on the ISO standard, ISO 17294-2:2016 [26] Assuming that the uranium isotopes are present in their natural isotopic abundances in the environment (^{234}U = 0.0055%, ^{235}U = 0.72%, ^{238}U > 99%), the activity concentration of ^{234}U, ^{235}U and ^{238}U were determined [21].

2.2.5. Radium Determination

For the determination of ^{226}Ra and ^{228}Ra, between 1.5 and 4 L was taken for the analysis. Each sample was acidified with nitric acid to a pH between 0 and 1. Thirty (30) mL of concentrated hydrochloric acid and 50 mg barium carrier solution were added to the sample in the beaker. The sample solution was boiled for 10 min. Thirty (30) mL of 9 M sulphuric acid was added and further boiled for 30 min to form a precipitate. The solution was left to cool overnight to allow the precipitation and settling of barium sulphate. The solution was then filtered through a pre-weighed filter paper (Whatman GF/C, 47 mm) (Whatman plc., Maidstone, United Kingdom). The filter was washed with

10 mL of ethanol and 10 mL of diethyl ether. The filter paper was allowed to dry overnight in a desiccator. The filter paper was prepared in a tightly sealed container, and the daughter products ^{214}Pb, ^{214}Bi (^{226}Ra) and ^{228}Ac (^{228}Ra) were ingrown for more than 30 days to reach secular equilibrium with Ra. The measurements were made via HPGe gamma spectrometry. GESPECOR Monte-Carlo software (CID Media GmbH, Hasselroth, Germany) is typically used for correction for true coincidence summing and self-attenuation of the samples; however, these were not required in this instance [27].

2.2.6. Polonium and Lead Determination

For the determination of ^{210}Po and ^{210}Pb, samples were prepared for spontaneous deposition on a silver (Ag) disc. An aliquot of 500 mL of water sample was placed in a jar and acidified with 2 M HCl (pH of 1–2) followed by the addition of 0.5 g of ascorbic acid and 0.25 Bq of ^{209}Po tracer. A silver disc was fixed to a holder attached to the lid of the jar, which allowed the disc to be immersed in the solution. The solution was heated to 80 °C with stirring for 8 h. The disc was rinsed with water and methanol and dried at room temperature. The ^{210}Po activities were determined by counting the disks for 345,600 s using PIPS detectors in the Canberra Alpha Analyst (Mirion Technologies Inc., San Ramon, California, USA) integrated spectrometry system in conjunction with the Apex Alpha spectrometry software (Mirion Technologies Inc., San Ramon, California, USA) [28]. The water samples were stored for 6 months, to allow the ingrowth of the ^{210}Pb daughter product, ^{210}Po. The spontaneous deposition process was repeated with a new aliquot of ^{209}Po tracer. After analysing the measurements by alpha spectrometry, the ^{210}Pb activity concentrations were determined from the polonium activities using Bateman's equations [29].

2.3. Determination of the Annual Effective Ingestion Doses

The annual effective dose for each radionuclide was estimated using the following equation:

$$E_d = A_c \times C_a \times D_{coeff} \qquad (2)$$

where E_d is the annual effective dose due to ingestion (nSv); A_c is the radionuclide activity concentration measured in the water sample (Bq/L); C_a is the annual consumption of 31.7 L (per capita) reported by the Japanese Mineral Association [4]; and D_{coeff} is the dose coefficient provided by the ICRP (nSv/Bq) [30], whose values are given in Table 2. To get the total effective dose for a given sample, the effective doses for each radionuclide were added. The effective dose was estimated for each sample based on the activities of the radionuclides analysed. For measurements below the minimum detectable activity concentration (MDC), the MDC value was used for the dose estimation, which gave a maximum annual effective dose for each sample.

Table 2. Dose coefficient values used for this study (nSv/Bq).

Isotope	Dose Coefficient (nSv/Bq)
^{222}Rn [31] [1]	3.5×10^0
^{3}H	1.8×10^{-2}
^{14}C	5.8×10^{-1}
^{134}Cs	1.9×10^1
^{137}Cs	1.3×10^1
^{210}Po	1.2×10^3
^{210}Pb	6.9×10^2
^{226}Ra	2.8×10^2
^{228}Ra	6.9×10^2
^{234}U	4.9×10^1
^{235}U	4.7×10^1
^{238}U	4.5×10^1

[1] Specific to ^{222}Rn in drinking water, the value is the sum of weighted equivalent doses.

3. Results and Discussion

3.1. pH and Water Hardness

The pH of the 20 bottled water samples ranged from 6.2 to 8.3. The water hardness, which was equivalent to the $CaCO_3$ content, ranged from below the detection limit (<4 mg/L) to 147 mg/L. Only one sample (No. 18) was classified as hard water. Samples 1, 3 and 17 were classified as moderately hard water, and the remaining Japanese bottled water samples were classified as soft water. No apparent differences were observed between soft and hard water samples.

3.2. Radionuclide Activity Concentrations

The activity concentrations measured in the bottled water samples, referenced to the date of receipt at the EPA laboratory, are given in Table 3. ^{222}Rn was not expected to be present in bottled water, as during the bottling process radon gas is released from the product. The analysis was conducted to rule out any ingrowth from its parent radionuclide, ^{226}Ra. Elevated levels of ^{3}H and ^{14}C were not expected either, as sources of these radionuclides discharged into the catchments of the bottled water sources are not significant or present in the environment at levels above the limits of detection for these radionuclides. This was confirmed by our measurements, which showed ^{3}H and ^{14}C activity concentrations below the detection limits in all cases. There were no detectable quantities of ^{134}Cs and ^{137}Cs in the water samples either. This indicates that the bottled water is not affected by fallout originating from the FDNPP accident. The MDC of ^{222}Rn, ^{3}H, ^{14}C, ^{134}Cs and ^{137}Cs were determined as 60, 210, 160, 10 and 9 mBq/L, respectively. ^{40}K determined by gamma analysis had an MDC of 160 mBq/. Therefore, the quoted ^{40}K activity concentrations are based on the determination of stable K by ICP–MS and were calculated based on its natural abundance in the environment.

Table 3. Radionuclide activity concentration and standard uncertainty ($k = 1$) values in bottled water (mBq/L).

Sample	^{210}Po	^{210}Pb	^{226}Ra	^{228}Ra	^{234}U	^{235}U	^{238}U	^{40}K
1	$<9.4 \times 10^{-1}$	$(5.7 \pm 0.5) \times 10^0$	$<1.9 \times 10^2$	$(2.6 \pm 1.5) \times 10^1$	$(2.6 \pm 0.5) \times 10^1$	$(1.2 \pm 0.2) \times 10^0$	$(2.4 \pm 0.5) \times 10^1$	$(1.3 \pm 0.3) \times 10^{-1}$
2	$<7.4 \times 10^{-1}$	$(1.8 \pm 0.2) \times 10^0$	$<1.1 \times 10^2$	$<3.7 \times 10^1$	$<1.3 \times 10^{-1}$	$<5.8 \times 10^{-3}$	$<1.2 \times 10^{-1}$	$<7.7 \times 10^{-3}$
3	$<1.3 \times 10^0$	$(2.0 \pm 0.2) \times 10^0$	$<1.8 \times 10^2$	$<3.6 \times 10^2$	$(2.4 \pm 0.5) \times 10^0$	$(1.0 \pm 0.2) \times 10^0$	$(2.2 \pm 0.5) \times 10^0$	$(1.5 \pm 0.3) \times 10^{-2}$
4	$(2.6 \pm 0.4) \times 10^0$	$(7.4 \pm 0.7) \times 10^0$	$<2.0 \times 10^2$	$<3.9 \times 10^2$	$(2.6 \pm 0.5) \times 10^{-1}$	$(1.2 \pm 0.2) \times 10^{-2}$	$(2.4 \pm 0.5) \times 10^{-1}$	$(1.9 \pm 0.4) \times 10^{-2}$
5	$<1.2 \times 10^0$	$<1.7 \times 10^0$	$<1.7 \times 10^2$	$<3.4 \times 10^2$	$(1.3 \pm 0.3) \times 10^{-1}$	$(5.8 \pm 0.1) \times 10^{-3}$	$(1.2 \pm 0.3) \times 10^{-1}$	$(3.8 \pm 0.8) \times 10^{-2}$
6	$<1.3 \times 10^0$	$(5.3 \pm 0.5) \times 10^0$	$(8.5 \pm 3.9) \times 10^0$	$(2.5 \pm 1.1) \times 10^1$	$(7.9 \pm 0.2) \times 10^{-1}$	$(3.5 \pm 0.7) \times 10^{-2}$	$(7.3 \pm 0.2) \times 10^{-1}$	$(6.2 \pm 1.3) \pm 10^{-2}$
7	$<8.9 \times 10^{-1}$	$(3.8 \pm 0.3) \times 10^0$	$<2.3 \times 10^2$	$<4.2 \times 10^1$	$(5.2 \pm 1.1) \times 10^{-1}$	$(2.3 \pm 0.5) \times 10^{-2}$	$(4.8 \pm 1.0) \times 10^{-1}$	$(3.5 \pm 0.7) \times 10^{-2}$
8	$<1.2 \times 10^0$	$(5.3 \pm 0.5) \times 10^{-1}$	$<1.7 \times 10^2$	$<3.4 \times 10^1$	$(2.6 \pm 0.5) \times 10^{-1}$	$(1.2 \pm 0.2) \times 10^{-2}$	$(2.4 \pm 0.5) \times 10^{-1}$	$(4.9 \pm 1.0) \times 10^{-2}$
9	$<1.1 \times 10^0$	$(3.7 \pm 0.3) \times 10^0$	$<6.0 \times 10^2$	$<1.1 \times 10^2$	$(1.3 \pm 0.3) \times 10^{-1}$	$(5.8 \pm 1.2) \times 10^{-3}$	$(1.2 \pm 0.3) \times 10^{-1}$	$(2.5 \pm 0.5) \times 10^{-2}$
10	$<1.1 \times 10^0$	$(8.1 \pm 0.7) \times 10^{-1}$	$<1.1 \times 10^2$	$<3.9 \times 10^2$	$(1.3 \pm 0.3) \times 10^{-1}$	$(5.8 \pm 1.2) \times 10^{-3}$	$(1.2 \pm 0.3) \times 10^{-1}$	$(2.5 \pm 0.5) \times 10^{-2}$
11	$<5.7 \times 10^{-1}$	$(2.0 \pm 0.2) \times 10^0$	$<1.5 \times 10^2$	$<2.9 \times 10^2$	$(3.9 \pm 0.8) \times 10^{-1}$	$(1.7 \pm 0.4) \times 10^{-2}$	$(3.6 \pm 0.8) \times 10^{-1}$	$(2.4 \pm 0.5) \times 10^{-2}$
12	$(1.0 \pm 0.3) \times 10^0$	$(4.4 \pm 0.4) \times 10^0$	$<2.4 \times 10^2$	$<4.3 \times 10^1$	$(5.2 \pm 0.1) \times 10^{-1}$	$(2.3 \pm 0.5) \times 10^{-2}$	$(4.8 \pm 1.0) \times 10^{-1}$	$(3.2 \pm 0.7) \times 10^{-2}$
13	$(4.9 \pm 0.4) \times 10^0$	$(1.9 \pm 0.2) \times 10^1$	$(1.2 \pm 0.5) \times 10^1$	$<3.3 \times 10^2$	$(1.6 \pm 0.3) \times 10^0$	$(6.9 \pm 0.1) \times 10^{-2}$	$(1.5 \pm 0.3) \times 10^0$	$(5.1 \pm 1.1) \times 10^{-2}$
14	$(1.5 \pm 0.6) \times 10^0$	$(4.3 \pm 0.4) \times 10^0$	$<2.3 \times 10^2$	$(4.9 \pm 1.8) \times 10^1$	$<1.3 \times 10^{-1}$	$<5.8 \times 10^{-3}$	$<1.2 \times 10^{-1}$	$(2.9 \pm 0.6) \times 10^{-2}$
15	$<1.4 \times 10^0$	$(3.0 \pm 0.3) \times 10^0$	$<1.9 \times 10^2$	$<3.9 \times 10^2$	$(3.0 \pm 0.6) \times 10^0$	$(1.3 \pm 0.3) \times 10^{-1}$	$(2.8 \pm 0.6) \times 10^0$	$(2.5 \pm 0.5) \times 10^{-1}$
16	$<9.7 \times 10^{-1}$	$(4.5 \pm 0.4) \times 10^0$	$<1.9 \times 10^2$	$(1.9 \pm 1.0) \times 10^1$	$(1.4 \pm 0.3) \times 10^{-1}$	$(6.3 \pm 1.3) \times 10^{-2}$	$(1.3 \pm 0.3) \times 10^0$	$(8.4 \pm 1.7) \times 10^{-1}$
17	$<8.3 \times 10^{-1}$	$(2.4 \pm 0.2) \times 10^0$	$(1.3 \pm 0.6) \times 10^1$	$<3.2 \times 10^2$	$(2.6 \pm 0.5) \times 10^{-1}$	$(1.2 \pm 0.2) \times 10^{-2}$	$(2.4 \pm 0.5) \times 10^{-1}$	$(1.4 \pm 0.3) \times 10^{-1}$
18	$<1.4 \times 10^0$	$(2.6 \pm 0.2) \times 10^0$	$<1.6 \times 10^2$	$<3.2 \times 10^2$	$(2.8 \pm 0.6) \times 10^0$	$(1.2 \pm 0.2) \times 10^{-1}$	$(2.5 \pm 0.5) \times 10^0$	$(2.4 \pm 0.5) \times 10^{-1}$
19	$(1.9 \pm 1.5) \times 10^0$	$(6.9 \pm 0.6) \times 10^0$	$(1.2 \pm 0.4) \times 10^1$	$<2.5 \times 10^1$	$(1.7 \pm 0.4) \times 10^{-1}$	$(7.5 \pm 1.5) \times 10^{-2}$	$(1.6 \pm 0.3) \times 10^0$	$(7.2 \pm 1.5) \times 10^{-2}$
20	$(1.7 \pm 1.5) \times 10^0$	$(5.9 \pm 0.5) \times 10^0$	$<7.1 \times 10^2$	$(1.6 \pm 0.8) \times 10^1$	$(1.3 \pm 0.3) \times 10^{-1}$	$(5.8 \pm 1.2) \times 10^{-3}$	$(1.2 \pm 0.3) \times 10^{-1}$	$(2.5 \pm 0.5) \times 10^{-2}$

3.2.1. Polonium and Lead activity Concentrations

In Table 4, the minimum, maximum and median activity concentrations of ^{210}Po and ^{210}Pb of the detected (above MDC) concentrations are shown. The maximum estimated annual effective dose, determined using Equation (2), is also included, which is based on the maximum measured activities for each nuclide. Seven bottled water samples showed ^{210}Po concentrations above the MDC. For ^{210}Pb, 19 samples were above the MDC.

Table 4. Activity concentrations for polonium and lead measured in bottled water (mBq/L).

Isotope	Min	Max	Median	Maximum Annual Effective Dose [1] (nSv)
^{210}Po [2]	1.0 ± 0.26	4.9 ± 0.39	1.7 ± 0.34	186
^{210}Pb [3]	0.53 ± 0.050	19 ± 1.8	3.8 ± 0.34	421

[1] Based on measured activities; [2] minimum detectable activity concentrations (MDC) = 0.06 mBq/L; [3] MDC = 0.12 mBq/L.

3.2.2. Radium Isotope Activity Concentrations

In Table 5, the minimum, maximum and median values of the radium isotopes of the detected concentrations are shown. The maximum estimated annual effective dose using Equation (2) is also included, which is based on the measured activities. Four and five bottled water samples showed concentrations of ^{226}Ra and ^{228}Ra above the MDC, respectively.

Table 5. Activity concentrations for radium measured in bottled water (mBq/L).

Isotope	Min	Max	Median	Maximum Annual Effective Dose [1] (nSv)
^{226}Ra [2]	0.85 ± 0.39	13 ± 5.5	12 ± 4.3	100
^{228}Ra [3]	16 ± 8.2	49 ± 18	25 ± 11	589

[1] Based on measured activities; [2] MDC = 112 mBq/L; [3] MDC = 25 mBq/L.

3.2.3. Uranium Isotope Activity Concentrations

In Table 6, the minimum, maximum and median values of the uranium isotopes of the detected concentrations are shown. The maximum estimated annual effective dose, determined using Equation (2), is also included, which is based on the measured activities. Eighteen bottled water samples contained detectable amounts of total uranium, and two were below the limits of detection. The total uranium content of the bottled water was measured, and the activity concentrations were calculated based on their natural abundance in the environment.

Table 6. Activity concentrations for uranium analysed in bottled water (mBq/L).

Isotope	Min	Max	Median	Maximum Annual Effective Dose [1] (nSv)
^{234}U [2]	0.13 ± 0.030	26 ± 5.4	0.52 ± 0.11	3.3
^{235}U [3]	0.005 ± 0.002	1.2 ± 0.24	0.023 ± 0.005	0.14
^{238}U [4]	0.24 ± 0.050	24 ± 5.0	0.48 ± 0.099	2.8

[1] Based on measured activities; [2] MDC = 0.13 mBq/L; [3] MDC = 0.005 mBq/L; [4] MDC = 0.12 mBq/L.

3.2.4. Comparison of Activity Concentrations in Bottled Mineral Waters for Sale in Other Countries

The activity concentrations found in the bottled water samples in this study were compared to those determined in previous studies in different countries. Most studies included the analysis of radium and uranium. In general, most studies reported radium as the largest contributor to the ingestion dose, apart from Rozmaric et al. [20] who reported uranium isotopes as the main contributor in Croatian mineral waters. The activity concentrations measured in this work for ^{210}Po were 1.0–4.9 mBq/L. These values are comparable with results found in Croatia [20] but are lower than those reported in Italy [14,15] and Austria [10,19]. Activity concentrations for ^{210}Pb were 0.53–19 mBq/L, whereas studies in Austria [10,19] showed a broader range for these values but reported a similar geometric mean for ^{210}Pb activities. In contrast, values reported for Croatian waters [20] showed a lower range of activities. The activity concentrations for ^{226}Ra and ^{228}Ra ranged between 0.85 and 13 mBq/L and 16 and 49 mBq/L, respectively, which are comparable to the values found in Greece [12] and Pakistan [13]. Studies in Algeria [9], Croatia [20], Italy [14,15] and Poland [16] reported a much broader range of ^{226}Ra and ^{228}Ra activity concentrations in bottled water, but all geometric mean values are in agreement with the values reported in this study, with the exception of those for Algeria [9]. Algeria reported a mean value of 26 mBq/L. Studies in Austria [10,19] reported a broader range in radium activity concentrations and a higher mean value than this study. Studies in Malaysia [22] and Hungary [11] reported a very large range for ^{226}Ra, with some values reported above 3000 mBq/L. For uranium isotopes, the ranges of activities reported in Japanese bottled water in this study were 0.24–24 mBq/L and 0.13–26 mBq/L for ^{238}U and ^{234}U, respectively. Studies in Poland [16] reported a lower range in uranium activity concentrations, whereas Croatia [20] and Tunisia [18] reported similar activities. Studies in Italy [14,15] and Austria reported a broader range in their results. In both Italian studies, the geometric mean values for ^{234}U, ^{235}U and ^{238}U were much higher than the reported geometric mean values in this study [14,15].

It has been reported that the absorbed dose rates in air due to terrestrial radiation in western parts of Japan are higher than those in eastern parts of Japan [32]. This difference in dose rate distribution has been attributed to the presence in western Japan of areas with higher natural uranium and actinium series radionuclides, corresponding to granitic regions with enhanced natural radionuclide concentrations, relative to other areas characterised by andesite or andosol soils. To investigate a possible similar effect on the uranium content between waters sourced in western and eastern Japan, the median activity concentrations were statistically compared. The median values of ^{234}U, ^{235}U and ^{238}U in western parts of Japan (Nos. 14, 15, 16, 17, 18, 19 and 20) were evaluated as 0.17 mBq/L, 0.063 mBq/L and 1.3 mBq/L, respectively. The corresponding values in eastern parts of Japan were evaluated as 0.39 mBq/L, 0.017 mBq/L and 0.36 mBq/L, respectively. A Mann–Whitney U Test (with a critical value of U at $p < 0.05$) showed that the values for each radionuclide from western and eastern Japan were not significantly different from each other.

3.3. Dose Assessment of the Maximum Annual Effective Ingestion Doses from Bottled Water

According to the WHO, ^{40}K levels do not need to be measured when assessing the dose from drinking water. The potassium level in a healthy individual is kept constant by a range of physiological processes in order to regulate the functions of the body [2]. Therefore, the levels of ^{40}K were not included in the calculation of the annual effective ingestion dose.

Figure 3 presents an overview of the estimated maximum annual effective dose for each sample dose received from the radionuclides analysed in the bottled water samples. The highest dose value calculated was 10% of the guidance level recommended by the WHO. The average annual effective dose estimated for all samples was 5.6 μSv. There was little correlation between doses and locations across Japan. There were two bottled water products from the same location, i.e., 9 and 10 and 7 and 8, and these reported similar dose values. In contrast, samples 12 and 13 were not similar, though they were from the same location.

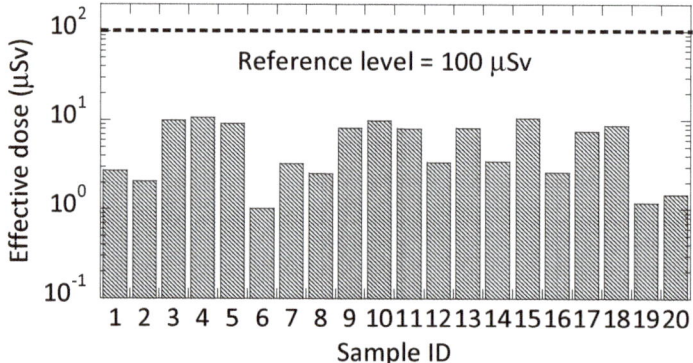

Figure 3. The maximum annual effective dose in each bottled water sample compared to the guidance level.

4. Conclusions

The activity concentrations of natural and artificial radionuclides in a wide range of bottled water produced in Japan were determined. The results showed that the highest activities were due to naturally occurring radionuclides, i.e., Ra and Pb isotopes. The results are comparable to results from other studies around the world. The total annual effective ingestion dose was assessed from the activity concentrations measured in this study and the average rate of consumption of bottled mineral water in Japan per capita. In all cases, the estimated doses were at least an order of magnitude below the WHO recommended guidance level of 0.1 mSv for the consumption of drinking water.

Author Contributions: Conceptualization, M.H. and K.K.; Methodology, M.H., K.K. and A.K.; Formal Analysis, A.K., M.H. and K.K.; Investigation, A.K., M.H. and K.K., Data Curation, A.K., K.K. and M.H.; Writing—original draft preparation, A.K.; Writing—review and editing, M.H., K.K., T.T., N.A., S.T., L.C. and L.L.V.; Funding acquisition, M.H. All authors have read and agreed to the published version of the manuscript.

Funding: This work was partially supported by the Hirosaki University Institutional Research Grant.

Conflicts of Interest: The authors declare no conflict of interest.

References

1. United Nations Scientific Committee on the Effects of Atomic Radiation (UNSCEAR). *UNSCEAR 2000 Report to the General Assembly, with Scientific Annexes, Volume I: SOURCES*; United Nations: New York, NY, USA, 2000.
2. World Health Organization (WHO). *Management of Radioactivity in Drinking-Water*; World Health Organization: Geneva, Switzerland, 2018.
3. World Health Organization (WHO). *Guidelines for Drinking-Water Quality, 4th edition, Incorporating the 1st Addendum*; World Health Organization: Geneva, Switzerland, 2017; pp. 203–218.
4. The Mineral Water Association of Japan. Data Sheets—Various Statistics of Mineral Waters. Available online: https://minekyo.net/publics/index/5/ (accessed on 1 April 2020).
5. The Federation of Electric Power Companies of Japan (FEPC). Nuclear Power Plants in Japan. Available online: https://www.fepc.or.jp/english/nuclear/power_generation/plants/index.html (accessed on 1 April 2020).
6. Shiraishi, K.; Kimura, S.; Sahoo, S.K.; Arae, H. Dose effect for Japanese due to 232Th and 238U in imported drinking water. *Health Phys.* **2004**, *86*, 365–373. [CrossRef] [PubMed]
7. Shozugawa, K.; Saito, T.; Hori, M.; Matsuo, M. High-sensitivity determination of radioactive cesium in Japanese foodstuffs: 3 years after the Fukushima accident. *J. Radioanal. Nucl. Chem.* **2016**, *307*, 2117–2122. [CrossRef]
8. Dávila Rangel, J.I.; López del Río, H.; García, F.M.; Torres, L.L.Q.; Villalba, M.L.; Sujo, L.C.; Cabrera, M.E.M. Radioactivity in bottled waters sold in Mexico. *Appl. Radiat. Isot.* **2002**, *56*, 931–936. [CrossRef]

9. Amrani, D. Natural radioactivity in Algerian bottled mineral waters. *J. Radioanal. Nucl. Chem.* **2002**, *252*, 597–600. [CrossRef]
10. Kralik, C.; Friedrich, M.; Vojir, F. Natural radionuclides in bottled water in Austria. *J. Environ. Radioact.* **2003**, *65*, 233–241. [CrossRef]
11. Somlai, J.; Horváth, G.; Kanyár, B.; Kovács, T.; Bodrogi, E.; Kávási, N. Concentration of 226Ra in Hungarian bottled mineral water. *J. Environ. Radioact.* **2002**, *62*, 235–240. [CrossRef]
12. Karamanis, D.; Stamoulis, K.; Ioannides, K.G. Natural radionuclides and heavy metals in bottled water in Greece. *Desalination* **2007**, *213*, 90–97. [CrossRef]
13. Fatima, I.; Zaidi, J.H.; Arif, M.; Tahir, S.N.A. Measurement of natural radioactivity in bottled drinking water in Pakistan and consequent dose estimates. *Radiat. Prot. Dosim.* **2007**, *123*, 234–240. [CrossRef] [PubMed]
14. Desideri, D.; Meli, M.A.; Feduzi, L.; Roselli, C.; Rongoni, A.; Saetta, D. ^{238}U, ^{234}U, ^{226}Ra, ^{210}Po concentrations of bottled mineral waters in Italy and their dose contribution. *J. Environ. Radioact.* **2007**, *94*, 86–97. [CrossRef] [PubMed]
15. Jia, G.; Torri, G. Estimation of radiation doses to members of the public in Italy from intakes of some important naturally occurring radionuclides (^{238}U, ^{234}U, ^{235}U, ^{226}Ra, ^{228}Ra, ^{224}Ra and ^{210}Po) in drinking water. *Appl. Radiat. Isot.* **2007**, *65*, 849–857. [CrossRef] [PubMed]
16. Kozłowska, B.; Walencik, A.; Dorda, J.; Przylibski, T.A. Uranium, radium and ^{40}K isotopes in bottled mineral waters from Outer Carpathians, Poland. *Radiat. Meas.* **2007**, *42*, 1380–1386. [CrossRef]
17. Palomo, M.; Peñalver, A.; Borrull, F.; Aguilar, C. Measurement of radioactivity in bottled drinking water in Spain. *Appl. Radiat. Isot.* **2007**, *65*, 1165–1172. [CrossRef] [PubMed]
18. Gharbi, F.; Baccouche, S.; Abdelli, W.; Samaali, M.; Oueslati, M.; Trabelsi, A. Uranium isotopes in Tunisian bottled mineral waters. *J. Environ. Radioact.* **2010**, *101*, 589–590. [CrossRef] [PubMed]
19. Wallner, G.; Jabbar, T. Natural radionuclides in Austrian bottled mineral waters. *J. Radioanal. Nucl. Chem.* **2010**, *286*, 329–334. [CrossRef]
20. Rožmarić, M.; Rogić, M.; Benedik, L.; Štrok, M. Natural radionuclides in bottled drinking waters produced in Croatia and their contribution to radiation dose. *Sci. Total Environ.* **2012**, *437*, 53–60. [CrossRef] [PubMed]
21. Currivan, L.; Kelleher, K.; Solodovnik, E.; McMahon, C. *Radioactivity in Bottled Water Produced in Ireland*; Technical Report; Radiological Protection Institute of Ireland: Dublin, Ireland, 2013.
22. Khandaker, M.U.; Nasir, N.L.M.; Zakirin, N.S.; Kassim, H.A.; Asaduzzaman, K.; Bradley, D.A.; Zulkifli, M.Y.; Hayyan, A. Radiation dose to the Malaysian populace via the consumption of bottled mineral water. *Radiat. Phys. Chem.* **2017**, *140*, 173–179. [CrossRef]
23. World Health Organization (WHO). *Hardness in Drinking-Water: Background Document for Development of WHO Guidelines for Drinking-Water Quality*; World Health Organization: Geneva, Switzerland, 2010.
24. International Organization for Standardization (ISO). *ISO 17025 General Requirements for the Competence of Testing and Calibration Laboratories*; ISO: Geneva, Switzerland, 2017.
25. International Organization for Standardization (ISO). *ISO 13164-4:2015—Water quality—Radon-222—Part 4: Test. Method Using Two-Phase Liquid Scintillation Counting*; ISO: Geneva, Switzerland, 2015.
26. International Organization for Standardization (ISO). *ISO 17294-2:2016—Water Quality—Application of Inductively Coupled Plasma Mass Spectrometry (ICP-MS)—Part 2: Determination of Selected Elements Including Uranium Isotopes*; ISO: Geneva, Switzerland, 2016.
27. Hosoda, M.; Kelleher, K.; Murray, M.; McGinnity, P.; Hanley, O.; Wong, J.; Currivan, L. Generation and Migration of ^{222}Rn in BaSO$_4$ Precipitate Samples and Implications for their Analysis for ^{226}Ra by Gamma Spectrometry. *Radiat. Environ. Med.* **2016**, *5*, 22–28.
28. Flynn, W.W. The Determination of Low Levels of Polonium-210 in Environmental Materials. *Anal. Chim. Acta* **1968**, *43*, 221–227. [CrossRef]
29. Ebaid, Y.Y.; Khater, A.E.M. Determination of 210 Pb in Environmental Samples. *J. Radioanal. Nucl. Chem.* **2006**, *270*, 609–619. [CrossRef]
30. ICRP. *ICRP Publication 72. Age-dependent Doses to the Members of the Public from Intake of Radionuclides—Part 5 Compilation of Ingestion and Inhalation Coefficients*; ICRP: Oxford, UK, 1996.

31. National Research Council (US). *Risk Assessment of Radon in Drinking Water*; National Academies Press (US): Washington, DC, USA, 1999; p. 76.
32. Omori, Y.; Hosoda, M.; Takahashi, F.; Sanada, T.; Hirao, S.; Ono, K.; Furukawa, M. Japanese Population Dose from Natural Radiation. *J. Radiol. Prot.* **2020**. Available online: https://iopscience.iop.org/article/10.1088/1361-6498/ab73b1/meta (accessed on 1 April 2020). [CrossRef] [PubMed]

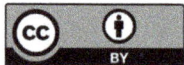

© 2020 by the authors. Licensee MDPI, Basel, Switzerland. This article is an open access article distributed under the terms and conditions of the Creative Commons Attribution (CC BY) license (http://creativecommons.org/licenses/by/4.0/).

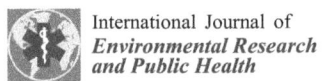

Article

Observation of Dispersion in the Japanese Coastal Area of Released ^{90}Sr, ^{134}Cs, and ^{137}Cs from the Fukushima Daiichi Nuclear Power Plant to the Sea in 2013

Hirofumi Tazoe [1,*], Takeyasu Yamagata [2], Kazuki Tsujita [3], Hisao Nagai [2], Hajime Obata [4], Daisuke Tsumune [5], Jota Kanda [6] and Masatoshi Yamada [1,7]

1. Department of Radiation Chemistry, Institute of Radiation Emergency Mediation, Hirosaki University, Hirosaki 036-8652, Japan; myamada@hirosaki-u.ac.jp
2. College of Humanities and Sciences, Nihon University, Tokyo 156-8550, Japan; yamagata@chs.nihon-u.ac.jp (T.Y.); hnagai@chs.nihon-u.ac.jp (H.N.)
3. Graduate School of Basic Integrated Sciences, Nihon University, Tokyo 156-8550, Japan; kaz.tsujita.chs@gmail.com
4. Atmosphere and Ocean Research Institute, University of Tokyo 277-8564, Japan; obata@aori.u-tokyo.ac.jp
5. Environmental Science Research Laboratory, Central Research Institute of Electric Power Industry, Tokyo 270-1194, Japan; tsumune@criepi.denken.or.jp
6. Department of Ocean Sciences, Graduate Faculty of Marine Science, Tokyo University of Marine Science and Technology, Tokyo 108-8477, Japan; jkanda@kaiyodai.ac.jp
7. Marine Ecology Research Institute, Chiba 299-5105, Japan
* Correspondence: tazoe@hirosaki-u.ac.jp; Tel.: +81-172-39-5503

Received: 30 September 2019; Accepted: 22 October 2019; Published: 24 October 2019

Abstract: The March 2011 earthquake and tsunami resulted in significant damage to the Fukushima Daiichi Nuclear Power Plant (FDNPP) and the subsequent release of radionuclides into the ocean. Here, we investigated the spatial distribution of strontium-90 (^{90}Sr) and cesium-134/cesium-137 ($^{134, 137}$Cs) in surface seawater of the coastal region near the FDNPP. In the coastal region, ^{90}Sr activity was high, from 0.89 to 29.13 mBq L^{-1}, with detectable FDNPP site-derived ^{134}Cs. This indicated that release of ^{90}Sr from the power plant was ongoing even in May 2013, as was that of ^{134}Cs and ^{137}Cs. ^{90}Sr activities measured at open ocean sites corresponded to background derived from atmospheric nuclear weapons testing fallout. The FDNPP site-derived ^{90}Sr/^{137}Cs activity ratios in seawater were much higher than those in the direct discharge event in March 2011, in river input, and in seabed sediment; those ratios showed large variability, ranging from 0.16 to 0.64 despite a short sampling period. This FDNPP site-derived ^{90}Sr/^{137}Cs activity ratio suggests that these radionuclides were mainly derived from stagnant water in the reactor and turbine buildings of the FDNPP, while a different source with a low ^{90}Sr/^{137}Cs ratio could contribute to and produce the temporal variability of the ^{90}Sr/^{137}Cs ratio in coastal water. We estimated the release rate of ^{90}Sr from the power plant as 9.6 ± 6.1 GBq day^{-1} in May 2013 on the basis of the relationship between ^{90}Sr and ^{137}Cs activity (^{90}Sr/^{137}Cs = 0.66 ± 0.05) and ^{137}Cs release rate.

Keywords: Fukushima Daiichi Nuclear Power Plant; strontium-90; cesium-137; seawater monitoring; contaminated water

1. Introduction

Large amounts of radionuclides, such as cesium-134 (^{134}Cs), cesium-137 (^{137}Cs), and iodine-131 (^{131}I), were dispersed into the terrestrial and aquatic environments as a result of an accident at the Fukushima Daiichi Nuclear Power Plant (FDNPP) of the Tokyo Electric Power Company (TEPCO) in March 2011. Atmospheric release of strontium-90 (^{90}Sr) in March 2011 was two to four orders of magnitude lower than that of ^{137}Cs on the basis of an analysis of highly contaminated soils (<1.1 Bq g^{-1}) and vegetation (0.026–1.1 Bq g^{-1}) collected from a contaminated area in Japan [1]. These ^{90}Sr/^{137}Cs activity ratios were much lower than the ratio for the estimated nuclear fuel compositions (^{90}Sr/^{137}Cs = 0.74) found in the reactor obtained by the ORIGEN2 code [2]. Atmospheric ^{90}Sr release (0.01–0.14 PBq [3]) was estimated at less than 0.027% of the total amount in the nuclear fuel (5.2 × 10^2 PBq [2]) at FDNPP reactor units 1, 2, and 3. Most of the ^{90}Sr remained in the reactor, although some of it had dissolved in stagnant water in the reactor and turbine buildings. Observed ^{90}Sr and ^{137}Cs concentrations in the stagnant water were 140 MBq L^{-1} and 2.8 GBq L^{-1}, respectively, on 27 March 2011 [4]. Hence, ^{137}Cs concentrations were 20 times higher than ^{90}Sr concentrations, and 1.6% of the ^{90}Sr core inventory was dissolved into stagnant water [2], which was the most likely candidate for pollution to the ocean. ^{90}Sr in seawater could be a useful tracer specific to the radionuclide contaminants directly released from the FDNPP into the ocean.

Analytical results of the stagnant water sampled from a turbine building in February 2012 indicated that ^{137}Cs activity decreased to 240 MBq L^{-1}, while ^{90}Sr concentration remained high (170 MBq L^{-1}) [5]. Highly contaminated stagnant water was decontaminated and stored in storage tanks on the FDNPP site. Some decontaminated water was transferred into reactors for cooling purposes after distillation or reverse osmosis processes. Before 2015, the decontamination system was optimized to remove Cs; hence, the treated water had significantly higher ^{90}Sr activity (150 MBq L^{-1}) than ^{137}Cs activity (3.9 kBq L^{-1}) [5]. This treated water in the storage tanks was a potential source for ^{90}Sr contamination in the environment.

In observation wells between the reactor buildings and the harbor, groundwater was also monitored by TEPCO after a leakage event of contaminated water in December 2012 [4]. In particular, ^{90}Sr activity in groundwater in the wells near the seawater intake for reactor units 1 and 2 were significantly higher than the ^{137}Cs activity (e.g., ^{90}Sr: 5 × 10^6 Bq L^{-1}; ^{137}Cs: 2.1 × 10^2 Bq L^{-1} at the no. 1–2 wells on 5 July 2013 [6]). The ^{90}Sr-enriched groundwater might have resulted from leakage of the decontamination system or from stagnant water. Due to these existing contamination sources, it is necessary to observe the ^{90}Sr behavior in the aquatic environment near the FDNPP.

Kanda [7] indicated that continuous release of ^{137}Cs from the FDNPP harbor to the ocean was occurring in 2012 based on time series seawater monitoring data. Due to the high ^{90}Sr/^{137}Cs activity ratio in the stagnant water, ^{90}Sr release from the FDNPP should also be evaluated. TEPCO has continued seawater monitoring for ^{90}Sr, ^{134,137}Cs, and other radionuclides near the FDNPP [3,6]. However, only a few ^{90}Sr data were obtained within small areas, particularly after 2012 (Figure 1). This limited monitoring cannot evaluate how much ^{90}Sr was released or its impact on the coastal environment and open ocean.

Time series seawater monitoring by TEPCO of ^{90}Sr near the FDNPP was infrequent compared to that for radiocesium [3,6]. Povinec et al. [3] showed that the ^{90}Sr/^{137}Cs ratio in seawater at a monitoring point near FDNPP increased gradually from 0.01 to 1 between April 2011 and February 2012 (Figure 1), which clearly related with decontamination of stagnant water. The transient increase of ^{90}Sr in seawater at the T2 site observed in December 2011 could reflect the leakage event from the ^{137}Cs decontamination system [4]. After 2012, the ^{90}Sr/^{137}Cs ratio remained at a constant value around 0.5 at the T2 site with large variability. ^{90}Sr/^{137}Cs activity ratios in stagnant water have varied depending on the decontamination of $^{134,\,137}$Cs. The agreement between the temporal variation of ^{90}Sr/^{137}Cs activity ratio and decontamination of the stagnant water supported the idea that the most probable candidate was the continuous release from reactor buildings of the FDNPP.

The behavior of ^{137}Cs in seawater and biota after the accident has been well documented [7–11]. High-density sampling of surface seawater to determine radiocesium activity [12] has been carried out. Kumamoto et al. [13] reported detailed vertical distributions of Fukushima-derived radiocesium along the 149 °E meridian in the western North Pacific. However, distributions of ^{90}Sr derived from the FDNPP in the sea have been studied to a significantly lesser extent [3,6,14–17]. Castrillejo et al. [17]

suggested that continuous release of ^{90}Sr from the FDNPP was occurring in September 2013 based on simultaneous observations of ^{90}Sr and ^{137}Cs. The estimated release rate of ^{90}Sr was 2.3–8.5 GBq day^{-1}, which was 2–3 orders of magnitude larger than river inputs.

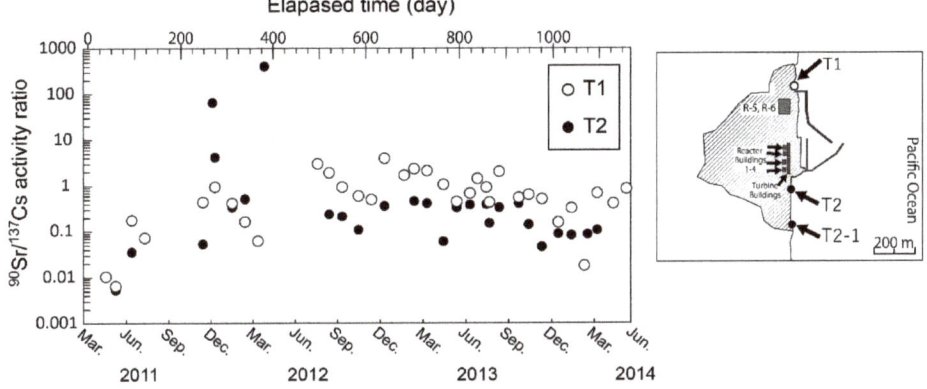

Figure 1. Temporal variations of strontium-90/cesium-137 (^{90}Sr/^{137}Cs) activity ratio in seawater from monitoring sites T1 and T2 (T2-1) in the Fukushima Daiichi Nuclear Power Plant (FDNPP) site [6]. T1 and T2 (T2-1) sites are located north and south of the discharge channel of the FDNPP, respectively.

It is still necessary to investigate the amount of released ^{90}Sr, including its subsequent dispersion from the FDNPP site to the ocean. Simultaneous determinations of ^{90}Sr and ^{137}Cs in seawater are important for monitoring the release of radionuclides from the reactor buildings and contaminated water from the storage tanks. By comparing ^{90}Sr behavior with that of ^{137}Cs in the ocean, we studied the input source to the sea and the environmental migration processes of both radionuclides, such as fluvial input, desorption from sediment, and atmospheric deposition. Accumulating environmental data and understanding the dispersion to the coastal and open oceans are necessary to respond to any accidental release during decommissioning of the FDNPP—work that will require more than 30 years. Our aim in this study is to determine the distributions of ^{90}Sr, ^{134}Cs, and ^{137}Cs in 2013 and evaluate the continuous release of radionuclides from the FDNPP to the ocean based on the comprehensive analysis of seawater.

2. Surface Current System off Fukushima Coast

The Kuroshio and Oyashio currents are generated in the mixed region around 36 °N off the Ibaraki Prefecture coast in the subject area (Figure 2a,b). The warm (16.5–22.0 °C) and saline (34.4–34.8 psu) Kuroshio flows northeastward off the Boso Peninsula. The Oyashio current, off the Fukushima Prefecture coast, intrudes southward into the mixing region. The southward intrusion (9.5–10.5 °C, salinity 33.4–33.8 psu) reaches 36.5 °N, 141.3 °E, and is called the First Branch of the Oyashio [18]. The coastal currents near Fukushima Prefecture are variable on a time scale different from those of the Kuroshio and Oyashio currents. Coastal water is at a higher temperature (10.8–12.7 °C) and lower salinity (33.2–33.4 psu) relative to the first branch of the Oyashio current. Current meter observations made between 1971 and 1981 [19] indicated that the along-shore (north–south component) currents were dominant in this coastal area. The direction of the currents varied approximately every 3–4 days because of changes in the synoptic-scale wind fields [19]. The spread of radionuclides from the direct-release event in April 2011 depended on the coastal current system. Model simulation of directly released Cs employed the Regional Ocean Modeling System (ROMS), which indicated that the plume was southwardly advected to the coastal region [20].

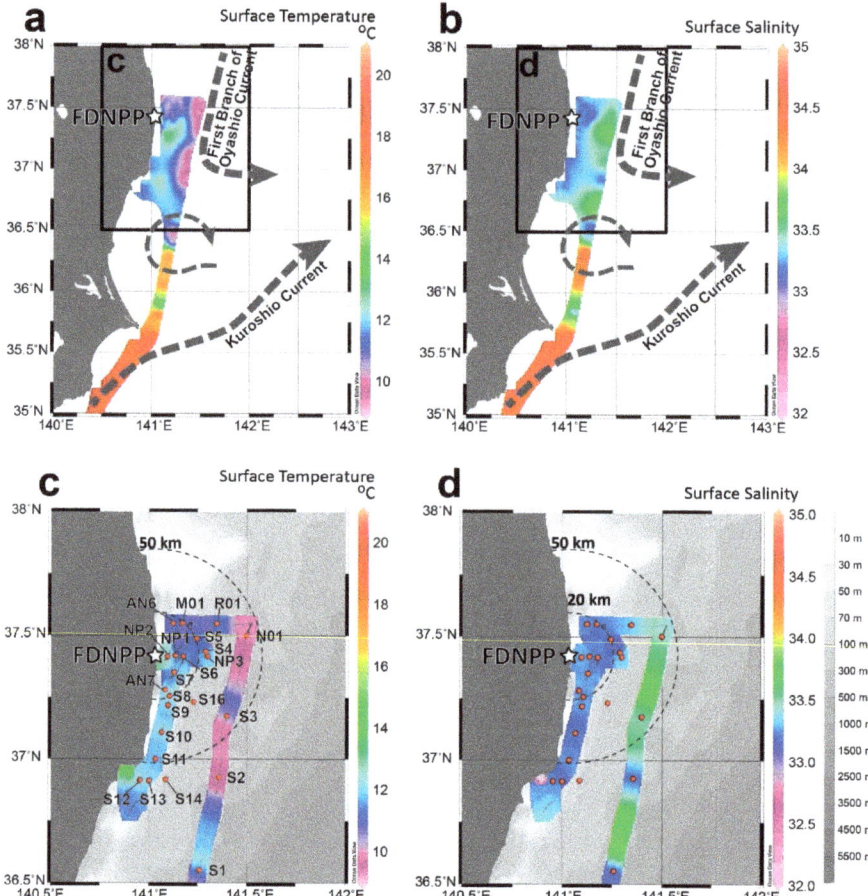

Figure 2. Maps showing sampling locations. (**a**) Surface temperature and (**b**) salinity had two boundary currents (dashed arrows), the warm northeastwardly Kuroshio current south of the Boso Peninsula and the cold southerly first branch of the Oyashio current off the Fukushima coast. (**c**,**d**) Sampling locations are marked by red circles and located near the coast of Fukushima Prefecture.

3. Materials and Methods

Seawater samples for the analysis of ^{90}Sr, ^{134}Cs, and ^{137}Cs were obtained during the UM13-5 cruise from 14 to 23 May 2013 undertaken by the RTV *Umitaka–Maru* of the Tokyo University of Fisheries, Japan. Seawater sampling sites were located in the offshore region in the first branch of the Oyashio current and the coastal region near Fukushima Prefecture (Figure 2c,d). Most of the coastal sites were south of the FDNPP and close to Iwaki city. The closest observation site to the FDNPP was NP-2, located approximately 6 km east of it. During the sampling period, most of the influence from the FDNPP could be detected in the region associated with the southerly coastal current.

During the cruise, surface seawater samples were collected by an underway sampling system, whose inlet was located on the bottom of the ship, at a depth 5 m below the surface. Collected samples were filtered through a 0.5 μm pore polypropylene cartridge filter (TCW-05N-PPS, Advantec, Tokyo, Japan). Filtered water samples were stored in 20 L polyethylene bags and ^{90}Sr and radiocesium analyses were carried out separately on land.

We conducted ^{134}Cs and ^{137}Cs analyses based on Aoyama et al. [21]. First, 20 L of a filtered seawater sample was acidified to pH 1.6 with HNO$_3$. Next, 0.26 g of CsCl was added and the solution was adsorbed on ammonium phosphomolybdate (AMP) [21]. Then, AMP was collected by filtering through a 0.45 µm pore mixed cellulose esters membrane (A045A047A, Advantec, Tokyo, Japan). After drying the AMP/Cs compound, gamma rays were counted for 80,000–200,000 s with a lead-shielded HPGe detector (EGPC 250-P 15, EURISYS MEASURES, NV, USA), 604.7 keV for ^{134}Cs and 661.7 keV for ^{137}Cs, at the Nihon University in Tokyo. Since the detector was slightly contaminated by atmospherically released ^{134}Cs and ^{137}Cs at the time of the accident of the FDNPP, the background was determined before and after this counting period and subtracted from the detected signals for seawater samples. Cs yield was determined gravimetrically based on AMP weight. The typical minimum detectable concentrations (MDCs) of ^{134}Cs and ^{137}Cs were 0.5 mBq L^{-1} and 0.4 mBq L^{-1}, respectively.

For ^{90}Sr analysis, we added 150 g of (NH$_4$)$_2$C$_2$O$_4$ H$_2$O to 20 L of filtered seawater and shook the solution vigorously. Sr was precipitated with Ca oxalate. Oxalate precipitate was decomposed to carbonate at 550 °C in a muffle oven. Then, the precipitate was dissolved in HCl and diluted to about 200 mL with Milli-Q water. A small portion of sample solution was used for determination of stable Sr yield by ICP-OES (SPECTROBLUE TI, SPECTRO Analytical Instruments GmbH, Kleve, Germany). After secular equilibrium between ^{90}Sr and yttrium-90 (^{90}Y) (>2 weeks), ^{90}Y with stable Y carrier (0.1 mg) was "milked" from the ^{90}Sr by precipitating the Fe hydroxide and purified by solid phase extraction using DGA Resin (DN1ML-R50-S) purchased from Eichrom Technologies, LLC. (IL, USA). Detailed chemical separation and beta counting procedures are described elsewhere [22,23]. Beta particles were counted by a low background 2π gas flow proportional counter (LB-4200, Canberra, NV, USA) during 120 min intervals for more than 20 h. Typical Sr and Y yields were 82 ± 9 % and 95 ± 5 %, respectively.

4. Results

Activities of ^{90}Sr, ^{134}Cs, and ^{137}Cs in surface seawater samples collected in May 2013 are summarized in Table 1. Mean ^{90}Sr activity of 0.80 ± 0.11 mBq L^{-1} at offshore sites (S1, S2, S3, and N01) was slightly lower than the estimated value (1.0 ± 0.1 mBq L^{-1} [3]) based on long-term monitoring for surface water of the western North Pacific. Around sites S2, S3, and N01, cool surface water (9.4–10.4 °C) from the southerly first branch of the Oyashio current was present. ^{134}Cs activities were lower than the MDC (<0.5 mBq L^{-1}) at the offshore sites. In this study, we used values obtained at the offshore sites as the background level originating from atmospheric nuclear weapons testing. Compared to ^{137}Cs and ^{90}Sr, ^{134}Cs has a relatively short half-life (2.06 years compared to 30.17 years for ^{137}Cs and 28.8 years for ^{90}Sr).

High ^{90}Sr activities were observed along the coastal region with higher temperatures (10.86–12.89 °C) and higher salinity (33.23–33.35 psu). The highest ^{90}Sr activity (29.13 ± 0.35 mBq L^{-1}) was found at AN7, approximately 16 km south of the FDNPP, with 22.4 ± 0.6 mBq L^{-1} for ^{134}Cs activity and 44.7 ± 0.4 mBq L^{-1} for ^{137}Cs activity. At the NP-2 site closest to the FDNPP (5 km offshore) in this sampling campaign, we also found high ^{90}Sr activity (21.81 ± 0.28 mBq L^{-1}). Furthermore, at S12 off Iwaki City, 57 km south of the FDNPP, relatively high ^{90}Sr activity (9.86 ± 0.22 mBq L^{-1}) was found. Distributions of radiocesium activities in surface seawater showed similar trends to those of ^{90}Sr. The maximum radiocesium activities were obtained at AN7; in particular, ^{137}Cs activities ranged from 1.4 mBq L^{-1} at S2 to 44.7 mBq L^{-1} there. In the coastal region, ^{134}Cs activities were in agreement with ^{137}Cs activities corrected to 11 March 2011, which indicated that this radiocesium was derived from the Fukushima accident (^{134}Cs/^{137}Cs = 0.99 ± 0.03 [11]).

Table 1. ^{90}Sr, ^{134}Cs, and ^{137}Cs activities and hydrographic data in seawater collected on the Fukushima Prefecture coast in May 2013. Uncertainties represent 1σ error.

ID	Sampling Date and Time (year/month/day)	Latitude	Latitude	Temperature (°C)	Salinity (psu)	^{90}Sr Activity (mBq L^{-1})	^{134}Cs Activity (mBq L^{-1})	^{137}Cs Activity (mBq L^{-1})
S1	2013/5/14 16:41	36°33.15′ N	141°15.60′ E	11.41	33.16	0.87 ± 0.06	<0.4	1.9 ± 0.1
S2	2013/5/14 18:39	36°55.62′ N	141°21.48′ E	9.43	33.21	0.66 ± 0.05	<0.4	1.4 ± 0.1
S3	2013/5/14 19:54	37°10.50′ N	141°23.88′ E	10.37	33.51	0.75 ± 0.06	<0.4	1.8 ± 0.1
S4	2013/5/14 20:47	37°26.13′ N	141°17.46′ E	9.88	33.64	1.03 ± 0.06	<0.4	1.5 ± 0.1
N01	2013/5/14 23:12	37°29.33′ N	141°14.75′ E	9.72	33.46	0.90 ± 0.07	<0.4	2.0 ± 0.2
R01	2013/5/15 5:39	37°25.20′ N	141° 8.26′ E	11.02	33.31	3.09 ± 0.07	4.1 ± 0.4	7.7 ± 0.3
AN6	2013/5/15 7:53	37°21.09′ N	141° 7.80′ E	10.86	33.24	2.94 ± 0.13	6.9 ± 0.4	6.9 ± 0.2
M01	2013/5/16 2:28	37°15.42′ N	141° 6.40′ E	10.37	33.24	0.92 ± 0.07	1.0 ± 0.3	3.8 ± 0.2
NP3	2013/5/16 8:05	37°13.11′ N	141° 5.94′ E	11.90	33.35	6.25 ± 0.08	7.2 ± 0.5	14.5 ± 0.3
S5	2013/5/16 6:36	37° 6.60′ N	141° 4.02′ E	11.22	33.17	0.89 ± 0.06	1.4 ± 0.3	3.5 ± 0.2
S6	2013/5/16 6:08	36°59.97′ N	141° 2.16′ E	11.09	33.26	3.46 ± 0.08	8.6 ± 0.5	18.2 ± 0.3
NP2	2013/5/16 22:05	36°54.93′ N	140°57.36′ E	12.41	33.26	21.81 ± 0.28	17.5 ± 1.2	39.0 ± 1.2
NP1	2013/5/17 3:48	36°54.87′ N	141° 0.06′ E	11.08	33.21	0.99 ± 0.07	1.4 ± 0.2	3.8 ± 0.1
S7	2013/5/17 11:27	36°55.05′ N	141° 5.35′ E	11.98	33.28	14.17 ± 0.23	7.9 ± 0.4	16.5 ± 0.3
S8	2013/5/17 12:08	37°16.94′ N	141° 5.14′ E	12.10	33.26	10.63 ± 0.27	14.4 ± 0.5	29.8 ± 0.4
S9	2013/5/17 12:40	37°14.00′ N	141°13.80′ E	11.95	33.24	21.74 ± 0.38	20.2 ± 0.5	39.8 ± 0.4
S10	2013/5/17 14:05	37°32.91′ N	141°20.85′ E	12.04	33.21	3.84 ± 0.12	7.2 ± 0.4	15.7 ± 0.3
S11	2013/5/17 15:11	37°33.03′ N	141°10.41′ E	11.74	33.24	3.68 ± 0.08	5.9 ± 0.4	12.5 ± 0.3
S12	2013/5/17 16:15	37°24.99′ N	141°17.99′ E	12.36	33.26	9.86 ± 0.22	11.9 ± 0.5	24.0 ± 0.3
S13	2013/5/19 0:57	37°33.03′ N	141° 7.56′ E	12.32	33.23	8.92 ± 0.25	7.7 ± 0.4	16.1 ± 0.3
S14	2013/5/19 5:09	37°24.99′ N	141°10.68′ E	12.69	33.30	4.56 ± 0.08	6.0 ± 0.4	13.3 ± 0.3
AN7	2013/5/20 8:45	37°24.99′ N	141° 5.88′ E	12.20	33.33	29.13 ± 0.35	22.4 ± 0.6	44.7 ± 0.4
S16	2013/5/20 23:05	37°30.00′ N	141°30.00′ E	12.16	33.26	2.10 ± 0.06	2.6 ± 0.3	5.7 ± 0.2

5. Discussion

5.1. Dispersion of High ^{90}Sr and $^{134,\,137}$Cs Activity Plume

The high activities of ^{90}Sr and ^{137}Cs in the coastal region (Figure 3) can be explained by the release at the time of the FDNPP accident and the physical processes that later occurred in the ocean. In the coastal region, high ^{90}Sr activity seawater samples with high ^{134}Cs and ^{137}Cs activities were mainly collected from south of the FDNPP (NP2, and AN7) to off Iwaki (S12 and S6), which reflects the southward transport of seawater along the Fukushima coast by the coastal currents. Higher ^{90}Sr activity in seawater (>8 mBq L^{-1}) was found where the salinity was 33.23–33.33 psu and 11.95–12.41 psu. In the coastal region, no clear correlation between ^{90}Sr and salinity or ^{90}Sr and temperature was observed.

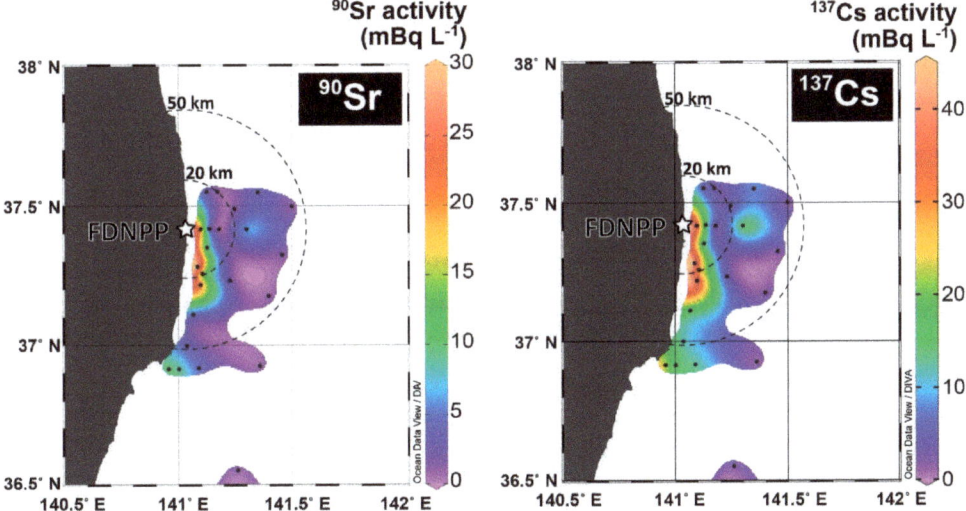

Figure 3. Distribution of ^{90}Sr and ^{137}Cs activities in surface seawater collected in May 2013.

The distributions of ^{90}Sr and ^{137}Cs activities in May 2013 observed in this study correspond to those of a model simulation of the direct-release event between 26 March and 6 April 2011 [20]. The ^{137}Cs released from the FDNPP from 26 March was initially advected southward, then transported to the Ibaraki coast. This simulation suggested that the ^{137}Cs concentration decreased in May due to advection and diffusion in the open ocean. The coastal currents are variable in this region and sometimes flow northward. Oikawa et al. [16] compiled monitoring data for seawater in the coastal region by the Ministry of Education, Culture, Sports, Science and Technology, Japan (MEXT) and suggested that the activities of ^{90}Sr in surface water decreased slowly over time in 2011 and reached the background level by the end of December 2011. However, because of a lack of sampling sites for ^{90}Sr, the ^{90}Sr plume could have been missed in previous observations. The distribution of our results indicates that the released ^{90}Sr plume from the FDNPP site (leakage of contaminated water from storage tanks) could move to the coastal region south of the FDNPP, carried by the southward coastal current.

Both activities decreased rapidly from NP2 toward the eastern sites (S6, NP1, and NP3), which indicate that the eastward dispersion was limited because of the effect of the southern coastal current during this sampling period. Compared with the pre-Fukushima accident, offshore ^{90}Sr activities in the north Pacific Ocean (1.0 ± 0.1) [3] and the activities measured in May 2013 indicate that the influences of the Fukushima-derived ^{90}Sr on open ocean sites in the mixed region between the Oyashio and Kuroshio currents were negligibly small, as were those of ^{134}Cs and ^{137}Cs. However, if any accidental releases from the FDNPP site were to occur during the decommissioning of the reactors, coastal areas could be exposed to a high activity plume.

In September 2017, low ^{90}Sr (1.0–1.8 mBq L^{-1}) and high ^{137}Cs (9–43 mBq L^{-1}) activities were obtained at low salinity (4–28 psu) in groundwater and beach seawater samples from Sendai Bay, located north of the FDNPP [17]. ^{90}Sr/^{137}Cs ratios ranged from 0.036 to 0.19. The ^{137}Cs activity in low salinity samples was affected by atmospheric fallout from the FDNPP accident that was deposited on land, while ^{90}Sr activity was not sensitive to terrestrial input. Therefore, the relationship between ^{90}Sr and ^{137}Cs can be a useful indicator for river input.

The mouth of the Ukedo River is located between collection sites NP2 and AN6. ^{137}Cs activity at NP2 (39.0 mBq L^{-1}) was more than five times higher than that at AN6 (6.9 mBq L^{-1}), though their salinities were comparable (33.24 and 33.26 psu). Dissolved ^{137}Cs activity in the Ukedo River, which drains a highly contaminated area, ranged from 200 to 1100 Bq L^{-1} in August and November 2012 [6]. ^{90}Sr activity in the Ukedo River was not available but the reported ^{90}Sr/^{137}Cs ratio for river water in the Fukushima Prefecture [6] was less than 0.04. The contribution to ^{90}Sr activity in seawater by input from the Ukedo River should be minor.

5.2. ^{90}Sr/^{137}Cs Activity Ratios Derived from the FDNPP Accident

The ^{90}Sr/^{137}Cs activity ratios in seawater are different according to timing of any release or leakage event (e.g., direct discharge event from late March to early April 2011 [3,15]). Since Sr and Cs are highly soluble in seawater, the ^{90}Sr/^{137}Cs activity ratio depends on the source, which could be a useful tracer for the source. The most possible source of ^{90}Sr and ^{137}Cs is stagnant water in the reactor building of unit 2. The ^{90}Sr/^{137}Cs ratio of open ocean seawater [3], seawater monitoring data near the FDNPP [6], stagnant water [4], atmospheric input [1], seabed sediment [24], and river water [6] are summarized with our data in Figure 4.

The ^{90}Sr activity of 0.80 ± 0.11 mBq L^{-1} was obtained at the offshore sites, S1, S2, S3, and N01 (Table 2). To evaluate FDNPP site-derived ^{90}Sr, measured ^{90}Sr activity was subtracted from this value as the background value for North Pacific seawater. The measured ^{134}Cs was a pure FDNPP site-derived component because of its short half-life ($T_{1/2}$ = 2.06 yr). The FDNPP site-derived ^{134}Cs/^{137}Cs ratio was reported to be 0.99 ± 0.03 [11] in March 2011. FDNPP site-derived ^{137}Cs was calculated on the basis of measured ^{134}Cs activity and the FDNPP site-derived ^{134}Cs/^{137}Cs ratio.

Table 2. FDNPP site-derived ^{90}Sr (^{90}Sr$_{corr.}$) and ^{137}Cs (^{137}Cs$_{corr.}$) activities and ^{90}Sr$_{corr.}$/^{137}Cs$_{corr.}$ activity ratios.

ID	^{90}Sr$_{corr.}$ Activity (mBq L^{-1})	^{137}Cs$_{corr.}$ Activity (mBq L^{-1})	^{90}Sr$_{corr.}$/^{137}Cs$_{corr.}$
S6	2.66 ± 0.13	17.0 ± 1.0	0.16 ± 0.01
S7	9.83 ± 0.28	15.6 ± 0.8	0.63 ± 0.04
S8	13.37 ± 0.25	28.5 ± 1.0	0.47 ± 0.02
S9	20.94 ± 0.39	40.0 ± 1.0	0.52 ± 0.02
S10	3.04 ± 0.16	14.2 ± 0.8	0.21 ± 0.02
S11	2.88 ± 0.13	11.7 ± 0.8	0.25 ± 0.02
S12	9.07 ± 0.24	23.5 ± 1.0	0.39 ± 0.02
S13	8.12 ± 0.27	15.2 ± 0.8	0.53 ± 0.03
S14	3.76 ± 0.13	11.9 ± 0.8	0.32 ± 0.02
AN7	28.33 ± 0.37	44.3 ± 1.2	0.64 ± 0.02
S16	1.30 ± 0.12	5.1 ± 0.6	0.25 ± 0.04
R01	2.30 ± 0.12	8.1 ± 0.8	0.28 ± 0.03
NP3	5.46 ± 0.13	14.2 ± 1.0	0.38 ± 0.03
AN6	2.15 ± 0.16	5.9 ± 0.6	0.36 ± 0.05
NP2	21.02 ± 0.30	34.6 ± 2.4	0.61 ± 0.04

The ^{90}Sr$_{corr}$/^{137}Cs$_{corr}$ ratio estimated from the slope of a linear regression fitting was 0.66 ± 0.05 in Figure 5. ^{90}Sr$_{corr}$ activities strongly correlated with those of ^{137}Cs$_{corr}$ (R^2 = 0.919), as described in similar contour maps of ^{90}Sr and ^{137}Cs (Figure 3). The high correlation between ^{90}Sr and ^{137}Cs indicates that ^{90}Sr and ^{137}Cs were derived from a common source. However, the low ^{90}Sr activity samples (<10 mBq L^{-1}) showed larger variability in ^{90}Sr/^{137}Cs activity ratio (0.34 ± 0.14) relative to those for high ^{90}Sr activity samples (>10 mBq L^{-1}: ratio of 0.56 ± 0.08). If multiple sources to seawater exist, such as stagnant water, storage water, and groundwater, contributions from each source could yield temporal and spatial variations. To distinguish these components, detailed ^{134,137}Cs and ^{90}Sr distributions should be investigated. Castrillejo et al. [17] found a short-term transition of ^{90}Sr/^{137}Cs ratio from 0.14 to 0.36 and an abrupt increase in ^{137}Cs activity in the vicinity of the FDNPP (observation site St. 1 (or NP0)) in September 2013. ^{90}Sr and ^{137}Cs release from the FDNPP could be related to the tidal cycle and weather conditions, which caused a temporal variation of the released ^{90}Sr/^{137}Cs ratio from the FDNPP site.

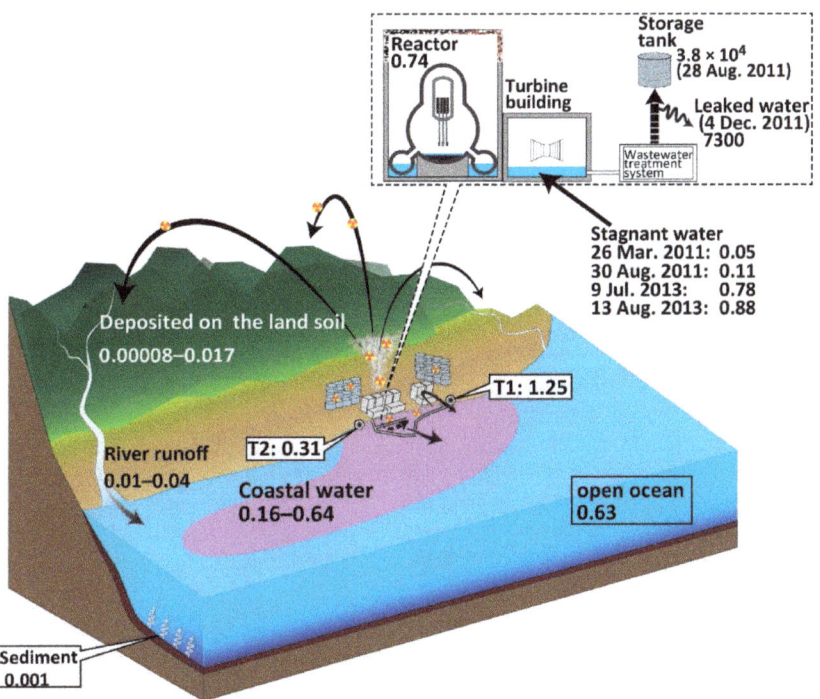

Figure 4. The ^{90}Sr/^{137}Cs activity ratios in the environment and the FDNPP site. The ^{90}Sr/^{137}Cs activity ratio in seawater near the FDNPP was consistent with those from the monitoring points, T1 and T2 [12]. Soil [4] and sediment [24] samples had extremely low ^{90}Sr/^{137}Cs activity ratios.

The slope of a linear regression fitting (0.66) was similar to the reported ^{90}Sr/^{137}Cs activity ratios in stagnant water of 0.78 and 0.88, respectively, in July and August of 2013 [5]. The stagnant water samples were collected from the sampling line behind the mixing point of water from each reactor building [4,5] (Figure 5). These radionuclides were thought to mainly be derived from the reactor building of unit 2 on the basis of the initial data for stagnant water in the unit 2 turbine building [2], which was severely damaged. The ^{90}Sr/^{137}Cs activity ratio in stagnant water varied depending on the decontamination of ^{134,137}Cs, and gradually increased from the direct-release event in March 2011 (0.0256 ± 0.0006 [15]). The ^{90}Sr/^{137}Cs activity ratio of seawater in this study is slightly lower than that of stagnant water, although the most possible source candidate is the continuous release of stagnant water from the FDNPP.

The discrepancy between our data and monitoring data at T1 (1.25 ± 0.71) implies multiple sources exist at the FDNPP site. The higher ^{90}Sr/^{137}Cs at the T1 site could reflect a contribution from

^{90}Sr-rich groundwater. Groundwater around the reactor buildings had a ^{90}Sr/^{137}Cs activity ratio (2.4×10^4 [5]) that was 5 orders of magnitude higher than the seawater value observed in this study. The decontaminated water in storage tanks in the FDNPP was also observed to have high ^{90}Sr/^{137}Cs activity ratios.

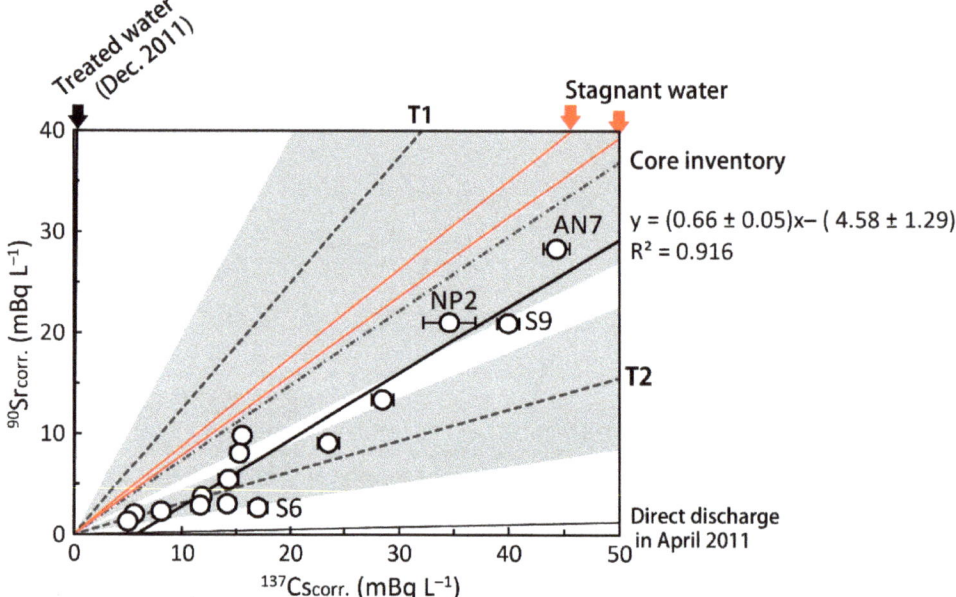

Figure 5. FDNPP site-derived ^{90}Sr and ^{137}Cs activities in surface seawater with ^{90}Sr/^{137}Cs ratio for possible sources. The lower and upper red solid lines show ^{90}Sr/^{137}Cs ratios for stagnant water in the reactor building in July 2013 (0.78) and August 2013 (0.88), respectively [6]. Core inventory (0.74) was estimated by the ORIGEN2 code [2]. Shaded areas were averaged monitoring data at T1 (1.25 ± 0.71) and T2-1 (0.31 ± 0.14) sites from January 2013 to October 2013.

The fitted regression line had an x-intercept of 5.8 mBq L^{-1}. A very low ^{90}Sr/^{137}Cs ratio (0.16) was observed at S6 without a change in salinity. These results indicate that there is a missing source for the site with a low ^{90}Sr/^{137}Cs ratio. In the coastal region, salinities ranged from 33.2 to 33.3 psu and showed no correlation with activities of ^{90}Sr and $^{134, 137}$Cs. Atmospherically deposited ^{90}Sr on land soil in March 2011 was at a lower level (<1.1 Bq g^{-1}) than ^{137}Cs, where the ^{90}Sr/^{137}Cs activity ratio was considered to be 0.00008–0.017 [1] (Figure 5). Higher mobility of ^{90}Sr has been recognized, but ^{90}Sr activity in water of the Fukushima River was less than 4 mBq L^{-1} in 2012 [6]. ^{137}Cs activity ranged from 12 to 190 mBq L^{-1}, which yielded a low ^{90}Sr/^{137}Cs activity ratio of 0.01–0.04 [6]. Considering the ^{90}Sr/^{137}Cs activity ratio in seawater, riverine input from the land to the ocean was minor for ^{90}Sr, though dissolved ^{90}Sr activity in the Ukedo River was never reported.

A possible supply process for ^{137}Cs is the release from seabed sediments. Some amount of Cs could be scavenged by seabed sediments through adsorption onto particles, such as clay minerals [25–27] during the direct discharge event. The sedimentary ^{137}Cs inventory of 100–200 TBq represents only 1%–3% of the total discharge from the FDNPP to the Pacific Ocean in 2011 [28,29]. Approximately 80% of the total ^{137}Cs sedimentary inventory was found in coastal sediments at less than 150 m water depth [29]. The highest ^{90}Sr activity of 63 Bq kg-dry^{-1} in seabed sediments was observed near the south discharge gate of the FDNPP site (T2 monitoring point) in September 2011 [6]. Sedimentary ^{90}Sr/^{137}Cs activity ratios observed after the accident ranged from 0.001 to 0.08, which were lower than those in seawater. ^{137}Cs could be attributed to the direct discharge event in late March to April 2011 [20].

The extremely low ^{90}Sr/^{137}Cs ratio indicates that the contribution of ^{90}Sr in seawater from the soil and seafloor sediments is less than that of ^{137}Cs, even if there is a higher mobility for Sr than for Cs in the soil and sediments.

Another possible low ^{90}Sr/^{137}Cs source is contaminated water that remained in a tunnel for pipes and cables, which were connected to the turbine buildings of units 2 and 3. Contaminated water in the turbine and reactor buildings was released into the ocean via the tunnel and cracks resulting from the earthquake and tsunami. During this direct release event, the ^{90}Sr/^{137}Cs ratio was very low 0.0256 ± 0.0006 [15] (Figure 5). ^{137}Cs activity at T1 reached 68 kBq L^{-1} [20]. After the direct release was stopped in early April 2011 by sealing cracks and the tunnel entrance, contaminated water could have been left in the tunnel until July 2015. Such highly contaminated water could be the source of the low ^{90}Sr/^{137}Cs ratio.

The ^{90}Sr/^{137}Cs activity ratio of 0.66 ± 0.05 observed in this study was higher than data at the monitoring point, T2-1, near the south discharge gate (0.31 ± 0.14) [6] from January to December 2013, but was lower than that at T1 near the north discharge gate (1.25 ± 0.71) [6] (Figure 5). A large variation of ^{90}Sr/^{137}Cs at T1 was observed, which might reflect the local input processes of ^{90}Sr and ^{137}Cs. A much higher ^{90}Sr/^{137}Cs activity ratio (e.g., ^{90}Sr activity of 7.5 Bq L^{-1} and ^{90}Sr/^{137}Cs activity ratio of 3.2 on 26 June 2013) was observed by TEPCO in the harbor [6] than the coastal region as observed in this study. The variation in ^{90}Sr/^{137}Cs activity ratios might reflect the spatial and temporal heterogeneities of released water.

As mentioned above, the similarity of the ^{90}Sr/^{137}Cs activity ratio between seawater and the stagnant water supported the idea that the most likely candidate was the continuous release from the reactor buildings of the FDNPP. Both high ^{90}Sr activity and ^{90}Sr/^{137}Cs activity ratio in the coastal region reflect the input of the stagnant water. Variability of ^{90}Sr/^{137}Cs activity ratios in seawater is an important indicator to understand the status of the release of contaminated water from the FDNPP. Unfortunately, the contribution of underground water near the reactor buildings, and released from sediments to the harbor water, could not be distinguished from the release of the reactor buildings on the basis of seawater obtained from outside of the harbor. More detailed temporal and spatial data in the harbor and for other radionuclides such as tritium (^{3}H) and iodine-129 (^{129}I) are necessary.

5.3. Estimation of ^{90}Sr Input to the Ocean from the FDNPP

The continuous release from the FDNPP was the main source to the Fukushima coast. The amount of ^{137}Cs released daily to the ocean was estimated to be from 8.1 GBq day^{-1} [7] to 30 GBq day^{-1} [8] in 2012 on the basis of simulation of the ^{137}Cs activities of seawater in the harbor and at the north discharge gate, respectively. We examined the amount of released ^{90}Sr based on that of ^{137}Cs in 2013 by using Equation (1):

$$N_{Sr-90} = N_{Cs-137} \times \left(\frac{C_{Sr-90}}{C_{Cs-137}}\right)_{SW} = C_{Cs-137} \times F \times \left(\frac{C_{Sr-90}}{C_{Cs-137}}\right)_{SW} \tag{1}$$

where N, C, and F represent release rate, activity, and conversion factor from activity to daily release rate of ^{137}Cs, respectively. For the estimation of daily released ^{137}Cs, the activities of ^{137}Cs at T2-1 300 m south of the south discharge gate were used (Table 3) [6]. Most of the ^{137}Cs activities were lower than the MDA (1.2–1.5 Bq L^{-1}). To avoid overestimation of the averaged ^{137}Cs activity, we used only precise analysis data. The ^{137}Cs activity at the T2-1 site ranged from 0.14 to 0.98 Bq L^{-1} and showed considerable variation (mean value = 0.60 ± 0.35 Bq L^{-1}). The conversion factors, F, from activity to daily release rate of ^{137}Cs were obtained on the basis of the amount of released ^{137}Cs in the direct release event of March 2011 and ^{137}Cs activities at the T2-1 site [7,20]. The conversion factor applied was 25.5 × 10^9 [20] for the T2-1 site.

Table 3. Estimation of the release rates for ^{90}Sr and ^{137}Cs into the ocean from the FDNPP site in May 2013. C: activity; F: conversion factor; N: release rate.

Monitoring Point	C_{Cs-137} (Bq L^{-1}) (Jan. to Oct. 2013)	F (×10^9 L day^{-1})	N_{Cs-137} (GBq day^{-1})	$(\frac{C_{Sr-90}}{C_{Cs-137}})_{SW}$	N_{Sr-90} (GBq day^{-1})
T2-1	0.60 ± 0.35 [6]	25.5 [20]	15.3 ± 8.9	0.63 ± 0.05	9.6 ± 6.1

The resulting daily released amount of ^{90}Sr was 9.1 ± 6.1 GBq day^{-1} during our sampling campaign in May 2013. The observed ^{90}Sr activity in the coastal region was too low to disturb the ecological system and affect the background radiation dose, as mentioned above. Continuous release could increase the inventory of ^{90}Sr in the Pacific Ocean. If the constant release (9.1 GBq day^{-1}) continued over the year, the annual release rate would be estimated at 3.3 TBq yr^{-1}, which is small relative to the inventory of 105 PBq in the ocean [3]. However, ^{90}Sr in seawater should be closely observed to detect any unexpected release from the nuclear reactor buildings and the contaminated water storage tanks. This estimation needs to assume a stable release rate from the single source. As discussed above, the low ^{90}Sr/^{137}Cs source contributed to seawater around the FDNPP. Therefore, this result could be overestimated.

In this study, the ^{90}Sr/^{137}Cs activity ratio of 0.66 ± 0.05, which was influenced by continuous release from the FDNPP, was distinguished based on precise ^{90}Sr analysis. Buesseler et al. [11,30] suggested that the possible source of ^{137}Cs was not only continuous release from the FDNPP but also the input from subsurface groundwater [31], river water [32], and desorption from the marine sediments in the coastal region [29,30,33]. The environmental migration of ^{137}Cs through particulate and dissolved fluvial inputs, and remineralization from the sediments contaminated by direct discharge of stagnant water from 26 March to 6 April 2011, must also be taken into consideration. ^{90}Sr/^{137}Cs activity ratios could fluctuate according to the source in the FDNPP area and remobilization of ^{137}Cs in coastal water. In addition to monitoring for ongoing release from the reactor buildings and possible leakage of stored contaminated water in tanks, continuous measurement of ^{90}Sr is necessary for investigation of the migration of ^{137}Cs in the marine environment. A combination of other fission product nuclides, ^{129}I and ^{3}H activity, will provide precise information for the current status of leakages from stagnant water, groundwater, and stored water in tanks.

5.4. Estimation of Effective Dose Rate by Ingestion from Marine Products

^{90}Sr dispersion to the coastal area is the most serious issue for fisheries due to its radiotoxicity. We estimated the dose impact to human health from marine products. The highest ^{90}Sr activity (29.13 mBq L^{-1} at AN7; Table 1) was comparable to typical levels for North Pacific surface seawater in the early 1960s during nuclear weapons testing [34]. Taking into consideration the processes in the food chain and the highest activity in the coastal water observed in this study (29.13 mBq L^{-1} at AN-7), we obtained Equation (2):

$$D = C \times CF \times IR \times F \tag{2}$$

where D is representative of the annual dose rate. C, CF, IR, and F are representative of the ^{90}Sr activity in seawater, the concentration factor from seawater to marine products (5–10 [35]), the intake rate of marine products (28.4 kg yr^{-1} [36]), and dose coefficient (2.8 × 10^{-8} Sv/Bq [37]), respectively. It should be noted that these concentrations are quite small (0.23 μSv yr^{-1}) compared with the International Commission on Radiological Protection (ICRP) limit of 1 mSv yr^{-1} for a member of the general public. Much higher ^{90}Sr activities were observed at monitoring points near the south (150–670 mBq L^{-1}) and north (260–5800 mBq L^{-1}) discharge gates [6]. Even this anomalously high ^{90}Sr activity (5800 mBq L^{-1}) close to the FDNPP would contribute 46 μSv yr^{-1} to the annual effective dose rate by marine products.

6. Conclusions

^{90}Sr is useful as a tracer for continuous releases from the FDNPP site. We reported ^{90}Sr data in seawater along with ^{134}Cs and ^{137}Cs in samples collected in the coastal area off Fukushima Prefecture. Released ^{90}Sr was dispersed along the Fukushima coast, and the highest ^{90}Sr activity was 29.13 mBq L^{-1} at a sampling site 16 km south of the FDNPP. FDNPP site-derived ^{90}Sr/^{137}Cs ranged from 0.16 to 0.64 and the slope of a linear regression fitting of the relationship of Fukushima site-derived ^{90}Sr and ^{137}Cs was 0.66 ± 0.05, which was similar to the ratio of contaminated water in the FDNPP reactor and turbine buildings. These results suggest that the major contamination source is contaminated water in the FDNPP buildings. On the other hand, the ^{137}Cs-rich source could also affect seawater and cause temporal and spatial variations. The estimated release rate of ^{90}Sr (9.6 ± 6.1 GBq day^{-1}) was small relative to the inventory of ^{90}Sr in the Pacific Ocean. Release of ^{90}Sr has been controlled by the water shielding wall between the reactor buildings and the harbor since 2015. However, our results imply that if any accidental release of radionuclides, including ^{90}Sr from the FDNPP, occurs during decommissioning of the reactors, the coastal area can be exposed to a high activity plume.

Author Contributions: Conceptualization, H.T. and M.Y.; methodology, H.T. and H.O.; investigation, H.T; data curation, H.T., T.Y., K.T., and H.N.; writing—original draft preparation, H.T.; writing—review and editing, H.O, D.T., and J.K.; visualization, H.T.; supervision, M.Y.; project administration, H.T.; funding acquisition, H.T. All authors interpreted the data. All authors provided final approval of the version of the manuscript for publication and agreed to be accountable for all aspects of the work.

Funding: This work was supported by JSPS KAKENHI (grant numbers: 24110004 and 26340019).

Acknowledgments: We would like to thank the captain, crew, and scientific party of the UM-13-5 cruise by the RTV *Umitaka-Maru* for their collaboration in sampling.

Conflicts of Interest: The authors declare no conflicts of interest.

References

1. Steinhauser, G.; Schauer, V.; Shozugawa, K. Concentration of strontium-90 at selected hot spots in Japan. *PLoS ONE* **2013**, *8*, e57760. [CrossRef] [PubMed]
2. Nishihara, K.; Yamagishi, I.; Yasuda, K.; Ishimori, K.; Tanaka, K.; Kuno, T.; Inada, S.; Gotoh, Y. Radionuclide release to stagnant water in Fukushima 1 Nuclear Power Plant. *J. At. Energy Soc. Jpn.* **2012**, *11*, 13–19. [CrossRef]
3. Povinec, P.P.; Hirose, K.; Aoyama, M. Radiostrontium in the western North Pacific: Characteristics, behavior, and the Fukushima impact. *Environ. Sci. Technol.* **2012**, *46*, 10356–10363. [CrossRef] [PubMed]
4. Japan Atomic Energy Agency—JAEA. Results of Radiological Analysis for Stagnant Water and Treated Water. Available online: https://www.meti.go.jp/earthquake/nuclear/decommissioning/committee/osensuitaisakuteam/2015/pdf/0730_3_4c.pdf (accessed on 15 September 2019). (In Japanese).
5. Tokyo Electric Power Company—TEPCO. Report to NISA upon the Additional Directive Document Regarding the Leak of Water Containing Radioactive Material from the Water Desalination Apparatus (Evaporative Concentration Apparatus) of Fukushima Daiichi Nuclear Power Plant (Update). 2012. Available online: http://www.tepco.co.jp/en/press/corp-com/release/2012/12013108-e.html (accessed on 23 October 2019).
6. Japan Atomic Energy Agency—JAEA. Database for Radioactive Substance Monitoring Data. Available online: https://emdb.jaea.go.jp/emdb/en/ (accessed on 12 September 2019).
7. Kanda, J. Continuing ^{137}Cs release to the sea from the Fukushima Dai-ichi Nuclear Power Plant through 2012. *Biogeosciences* **2013**, *10*, 6107–6113. [CrossRef]
8. Tsumune, D.; Tsubono, T.; Aoyama, M.; Uematsu, M.; Misumi, K.; Maeda, Y.; Yoshida, Y.; Hayami, H. One-year, regional-scale simulation of Cs-137 radioactivity in the ocean following the Fukushima Dai-Ichi Nuclear Power Plant accident. *Biogeosciences* **2013**, *10*, 5601–5617. [CrossRef]
9. Honda, M.; Kawakami, H.; Watanabe, S.; Saino, T. Concentration and vertical flux of Fukushima-derived radiocesium in sinking particles from two sites in the Northwestern Pacific Ocean. *Biogeosciences* **2013**, *10*, 3525–3534. [CrossRef]

10. Buesseler, K.O.; Jayne, S.R.; Fisher, N.S.; Rypina, I.I.; Baumann, H.; Baumann, Z.; Breier, C.F.; Douglass, E.M.; George, J.; MacDonald, A.M.; et al. Fukushima-derived radionuclides in the ocean and biota off Japan. *Proc. Natl. Acad. Sci. USA* **2012**, *109*, 5984–5988. [CrossRef]
11. Buesseler, K.O.; Aoyama, M.; Fukasawa, M. Impacts of the Fukushima Nuclear Power Plants on marine radioactivity. *Environ. Sci. Technol.* **2011**, *45*, 9931–9935. [CrossRef]
12. Aoyama, M.; Uematsu, M.; Tsumune, D.; Hamajima, Y. Surface pathway of radioactive plume of TEPCO Fukushima NPP1 released Cs-134 and Cs-137. *Biogeosciences* **2013**, *10*, 3067–3078. [CrossRef]
13. Kumamoto, Y.; Aoyama, M.; Hamajima, Y.; Aono, T.; Kouketsu, S.; Murata, A.; Kawano, T. Southward spreading of the Fukushima-derived radiocesium across the Kuroshio Extension in the North Pacific. *Sci. Rep.* **2014**, *4*, 4274. [CrossRef]
14. Ministry of Education. Culture, Sports, Science and Technology—Japan MEXT Readings of Environmental Radioactivity Level (English Version). Available online: http://radioactivity.mext.go.jp/en/ (accessed on 30 September 2019).
15. Casacuberta, N.; Masque, P.; Garcia-Orellana, J.; Garcia-Tenorio, R.; Buesseler, K.O. Sr-90 and Sr-89 in seawater off Japan as a consequence of the Fukushima Dai-ichi nuclear accident. *Biogeosciences* **2013**, *10*, 3649–3659. [CrossRef]
16. Oikawa, S.; Takata, H.; Watabe, T.; Misonoo, J.; Kusakabe, M. Distribution of the Fukushima-derived radionuclides in seawater in the Pacific off the coast of Miyagi, Fukushima, and Ibaraki Prefectures, Japan. *Biogeosciences* **2013**, *10*, 5031–5047. [CrossRef]
17. Castrillejo, M.; Casacuberta, N.; Breier, C.F.; Pike, S.M.; Masque, P.; Buesseler, K.O. Reassessment of ^{90}Sr, ^{137}Cs, and ^{134}Cs in the Coast off Japan Derived from the Fukushima Dai-ichi Nuclear Accident. *Environ. Sci. Technol.* **2016**, *50*, 173–180. [CrossRef] [PubMed]
18. Okuda, K.; Yasuda, I.; Hiroe, Y.; Shimizu, Y. Structure of subsurface intrusion of the Oyashio water into the Kuroshio Extension and formation process of the North Pacific Intermediate Water. *J. Oceanogr.* **2001**, *57*, 121–140. [CrossRef]
19. Nakamura, Y. Studies on the fishing ground formation of Sakhalin Surf Clam and the hydraulic environment in coastal region. *Fukushima Suisan Shikenjo Res. Rep.* **1991**, 1–118. (In Japanese)
20. Tsumune, D.; Tsubono, T.; Aoyama, M.; Hirose, K. Distribution of oceanic Cs-137 from the Fukushima Dai-ichi Nuclear Power Plant simulated numerically by a regional ocean model. *J. Environ. Radioact.* **2012**, *111*, 100–108. [CrossRef]
21. Aoyama, M.; Hirose, K.; Miyao, T.; Igarashi, Y. Low-level ^{137}Cs measurements in deep seawater samples. *Appl. Radiat. Isot.* **2000**, *53*, 159–162. [CrossRef]
22. Tazoe, H.; Obata, H.; Yamagata, T.; Karube, Z.; Nagai, H.; Yamada, M. Determination of strontium-90 from direct separation of yttrium-90 by solid phase extraction using DGA Resin for seawater monitoring. *Talanta* **2016**, *15*, 219–227. [CrossRef]
23. Tazoe, H.; Obata, H.; Tomita, M.; Namura, S.; Nishioka, J.; Yamagata, T.; Karube, Z.; Yamada, M. Novel method for low level Sr-90 activity detection in seawater by combining oxalate precipitation and chelating resin extraction. *Geochem. J.* **2017**, *51*, 193–197. [CrossRef]
24. Kusakabe, M.; Oikawa, S.; Takata, H.; Misonoo, J. Spatiotemporal distributions of Fukushima-derived radionuclides in nearby marine surface sediments. *Biogeosciences* **2013**, *10*, 5019–5030. [CrossRef]
25. Santschi, P.H.; Bower, P.; Nyffeler, U.P.; Azevedo, A.; Broecker, W.S. Estimates of the resistance to chemical transport posed by the deep-sea boundary layer. *Limnol. Oceanogr.* **1983**, *28*, 899–912. [CrossRef]
26. Nyffeler, U.P.; Li, Y.H.; Santschi, P.H. A kinetic approach to describe trace-element distribution between particles and solution in natural aquatic systems. *Geochim. Cosmochim. Acta* **1984**, *48*, 1513–1522. [CrossRef]
27. Lujanienė, G.; Vilimaitė-Šilobritienė, B.; Jokšas, K. Accumulation of ^{137}Cs in bottom sediments of the Curonian Lagoon. *Nucleonika* **2005**, *50*, 23–29.
28. Black, E.; Buesseler, K. Spatial variability and the fate of cesium in coastal sediments near Fukushima, Japan. *Biogeosci. Discuss.* **2014**, *11*, 7235–7271.
29. Otosaka, S.; Kato, Y. Radiocesium derived from the Fukushima Daiichi Nuclear Power Plant accident in seabed sediments: Initial deposition and inventories. *Environ. Sci. Proc. Impacts* **2014**, *16*, 978–990. [CrossRef]
30. Buesseler, K.O. Fukushima and ocean radioactivity. *Oceanography* **2014**, *27*, 92–105. [CrossRef]

31. Charette, M.A.; Breier, C.F.; Henderson, P.B.; Pike, S.M.; Rypina, I.I.; Jayne, S.R.; Buesseler, K.O. Radium-based estimates of cesium isotope transport and total direct ocean discharges from the Fukushima Nuclear Power Plant accident. *Biogeosciences* **2013**, *10*, 2159–2167. [CrossRef]
32. Nagao, S.; Kanamori, M.; Ochiai, S.; Tomihara, S.; Fukushi, K.; Yamamoto, M. Export of ^{134}Cs and ^{137}Cs in the Fukushima river systems at heavy rains by Typhoon Roke in September 2011. *Biogeosciences* **2013**, *10*, 6215–6223. [CrossRef]
33. Mitchell, P.; Condren, O.; Vintró, L.L.; McMahon, C. Trends in plutonium, americium and radiocaesium accumulation and long-term bioavailability in the western Irish Sea mud basin. *J. Environ. Radioact.* **1999**, *44*, 223–251. [CrossRef]
34. United Nations Scientific Committee on the Effects of Atomic Radiation—UNSCEAR. *Sources and Effects of Ionizing Radiation: Sources*; United Nations Publications: New York, NY, USA, 2000; Volume 1.
35. International Atomic Energy Agency (IAEA). *Sediment Distribution Coefficients and Concentration Factors for Biota in the Marine Environment*; Technical Reports Series No.422; IAEA: Vienna, Austria, 2004.
36. Ministry of Agriculture, Forestry and Fisheries. MAFF Annual Report Food Balance Sheet 2012. Available online: http://www.maff.go.jp/e/tokei/kikaku/nenji_e/88nenji/index.html#nse01372 (accessed on 15 September 2019).
37. International Commission on Radiological Protection. *Age-Dependent Doses to the Members of the Public from Intake of Radionuclides Part 5, Compilation of Ingestion and Inhalation Coefficients*; ICRP Publication 72; Pergamon Press: Oxford, UK, 1996.

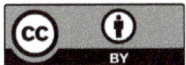

© 2019 by the authors. Licensee MDPI, Basel, Switzerland. This article is an open access article distributed under the terms and conditions of the Creative Commons Attribution (CC BY) license (http://creativecommons.org/licenses/by/4.0/).

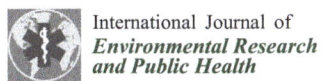

Article

Isotope Composition and Chemical Species of Monthly Precipitation Collected at the Site of a Fusion Test Facility in Japan

Naofumi Akata [1,*], Masahiro Tanaka [2], Chie Iwata [3], Akemi Kato [3], Miki Nakada [3], Tibor Kovács [4] and Hideki Kakiuchi [5]

[1] Department of Radiation Chemistry, Institute of Radiation Emergency Medicine, Hirosaki University, Hirosaki 036-8564, Japan
[2] Department of Helical Plasma Research, National Institute for Fusion Science, National Institutes of Natural Sciences, Toki 509-5292, Gifu, Japan; tanaka.masahiro@nifs.ac.jp
[3] Department of Engineering and Technical Services, National Institute for Fusion Science, National Institutes of Natural Sciences, Toki 509-5292, Gifu, Japan; iwata.chie@nifs.ac.jp (C.I.); kakemi@nifs.ac.jp (A.K.); nakada.miki@nifs.ac.jp (M.N.)
[4] Institute of Radiochemistry and Radioecology, University of Pannonia, H-820010 Egyetem Str, Veszprém, Hungary; kt@almos.uni-pannon.hu
[5] Department of Radioecology, Institute for Environmental Sciences, Aomori 039-3212, Japan; ckhsd@ies.or.jp
* Correspondence: akata@hirosaki-u.ac.jp; Tel.: +81-173-39-5405

Received: 6 September 2019; Accepted: 9 October 2019; Published: 14 October 2019

Abstract: The deuterium plasma experiment was started using the Large Helical Device (LHD) at the National Institute for Fusion Science (NIFS) in March 2017 to investigate high-temperature plasma physics and the hydrogen isotope effects towards the realization of fusion energy. In order to clarify any experimental impacts on precipitation, precipitation has been collected at the NIFS site since November 2013 as a means to assess the relationship between isotope composition and chemical species in precipitation containing tritium. The tritium concentration ranged from 0.10 to 0.61 Bq L^{-1} and was high in spring and low in summer. The stable isotope composition and the chemical species were unchanged before and after the deuterium plasma experiment. Additionally, the tritium concentration after starting the deuterium plasma experiment was within three sigma of the average tritium concentration before the deuterium plasma experiment. These results suggested that there was no impact by tritium on the environment surrounding the fusion test facility.

Keywords: tritium monitoring; fusion test facility; deuterium plasma experiment; monthly precipitation; chemical composition

1. Introduction

The sources of environmental tritium (^{3}H), a radioisotope of hydrogen that decays to ^{3}He with a half-life of 12.3 years, have been summarized by researchers [1–3]. Most naturally sourced tritium is produced by the interaction of cosmic rays with nitrogen (^{14}N) and oxygen (^{16}O) atoms in the upper atmosphere. The tritium production rate by cosmic rays is estimated as 0.25 atoms cm^{-2} s^{-1} [2]. The global production rate of natural tritium is 72 × 10^{15} Bq y^{-1} if it is assumed that surface area of the earth is 5.1 × 10^{14} m^2. On the other hand, anthropogenic ^{3}H arises from several sources. Atmospheric nuclear weapon testing from the 1950s to the early 1960s released significant amounts of tritium into the environment [2], and approximately 1.86 × 10^{20} Bq (650 kg) of tritium was released during 1945 to 1985 [4]. Tritium concentrations in precipitation were rapidly increased by these events, and many researchers found high tritium concentrations in precipitation [5,6]. Even now, residual artificial tritium is estimated to be approximately 10^{18} Bq. Nuclear facilities such as nuclear power reactors and nuclear fuel reprocessing plants also release tritium to the environment, and they have become the dominant anthropogenic source. Annual average amounts of released tritium from nuclear facilities worldwide to the atmosphere were estimated to be 11.7×10^{15} Bq during the period from 1998 to 2002 [4]. This amount corresponds to approximately 15 to 20% of the annual tritium production rate by cosmic rays. The amount of tritium on the earth was estimated at approximately $1.0–1.3 \times 10^{18}$ Bq and is dependent on the balance between production rate and radioactive decay rate. Accident-released tritium is also important for the natural environment. After the Chernobyl Nuclear Power Plant accident and the Fukushima Dai-ichi Nuclear Power Plant accident, elevated tritium in environmental samples was observed [7,8]. In the case of Japan, Nakasone et al. [9] concluded that tritium concentrations in monthly precipitation were increased by nuclear weapon testing and the Fukushima Dai-ichi Nuclear Power Plant accident. In the future, nuclear fusion reactors will have a large inventory of tritium as fuel. The fuel of nuclear fusion reactors would be the hydrogen isotopes, deuterium (D) and tritium (T). In the 1990s, the Tokamak Fusion Test Reactor (TFTR) in New Jersey, USA and the Joint European Torus (JET) in Oxfordshire, UK were used to carry out D–T plasma experiments. Although the inventory of tritium in these facilities was less than 10 g and tritium in the facilities was confined using a safety system, tritium concentrations in their surrounding environments were slightly increased [10]. The International Thermonuclear Experimental Reactor (ITER) is another international nuclear fusion research and engineering project, and a large experimental tokamak nuclear fusion device designed to study fusion plasmas of D–T reaction is now under construction in Saint-Paul-lès-Durance, France [11]. It is envisioned to be the next major step in the world's fusion programs. Within the ITER, a total inventory of about 2 to 3 kg (10^{18} Bq) will be necessary to implement the D–T reaction [12]. Therefore, it is important to understand the tritium level in a surrounding environment before and after facility operation starts [13].

The Large Helical Device (LHD) was constructed by the National Institute for Fusion Science (NIFS) at Toki City, Gifu Prefecture, and it is one of the world's largest magnetically confined helical type fusion experimental devices [14]. The deuterium plasma experiment using LHD was started there in March 2017 to investigate high-temperature plasma physics and the hydrogen isotope effects [14]. A small amount of tritium was produced by a fusion reaction in the deuterium plasma experiment. Although the deuterium and the tritium gases were exhausted from the vacuum vessel of the LHD and recovered by the exhaust detritiation system (EDS) [15], a part of the tritium was released into the environment through the main stack. In the first year of the deuterium plasma experiment, the annual tritium yield was permitted up to 3.7×10^{10} Bq for commissioning of the deuterium plasma experiment. The amount of tritium released from the stack was monitored, and the total amount of tritium released during the first year of the deuterium plasma experiment (from 6 March 2017 to 31 March 2018) was approximately 0.13×10^9 Bq [16]. This value was negligibly small compared with the permitted annual tritium yield (3.7×10^{10} Bq). The tritium concentrations in environmental samples (environmental water, air, vegetation, etc.) were monitored before and after the deuterium plasma experiment to assess the impact of released tritium [17–21]. The tritium concentration levels were within the background range of the environmental variation. As part of the environmental tritium monitoring, tritium concentration and chemical composition in monthly precipitation and radioactive materials in monthly total deposition samples were monitored.

In order to clarify the experimental impact on precipitation, precipitation has been collected at the NIFS site in Toki, Japan since November 2013 as a means to assess the relationship between isotope composition and chemical species in precipitation with tritium concentration. Partial data of tritium concentration and stable isotope ratio in precipitation before the deuterium plasma experiment have already been reported [21]. This paper reports isotope composition and chemical characteristics of monthly precipitation collected at Toki and discusses the impact of the first year of the deuterium plasma experiment in the LHD on the surrounding environment.

2. Materials and Methods

2.1. Overview of Study Site

The study sampling site was on the roof of a building at the NIFS at Toki City, Gifu Prefecture (35°19′ N, 137°10′ E). Figure 1 shows the sampling location. Toki City is located approximately 30 km northeast of Nagoya City in the central region of Japan. Toki is located in a small-scale basin, approximately 10 km in diameter, and it is surrounded by low elevation mountains. The Meteorological Agency has reported average weather conditions for 30 years (1981–2010) observed at the Tajimi AMeDAS (Automated Meteorological Data Acquisition System) site, which is located 6 km northwest of NIFS [22]. The average monthly precipitation was high in summer and low in winter, while the average wind speed was lower than 1.0 m s^{-1} in that time period. Average monthly temperature ranged from 2.9 to 27.4 °C [23].

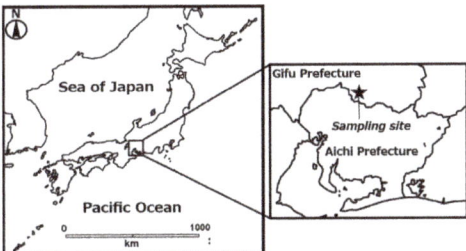

Figure 1. Maps showing location of the sampling site.

2.2. Sample Collection and Analysis

Monthly precipitation was collected at NIFS. Precipitation samples were collected from November 2013 to the end of 2017 using a precipitation sampler (ST-1F, Suntechno, Tokyo, Japan) with a 10 L polyethylene container that had been washed with pure water. After measuring sample weight, pH (B-211, Horiba, Kyoto, Japan) and electrical conductivity (EC) (E-771, Horiba) were measured. Approximately 1 L of sample water was distilled, and 800 mL of distilled sample water was electrolyzed to a volume of 65 mL to enrich its tritium content using an electrolytic enrichment system with a solid polymer electrolyte membrane (XZ001, De Nora Permelec Ltd. Fujisawa, Japan). After distilling the tritium-enriched sample water, 50 mL of sample water was mixed with the same volume of a liquid scintillation cocktail (Ultima Gold LLT, PerkinElmer, Waltham, MA, USA) in a 145 mL low diffusion polyethylene vial with an inner Teflon coating. Tritium radioactivity was measured with a low background liquid scintillation counter (LSC: LSC-LB5 or LSC-LB7, Hitachi, Tokyo, Japan) for 1500 min. Counting efficiencies were determined using standard tritium solution (SRM 4361C, NIST, Gaithersburg, MD, USA). The minimum detection level (MDL) of LSC-LB5 and LSC-LB7 with the electrolytic enrichment system was approximately 0.04 Bq L^{-1}. Measured values were corrected for radioactive decay to the middle of the sampling period [21].

A part of each sample was filtered using a 0.45 µm membrane filter (DISMIC 25CS045AS, ADVANTEC, Tokyo, Japan). The ionic species (Cl$^-$, NO$_3^-$, SO$_4^{2-}$, Na$^+$, Mg^{2+}, K$^+$, Ca^{2+}, NH$_4^+$) in the filtered samples were determined by ion chromatography (ICS-2100, Dionex, Sunnyvale, CA, USA). The Gard column and the Separation column produced by Dionex Inc. were used Ion Pac AG17 4 × 50 mm and Ion Pac AS19 4 × 250 mm for anion analysis and Ion Pac CG16 5 × 50 mm and Ion Pac CS16 5 × 250 mm for cation analysis. We used anion mixed standard solution and cation mixed standard solution (Kanto Chemical Co. Inc. Tokyo, Japan) for quality control. Stable isotope analysis was performed using both an isotope ratio mass spectrometer (Delta V Advantage, Thermo Fisher Scientific, Waltham, MA, USA) with a water equilibrium device (Nakano Electric Inc. Kyoto, Japan) and a cavity ring-down spectroscopy isotopic water analyzer (model L1102-i, Picarro Inc. Sunnyvale, CA, USA) with a CTC analytics autosampler (HTC-PAL, Leap Technologies, Carrboro, NC, USA). Measurement precision was better than ± 1.5‰ for δD and ± 0.15‰ for $\delta^{18}O$.

3. Results and Discussion

3.1. Tritium Concentration in Precipitation

Figure 2 shows the monthly variations of precipitation data collected at Toki during the sampling period; they are precipitation amount (A), pH (B), EC (C), and tritium concentration (D). Monthly precipitation amount ranged from 26 to 363 mm and was high in summer and low in winter. Annual precipitation amounts in 2014, 2015, 2016, and 2017 were 1515, 1435, 1550, and 1626 mm with the arithmetic mean value of 1532 mm. Average annual precipitation amount for 30 years (1981–2010) was 1626.7 mm [22], and the value in 2017 was comparable to the reported value, while those of 2014, 2015, and 2016 were slightly lower than the reported values. The pH data ranged from 4.3 to 6.9, and about 56% of the samples were in the range of acid rain with the pH < 5.0. The EC ranged from 5 to 28 μS cm^{-1}. There was no clear seasonal trend for either pH or EC.

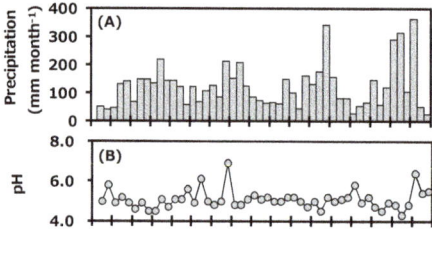
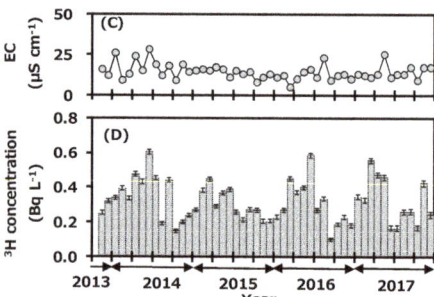

Figure 2. Monthly variations of precipitation amount (**A**), pH (**B**), electrical conductivity (EC) (**C**), and tritium concentration (**D**) in precipitation collected at Toki, Japan before (2013–2016) and after (2017) the first campaign of the deuterium plasma experiment.

The tritium concentration in the monthly precipitation ranged from 0.10 to 0.61 Bq L^{-1} and was high in spring and low in summer. Annual tritium concentrations (arithmetic mean ± standard deviation) in 2014, 2015, 2016, and 2017 were 0.35 ± 0.14, 0.30 ± 0.08, 0.30 ± 0.13, and 0.32 ± 0.13 Bq L^{-1}. Recent data for tritium concentration in monthly precipitation in Japan have been summarized [9,24,25]. It is known that the concentration of environmental tritium depends on the latitude of the sampling location; it is high at northern latitudes and low at southern latitudes [26,27]. For example, tritium concentration in monthly precipitation in Sapporo (northern Japan) during July 2015 to December 2017 ranged from 0.24 to 1.27 Bq L^{-1} [9], that of Rokkasho during April 2001 to March 2006 ranged from 0.16 to 1.23 Bq L^{-1} [28], that of Chiba during November 2013 to December 2017 ranged from 0.12 to 0.53 Bq L^{-1} [24], and that of Okinawa (southern Japan) during June 2014 to December 2017 ranged from 0.05 to 0.27 Bq L^{-1} [9]. The results of the present study were similar to those of Chiba, which is at a similar latitude. The seasonal trend for tritium concentration in precipitation was similar to the general background pattern observed in Japan, which is high in spring and low in summer [27]. The northwestern monsoon from the Asian continent blows into Japan during winter to spring. A relatively higher tritium concentration in precipitation was observed in inland continental areas due to recycling of tritium by evaporation and precipitation, the so-called continental effect [29]. On the other hand, high-pressure systems develop in the Pacific Ocean in summer and bring air masses to Japan from the ocean, which have slightly lower tritium concentration [28]. Tritium concentration in precipitation at Toki changed with meteorological conditions depending on the air-mass transportation course. The transfer of cosmogenic tritium from the upper atmosphere to the troposphere in spring also seemed to contribute to the seasonal pattern observed.

3.2. Stable hydrogen and Oxygen Isotope Composition in Precipitation

The seasonal variations of δD and δ^{18}O in monthly precipitation at Toki are shown in Figure 3A with the monthly precipitation amount, and the reported monthly average temperature at Tajimi AMeDas site [22] is shown in Figure 3B. δD and δ^{18}O in monthly precipitation ranged from −103.62 to −20.77‰ and −15.14 to −3.92‰, respectively. Although precipitation amount and average temperature had a clear seasonal trend, which was high in summer and low in winter, there was no clear seasonal change in δD and δ^{18}O. A weak seasonal change of δD and δ^{18}O in precipitation was reported to have been observed in the East Asian region [30]. The present results had a similar seasonal trend to this reported one.

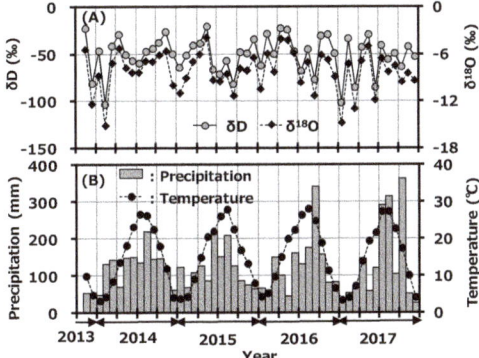

Figure 3. Variations of δD and δ^{18}O in monthly precipitation collected at Toki, Japan with monthly precipitation amount (**A**) and the reported monthly average temperature at the Tajimi AMeDas site (**B**).

In general, δD and δ^{18}O in global precipitation are well-related by the following equation.

$$dD = 8.0 \times \delta^{18}O + 10 \quad (1)$$

This equation, called the global meteoric water line (GMWL), is based on precipitation data collected worldwide [31]. Figure 4 shows the relationship between δD and δ^{18}O in monthly precipitation collected at Toki, Japan. The slope of the regression line (δD = 7.5 × δ^{18}O + 10.6) of precipitation at Toki was similar to the slope of the GMWL. Additionally, the reported equation based on observations in the Kanto area of Japan (Kumagaya, Saitama: δD = 7.4 × δ^{18}O + 9.6, r^2 = 0.868) [32] was also similar to our equation. Here, the intercept of GMWL is known as the deuterium excess (d-excess), and its equation is as follows [33].

$$d - excess = \delta D - 8 \times d^{18}O \quad (2)$$

The d-excess value is used as a convenient tool for describing conditions affecting evaporation in oceanic moisture source regions. There have been some reports about seasonality of d-excess in precipitation in Japan [34,35]. In general, high d-excess indicates lower relative humidity in the maritime air-mass source region [36]. Figure 5A shows the variation of d-excess in monthly precipitation collected at Toki with precipitation rate, and Figure 5B shows the reported monthly average temperature at the Tajimi AMeDas site [22]. The d-excess had clear seasonal variation and was high in winter and low in summer; d-excess and average temperature were negatively correlated (r^2 = 0.647). As mentioned before, the northwestern monsoon from the Asian continent blows onto the Japanese islands during winter to early spring and carries a dry air-mass with water vapor evaporated rapidly from the Japan

Sea. On the other hand, high-pressure systems develop in the Pacific Ocean in summer and bring air-masses from the southern maritime area. This seasonal variation is a general trend seen in Japan, and the present d-excess value was comparable to the reported value [35]. No impact was found from the deuterium plasma experiment on the environment.

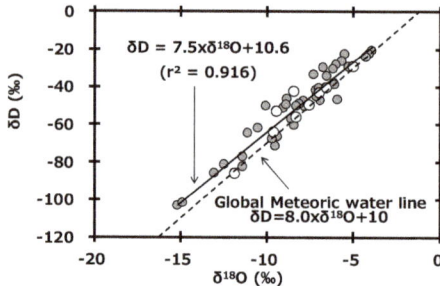

Figure 4. Relationship between δD and $\delta^{18}O$ in monthly precipitation collected at Toki, Japan and a plot of the global meteoric water line.

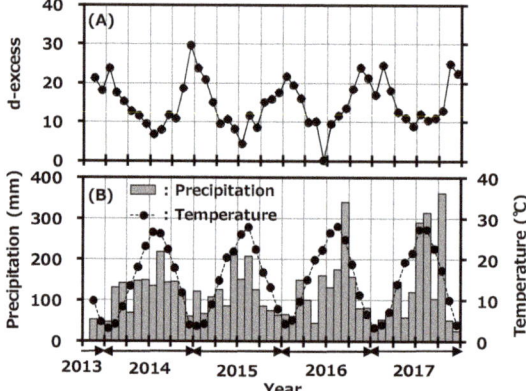

Figure 5. Variation of deuterium excess (d-excess) in monthly precipitation collected at Toki, Japan with monthly precipitation amount (**A**) and the reported monthly average temperature at the Tajimi Automated Meteorological Data Acquisition System (AMeDas) site (**B**).

3.3. Ion Concentrations in Precipitation

Concentrations of anions and cations in precipitation collected at Toki are shown in Figure 6. Concentration ranges of the anions were Cl^-, 0.19 to 1.06 mg L^{-1}; NO_3^-, 0.35 to 3.06 mg L^{-1}; and SO_4^{2-}, 0.41 to 2.35 mg L^{-1}. The ranges of cations were Na^+, 0.08 to 0.66 mg L^{-1}; NH_4^+, 0.03 to 0.68 mg L^{-1}; K^+, <0.05 to 0.20 mg L^{-1}; Mg^{2+}, <0.05 to 0.10 mg L^{-1}; and Ca^{2+}, 0.11 to 0.62 mg L^{-1}. Seasonal variations of Cl^-, Na^+, and Mg^{2+} were a high concentration in winter and a low one in summer. Those of NO_3^-, SO_4^{2-}, and NH_4^+ were a high concentration in spring and a low one in other seasons. The correlation coefficients of ion concentrations in monthly precipitation at Toki, Japan are shown in Table 1. The relationship between Na^+ and Cl^- concentrations was found to have a strong correlation ($r = 0.97$, $p < 0.01$), and the Na^+/Cl^- concentration ratio was similar to their ratio in seawater, and Mg^{2+} and Cl^- also showed a good correlation ($r = 0.81$, $p < 0.01$). It was suggested that Na^+, Cl^- and Mg^{2+} originated from seawater. A good correlation was found between NO_3^-, SO_4^{2-}, and NH_4^+ ($r > 0.80$, $p < 0.01$). It was reported that main anthropogenic sources of NH_4NO_3 are biomass burning, fossil fuel combustion, and gas to particle conversion, and those of $(NH_4)_2SO_4$ are biomass burning, fossil fuel combustion, vehicle exhaust, and gas to particle conversion [37]. In spring, the continental air-mass is coming to Japan. The present species concentration results indicated that NO_3^-, SO_4^{2-}, and NH_4^+ were transported from the Asian continent to Japan as long-range transported pollutants. In May 2017, NO_3^-, SO_4^{2-}, NH_4^+, and Ca^{2+} were seen to rapidly increase. The Japan Meteorological Agency reported that a large-scale Asian dust event known as *kosa* was observed on the 7th and the 8th of May 2017 near the sampling site [38]. From these results, NO_3^-, SO_4^{2-}, and NH_4^+ were thought to have been transported by the *kosa* in the chemical forms of NH_4NO_3 and $(NH_4)_2SO_4$. It seemed that there was no impact from the deuterium plasma experiment on the chemical species in the precipitation.

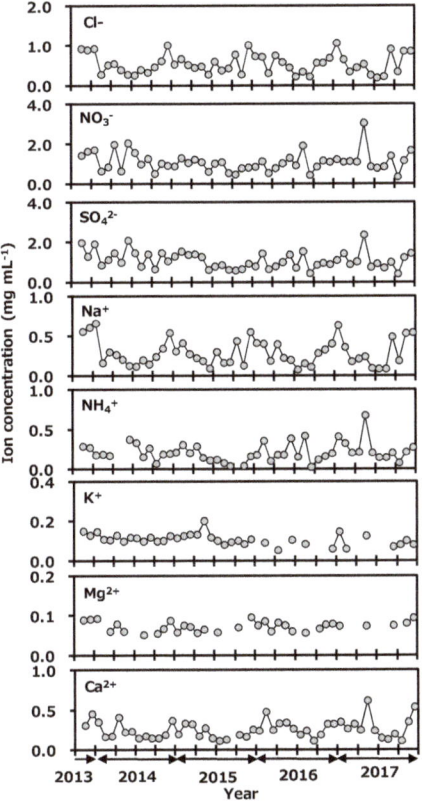

Figure 6. Variation of anion and cation concentrations in monthly precipitation collected at Toki, Japan.

Table 1. Correlation coefficients of ion species in monthly precipitation collected at Toki, Japan.

	SO_4^{2-}	NO_3^-	Na^+	NH_4^+	K^+	Mg^{2+}	Ca^{2+}
Cl^-	0.28	0.21	0.97	0.23	0.10	0.81	0.56
SO_4^{2-}		0.85	0.30	0.80	0.42	0.30	0.56
NO_3^-			0.20	0.84	0.26	0.28	0.62
Na^+				0.21	0.10	0.79	0.54
NH_4^+					0.19	0.11	0.60
K^+						0.04	0.17
Mg^{2+}							0.68

3.4. Environmental Assessment of Impact from the Deuterium Plasma Experiment

After starting the first campaign of the deuterium plasma experiment in April 2017, a part of the produced tritium was released into the atmosphere through the facility stack [16]. Here, the impact of the experiment on monthly precipitation is discussed. After starting the deuterium plasma experiment, tritium concentration in precipitation ranged from 0.17 to 0.47 Bq L^{-1}, which was similar to the concentration range before the experiment, and the seasonal variation was similar too (Figure 2). All data were within three sigma of the average tritium concentration before the deuterium plasma experiment [21]. From this result, it was suggested that there was no impact by tritium on the surrounding environment of the fusion test facility.

The survey of deuterium in precipitation is also important to assess the impact from the deuterium plasma experiment, because deuterium gas is used as fuel gas [21]. The unit of tritium concentration usually used is the tritium unit (1 TU = 0.118 Bq L^{-1}). Figure 7 shows the relationship between tritium concentration (TU) and δD in precipitation at Toki. The values were in the same area of the graph before and after the deuterium plasma experiment. This also suggested that there were no impacts by tritium and deuterium on the surrounding environment of the fusion test facility after the deuterium plasma experiment. Additionally, these results supported those reported by Tanaka et al [20]. A committed effective dose equivalent of 6.2 × 10^{-6} mSv y^{-1} was estimated for an annual consumption of drinking water having the highest tritium concentration in precipitation after starting the deuterium plasma experiment (0.47 Bq L^{-1}) by using a dose conversion factor of 1.8 × 10^{-11} Sv/Bq [39] and a daily water intake rate of 2.0 L [40]. This value was negligibly small compared with 1 mSv, which is the index of the annual dose limit for the general public.

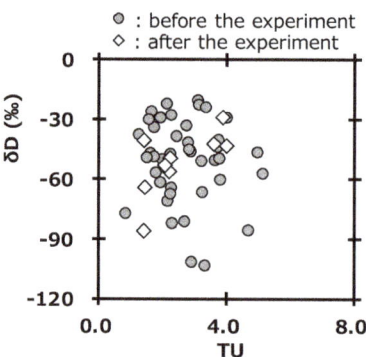

Figure 7. Relationship between tritium concentration (TU) and δD in precipitation at Toki.

4. Conclusions

The deuterium plasma experiment using the LHD was started in March 2017 to investigate high-temperature plasma physics and the hydrogen isotope effect. Although deuterium and tritium gas were exhausted from the vacuum vessel of the LHD and recovered by the exhaust detritiation system, a small amount of hydrogen gas was released into the atmosphere through the main stack. To assess the impact of released tritium to precipitation, monthly precipitation had been monitored at the NIFS site from November 2013 to establish background values for tritium, hydrogen, and oxygen stable isotope compositions and chemical species. The tritium concentration ranged from 0.10 to 0.61 Bq L^{-1} and was high in spring and low in summer. δD and δ^{18}O in monthly precipitation ranged from −103.62 to −20.77‰ and −15.14 to −3.92‰, respectively. There was no clear seasonal change in δD and δ^{18}O, and the findings were similar to reported seasonal data. The slope of the line showing the relationship between δD and δ^{18}O in monthly precipitation (δD = 7.5 × δ^{18}O + 10.6) was similar to the slope of GMWL. The d-excess showed clear seasonal variation, which was high in winter and low in summer; d-excess and average temperature were negatively correlated (r^2 = 0.647). As a result of ion species measurements, NO_3^-, SO_4^{2-}, and NH_4^+ were determined to have been transported from the Asian continent to Japan as NH_4NO_3 and $(NH_4)_2SO_4$.

Tritium concentration in precipitation after starting the deuterium plasma experiment was within three sigma of the average tritium concentration before the deuterium plasma experiment. There was no clear change in stable isotope composition and chemical species. From this, it seemed that there was no impact from tritium on the surrounding environment of the fusion test facility. The committed effective dose equivalent from drinking water to local residents after the deuterium plasma experiment was calculated to be negligibly small compared with the annual dose limit of 1 mSv. We plan to survey continuously until shutdown of LHD.

Author Contributions: Conceived and designed the survey: N.A., M.T., T.K., H.K. Performed experiments: N.A., C.I., A.K., M.N. Analyzed the data: N.A., C.I., M.N. Wrote the paper: N.A., T.K. Acquired the funding: N.A. Contributed to discussions: N.A., M.T., T.K., H.K.

Funding: This research was funded by the NIFS budget 10203004ULAA024, JSPS KAKENHI Grant Number 17K00559 and 17KK0015, and Hungarian National Research OTKA Grant No K128805.

Acknowledgments: The authors are grateful to T. Saze, H. Miyake and T Nishimura (National Institute for Fusion Science) for their important support and discussions.

Conflicts of Interest: The authors declare that they have no conflicts of interest.

References

1. Okada, S.; Momoshima, N. Overview of tritium: Characteristics, sources, and problems. *Health Phys.* **1993**, *65*, 595–609. [CrossRef] [PubMed]
2. United Nations Scientific Committee on the Effects of Atomic Radiation. *Sources and Effects of Ionizing Radiation, Volume I: Source*; UNSCEAR 2000 Report; Report to the General Assembly, Scientific Annexes; United Nations: New York, NY, USA, 2000.
3. Canadian Nuclear Safety Commission. *Investigation of the Environmental Fate of Tritium in the—Part of the Tritium Studies Projec*; INFO0792; Canadian Nuclear Safety Commission: Ottawa, ON, Canada, 2009.
4. United Nations Scientific Committee on the Effects of Atomic Radiation. *Sources and Effects of Ionizing Radiation*; UNSCEAR 2008; Report to General Assembly; Scientific Annexes Volume I; United Nations: New York, NY, USA, 2010.
5. Schell, W.R.; Sauzay, G.; Payne, B.R. Tritium injection and concentration distribution in the atmosphere. *J. Geophys. Res.* **1970**, *75*, 2251–2260. [CrossRef]
6. Morishima, H.; Kawai, H.; Koga, T.; Niwa, T. The trends of global precipitations. *J. Radiat. Res.* **1985**, *26*, 283–312. [CrossRef] [PubMed]
7. Salonen, L. Carbon-14 and tritium in air in Finland after the Chernobyl accident. *Radiochim. Acta* **1987**, *41*, 145–148. [CrossRef]
8. Matsumoto, T.; Maruoka, T.; Shimoda, G.; Obata, H.; Kagi, H.; Suzuki, K.; Yamamoto, K.; Mitsuguchi, T.; Hagino, K.; Tomioka, N.; et al. Tritium in Japanese precipitation following the March 2011 Fukushima Daiichi Nuclear Plant accident. *Sci. Total Environ.* **2013**, *445-446*, 365–370. [CrossRef] [PubMed]
9. Nakasone, S.; Ishimine, A.; Ishizu, Y.; Shiroma, Y.; Tanaka, M.; Akata, N.; Kakiuchi, H.; Sanada, T.; Furukawa, M. Recent tritium concentration of monthly precipitation in Japan. *Radiat. Prot. Dosim.* **2019**. [CrossRef]
10. Patel, B.; Campling, D.C.; Macheta, P.; Sandland, K.; Schofield, P.A. Health physics aspects of tritium operation at JET. *Fusion Eng. Des.* **1999**, *47*, 267–283. [CrossRef]
11. Holtkamp, N.; for the ITER Project Team. An overview of the ITER project. *Fusion Eng. Des.* **2007**, *82*, 427–434. [CrossRef]
12. Cristescu, I.R.; Cristescu, I.; Doerr, L.; Glugla, M.; Murdoch, D. Tritium inventories and tritium safety design principles for the fuel cycle of ITER. *Nuclear Fusion* **2007**, *47*. [CrossRef]
13. Stamoulis, K.C.; Karamanis, D.; Ioannides, K.G. Assessment of tritium levels in rivers and precipitation in north-western Greece before the ITER operation. *Fusion Eng. Des.* **2011**, *86*, 206–213. [CrossRef]
14. Takeiri, Y. Advanced helical plasma research towards a steady-state fusion reactor by deuterium experiment in large helical device. *Atmos* **2018**, *6*, 69. [CrossRef]

15. Tanaka, M.; Suzuki, N.; Kato, H.; Kondo, T.; Yokosawa, M.; Kawamata, T.; Ikeda, M.; Meguro, T.; Tanaka, T.; Sonoi, K. Design and commissioning of exhaust detritiation system for the large helical device. *Fusion Eng. Des.* **2018**, *127*, 275–283. [CrossRef]
16. National Institute for Fusion Science. *Annual Report for FY 2017 on the Activities of Radiation Safety in LHD Deuterium Plasma Experiment*; National Institute for Fusion Science: Toki, Japan, 2018. (In Japanese)
17. Akata, N.; Kakiuchi, H.; Tamari, T.; Tanaka, M.; Kawano, T.; Miyake, H.; Uda, T.; Nishimura, K. FWT and OBT concentrations in pine needle samples collected at Toki, Japan (1998–2012). *Radiat. Prot. Dosim.* **2015**, *187*, 210–214. [CrossRef] [PubMed]
18. Tanaka, M.; Uda, T. Variation of atmospheric tritium concentration in three chemical forms at Toki, Japan: 2004–12. *Radiat. Prot. Dosim.* **2015**, *187*, 187–191. [CrossRef] [PubMed]
19. Akata, N.; Tanaka, M.; Kato, H.; Yamanishi, H.; Kakiuchi, H.; Hayashi, H.; Miyake, H.; Nishimura, K. Long-term monitoring of tritium concentration in environmental water samples collected at Tono area, Japan. *Plasma Fusion Res.* **2016**, *11*, 1305032. [CrossRef]
20. Tanaka, M.; Akata, N.; Iwata, C. Environmental tritium around a fusion test facility, Japan. *Radiat. Prot. Dosim.* **2019**. [CrossRef]
21. Akata, N.; Hasegawa, H.; Sugihara, S.; Tanaka, M.; Furukawa, M.; Kurita, N.; Kovács, T.; Shiroma, Y.; Kakiuchi, H. Tritium, hydrogen and oxygen isotope compositions in monthly precipitation samples collected at Toki, Japan. *Radiat. Prot. Dosim.* **2019**. [CrossRef]
22. Japan Meteorological Agency. Automated Meteorological Data AcquistionSystem (AMeDAS). Available online: http://www.data.jma.go.jp/obd/stats/etrn/index.php (accessed on 8 August 2019).
23. Akata, N.; Shiroma, Y.; Ikemoto, N.; Kato, A.; Hegedűs, M.; Tanaka, M.; Kakiuchi, H.; Kovács, T. Atmospheric concentration and deposition flux of cosmogenic beryllium-7 at Toki, central part of Japan. *Radiat. Environ. Med.* **2018**, *7*, 47–52.
24. Japan Chemical Analysis Center. Environmental Radioactivity and Radiation in Japan. Available online: http://search.kankyo-hoshano.go.jp (accessed on 8 August 2019).
25. Gusyev, M.A.; Morgenstern, U.; Nishihara, T.; Hayashi, T.; Akata, N.; Ichiyanagi, K.; Sugimoto, A.; Hasegawa, A.; Stewart, M.K. Evaluating anthropogenic and environmental tritium effects using precipitation and Hokkaido snowpack at selected coastal locations in Asia. *Sci. Total Environ.* **2019**, *659*, 1307–1321. [CrossRef]
26. Weiss, W.; Roether, W. The rates of tritium input to the world ocean. *Earth Planet. Sci. Lett.* **1980**, *49*, 435–446. [CrossRef]
27. Momoshima, N.; Okai, T.; Kaji, T.; Takashima, Y. Distribution and transformation of various chemical forms of tritium in the environment. *Radiochim. Acta* **1991**, *54*, 129–132. [CrossRef]
28. Akata, N.; Kakiuchi, H.; Shima, N.; Iyogi, T.; Momoshima, N.; Hisamatsu, S. Tritium concentrations in the atmospheric environment at Rokkasho, Japan before the final testing of the spent fuel reprocessing plant. *J. Environ. Radioact.* **2011**, *102*, 837–842. [CrossRef] [PubMed]
29. Lewis, R.R.; Fröhlich, K.; Hebert, D. Contribution to the tritium continental effect. *Isot. Environ. Health Stud.* **2008**, *23*, 266–268. [CrossRef]
30. Araguas-Araguas, L.; Froehlich, K.; Rozanski, K. Stable isotope composition of precipitation over southeast Asia. *J. Geophys. Res.* **1998**, *103*, 28721–28742. [CrossRef]
31. Craig, H. Isotope variations in meteoric waters. *Science* **1961**, *133*, 1702–1703. [CrossRef]
32. Yabusaki, S. Characteristics of stable isotopes in precipitation at Kumagaya City, Saitama Prefecture. *Bull. Geo-Environ. Sci.* **2010**, *12*, 121–125. (In Japanese)
33. Dansgaard, W. Stable isotopes in precipitation. *Tellus* **1964**, *16*, 436–468. [CrossRef]
34. Waseda, A.; Nakai, N. Isotopic compositions of meteoric and surface waters in Central and Northeast Japan. *Chikyukagaku* **1983**, *17*, 83–91. (In Japanese)
35. Tanoue, M.; Ichiyanagi, K. Deuterium excess in precipitation and water vapor origins over Japan: A review. *J. Jpn. Hydrol. Sci.* **2016**, *46*, 101–115. (In Japanese)
36. Hasegawa, H.; Akata, N.; Kawabata, H.; Sato, T.; Chikuchi, Y.; Hisamatsu, S. Characteristics of hydrogen and oxygen stable isotope ratios in precipitation collected in a snowfall region, Aomori Prefecture, Japan. *Geochem. J.* **2014**, *48*, 9–18. [CrossRef]
37. Ianniello, A.; Spataro, F.; Esposito, I.; Hu, M.; Zhu, T. Chemical characteristics of inorganic ammonium salts in $PM_{2.5}$ in the atmosphere of Beijing (China). *Atmos. Chem. Phys.* **2011**, *11*, 10803–10822. [CrossRef]

38. Observation Day of Kosa in Gifu Prefecture (1967–2018). Available online: http://www.data.jma.go.jp/gmd/env/kosahp/59chiten/632.html (accessed on 8 August 2019).
39. International Commission on Radiological Protection. *ICRP Publication 119; Compendium of Dose Coefficients Based on ICRP Publication 60*; Elsevier: Amsterdam, The Netherlands, 2011.
40. World Health Organization. *Guidelines for Drinking-Water Quality, Third Edition Incorporating the First and Second Addenda Volume I; Recommendation*; WHO: Geneva, Switzerland, 2008.

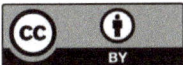

© 2019 by the authors. Licensee MDPI, Basel, Switzerland. This article is an open access article distributed under the terms and conditions of the Creative Commons Attribution (CC BY) license (http://creativecommons.org/licenses/by/4.0/).

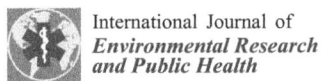

Article

Evaluation of Environmental Contamination and Estimated Radiation Exposure Dose Rates among Residents Immediately after Returning Home to Tomioka Town, Fukushima Prefecture

Masahiko Matsuo [1], Yasuyuki Taira [1,*], Makiko Orita [1], Yumiko Yamada [1], Juichi Ide [2], Shunichi Yamashita [3] and Noboru Takamura [1]

1. Department of Global Health, Medicine and Welfare, Atomic Bomb Disease Institute, Nagasaki University Graduate School of Biomedical Sciences, Nagasaki, Nagasaki Prefecture 852-8523, Japan; bb55b16008@ms.nagasaki-u.ac.jp (M.M.); orita@nagasaki-u.ac.jp (M.O.); yumiko@nagasaki-u.ac.jp (Y.Y.); takamura@nagasaki-u.ac.jp (N.T.)
2. Nuclear Safety Research Association, Tokyo 105-0004, Japan; j-ide@fukushima-power.com
3. Special Advisor to the President, Nagasaki University, Nagasaki, Nagasaki Prefecture 852-8521, Japan; shun@nagasaki-u.ac.jp
* Correspondence: y-taira@nagasaki-u.ac.jp; Tel.: +81-95-819-7171

Received: 2 April 2019; Accepted: 23 April 2019; Published: 26 April 2019

Abstract: On 1 April 2017, six years have passed since the Fukushima Daiichi Nuclear Power Station (FDNPS) accident, and the Japanese government declared that some residents who lived in Tomioka Town, Fukushima Prefecture could return to their homes. We evaluated environmental contamination and radiation exposure dose rates due to artificial radionuclides in the livelihood zone of residents (living space such as housing sites), including a restricted area located within a 10-km radius from the FDNPS, immediately after residents had returned home in Tomioka town. In areas where the evacuation orders had been lifted, the median air dose rates were 0.20 µSv/h indoors and 0.26 µSv/h outdoors, and the radiation exposure dose rate was 1.6 mSv/y. By contrast, in the "difficult-to-return zone," the median air dose rate was 2.3 µSv/h (20 mSv/y) outdoors. Moreover, the dose-forming artificial radionuclides (radiocesium) in the surface soil were 0.018 µSv/h (0.17 mSv/y) in the evacuation order-lifted areas and 0.73 µSv/h (6.4 mSv/y) in the difficult-to-return zone. These findings indicate that current concentrations of artificial radionuclides in soil samples have been decreasing in the evacuation order-lifted areas of Tomioka town; however, a significant external exposure risk still exists in the difficult-to-return zone. The case of Tomioka town is expected to be the first reconstruction model including the difficult-to-return zone.

Keywords: air dose rate; difficult-to-return zone; evacuation order-lifted areas; effective dose rate; external exposure risk; Fukushima Daiichi Nuclear Power Station accident; living space; radiocesium; surface soil; Tomioka town

1. Introduction

More than eight years have passed since 11 March 2011, the date of the 9.0-magnitude Great East Japan Earthquake, subsequent tsunami, and disaster at the Fukushima Daiichi Nuclear Power Station (FDNPS), which is operated by the Tokyo Electric Power Company. Various radionuclides were released from the FDNPS into the atmosphere, eventually being deposited on land and at sea in the surrounding areas [1]. The estimated total amount of iodine-131 (^{131}I) released ranged from about 100–500 petabecquerel (PBq), and that of cesium-137 (^{137}Cs) was generally in the range of 6–20 PBq [2]. For perspective, the estimated releases of ^{131}I and ^{137}Cs from the FDNPS were about

10% and 20%, respectively, of those estimated for the Chernobyl accident [2]. Although much of the released radionuclides was dispersed over the Pacific Ocean, a fraction was dispersed over the eastern mainland of Japan; these radionuclides were deposited on the ground by dry and/or wet atmospheric deposition through rain, fog, or snow, depending on the meteorological conditions [2,3]. These two radionuclides, together with cesium-134 (^{134}Cs), made the largest contribution by far in terms of public exposure [2]. Thus, the Japanese government, municipality and private companies have carried out the environmental and individual radiation monitoring including the external and internal exposure doses to confirm the radiation level affected areas by the FDNPS accident [4–6]. From these monitoring results, it is confirmed that artificial radionuclides with a relatively long half-life such as ^{134}Cs (half-life: 2.1 y) and ^{137}Cs (half-life: 30 y) still exist in the environmental samples including soils and plants in areas around the FDNPS [4–6].

During the eight years since the FDNPS accident, the levels of environmental radioactivity have been decreasing because of the natural decay of the radionuclides, meteorological conditions (weathering), and decontamination by the Japanese government and municipality including Tomioka Town [7–10]. The efforts of the Japanese government to reduce the estimated annual exposure dose rate to less than 20 mSv/y in the areas with an estimated annual exposure dose rate greater than 20 mSv/y (the restricted residence and difficult-to-return zones), and to reduce the estimated annual exposure dose rate closer to 1 mSv/y in the areas with an estimated annual exposure dose rate of less than 20 mSv/y (the evacuation order cancellation preparation zone and the evacuation order-lifted areas) are still ongoing; this is being done with the cooperation of local authorities and inhabitants through the implementation of effective decontamination work, which is being carried out according to the recommendations of the International Commission on Radiological Protection [4,11,12]. However, it is still necessary to evaluate the long-term behavior and exposure risk of radiocesium in the environmental samples such as soils by the radiation monitoring.

Tomioka town is located within a 20-km radius of the FDNPS. On 1 April 2017, with the Act on Special Measures Concerning Nuclear Emergency Preparedness, the Japanese government declared that residents who lived in approximately 88% of the gross area of the Tomioka town could return to their homes because the air dose rates were at low levels (estimated doses were expected to be less than 20 mSv/y) [4,5]. Although 1.5 years have passed since this "declaration of return," as of 1 October 2018, there were 12,341 evacuees of the Tomioka town, 2627 (21.3%) of whom still currently live outside of Fukushima Prefecture, 9714 (78.7%) living somewhere in Fukushima Prefecture, and the rate of residents who have returned home in Tomioka town is still extremely low, at 791 (6.4%) [6]. The reason for this limited number is thought to be anxiety regarding exposure to radiation derived from the accident [13,14]. In fact, the "difficult-to-return" zone, where the integrated dose rates are over 50 mSv/y, represents approximately 12% of the gross area of the Tomioka town; therefore, the risk of external and internal exposure while residents perform activities of daily living (ADL) remains a particular concern, and some means to reassure the public safety are required [4].

Our previous reports showed that the external and internal exposure dose rates among residents who had returned to Kawauchi village, which is adjacent to Tomioka town, were limited [15] (Figure 1). Nevertheless, long-term environmental monitoring, as well as efforts such as further decontamination and food monitoring, should continue around the FDNPS [16–19], including the Tomioka town. Especially, the external exposure risk on the livelihood zone of residents (returner's living space) such as housing sites is not evaluated unlike the data which the municipal government including the national and municipality government have reported by literature, database and website. Therefore, in the present study, to evaluate the amount of environmental contamination and calculate the contributory external radiation exposure doses of residents who had already returned or who planned to return in the future, we measured air dose rates and analyzed the concentrations of artificial radionuclides in soil samples collected in the residential areas of the Tomioka town using gamma spectrometry (Figure 1).

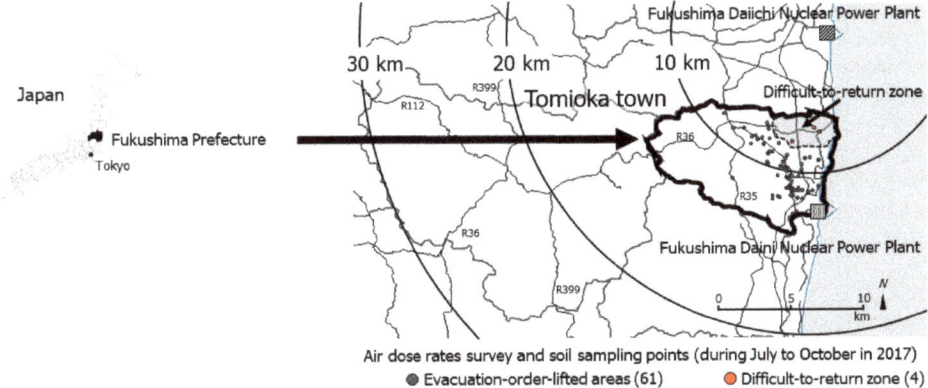

Air dose rates survey and soil sampling points (during July to October in 2017)
● Evacuation-order-lifted areas (61)   ○ Difficult-to-return zone (4)

Tomioka town is located within a 20-km radius from the Fukushima Daiichi Nuclear Power Station in an area that also includes a "difficult-to-return zone" and "evacuation order-lifted areas." The gray dotted circles are the sampling points in the evacuation order-lifted areas, and the red circles are the sampling points in the "difficult-to-return" zone.

Figure 1. Location of Tomioka town, Fukushima Prefecture.

2. Materials and Methods

2.1. Sampling Points

The FDNPS (37°25′ N, 141°02′ E) is located on the east coast of Honshu Island, approximately 200 km northeast of Tokyo. Tomioka town (public office: 37°20′ N, 141°0′ E) is located 8.5 km south of the FDNPS. In the present study, we measured air dose rates and collected soils from 65 sampling points in 45 residential areas where residents had returned home and near 20 assembly halls in Tomioka town between 11 July and 25 October 2017 (Figure 1).

2.2. Measurement of Air Dose Rates and Radionuclides

In the present study, the air dose rates were monitored in air 1 m above the ground at all sampling points using a NaI(Tl) scintillation survey meter (TCS-172B, Hitachi-Aloka Medical, Ltd., Tokyo, Japan), which can measure gamma rays (50 keV-3 MeV, ambient dose equivalent rate at 1cm depth: 0.00–30.0 μSv/h). We measured air dose rates with a time constant of 10. In the evacuation order-lifted areas, an additional radiation dose (radiocesium) including the natural dose was estimated using the following formula:

$$A_{ext} \text{ (mSv/y)} = [(C_{int} - 0.04 \text{ μSv/h}) \cdot 16\text{h} + (C_{ext} - 0.04 \text{ μSv/h}) \cdot 8 \text{ h}] \cdot 365 \text{ d} \cdot 0.001 \tag{1}$$

where C_{int} is the indoor air dose rate (μSv/h) and C_{ext} is the outdoor air dose rate (μSv/h). The fixed number (0.04 μSv/h) in the formula is defined as the natural dose in Japan, and 16 h and 8 h are defined as representing the indoor and outdoor ADL, respectively. This calculation was based on the method described by the Ministry of the Environment [8]. According to the monitoring information by the national and local authorities, the prevalent dose-forming artificial radionuclides from various samples have been mainly ^{134}Cs and/or ^{137}Cs in offsite areas around the FDNPS. [4,5].

At the same time, to evaluate the vertical distribution and external radiation exposure, 130 samples (65 sites × 2) of surface soil (0–5 and 5–10 cm below the surface) were collected at Tomioka town from July to October 2017. Soil sampling was carried out at all sampling sites using a core sampling technique (two core samples for each point). The size of the soil samples was 18.2 cm^2 (diameter of 4.8 cm) and the density of the soil layers (0–10 cm) ranged from 0.31 to 2.3 g/cm^3 (dry). The mass of the soil samples collected in each area ranged from 24.5 to 284 g. After collection, all samples were dried for 24 h in a fixed temperature dryer (105 °C). Next, the samples were sieved for pebbles and organic materials (>2 mm). After preparation, the samples were placed in plastic containers made of polypropylene and analyzed using a high purity germanium detector (ORTEC® GMX series, Ortec International Inc., Oak Ridge, TN, USA) coupled to a multi-channel analyzer (MCA7600, Seiko EG&G Co., Ltd., Chiba, Japan) for 3600–36,000 s. We set the measuring time to detect objective radionuclide levels. The target gamma ray peaks used for the measurements were 604.66 keV for ^{134}Cs (half-life: 2.1 y) and 661.64 keV for ^{137}Cs (half-life: 30 y). Decay corrections were made based on the sampling date. The detector efficiency calibration for different measurement geometries including the density and thickness of samples was performed using mixed activity standard volume sources (Japan Radioisotope Association, Tokyo, Japan); the relative detection efficiency of this instrument was 33.04%. Sample collection, processing, and analysis were executed in accordance with standard methods of the radioactivity measurement authorized by the Ministry of Education, Culture, Sports, Science, and Technology, Japan [20]. All measurements were performed at Nagasaki University, Nagasaki, Japan. The obtained data are expressed as average, range (minimum–maximum) and medians.

2.3. Effective Dose Rate

After the measurements, external effective dose rates (μSv/h and mSv/y) from soil samples were estimated from artificial radionuclide concentrations using the following formula:

$$H_{ext} = C \cdot D_{ext} \cdot f \cdot s \qquad (2)$$

where C is the activity concentration (median) of detected artificial radionuclides (^{134}Cs and ^{137}Cs) (kBq/m^2; estimated from the radiocesium concentration in Bq/kg, including soil particles (<2 mm) and collected surface soil (0.00182 m^2)), D_{ext} is the dose conversion coefficient reported as the kerma-rate in air at 1 m above the ground per unit activity per unit area ((μGy/h)/(kBq/m^2)), supposing that the air-kerma rate and the absorbed dose rate in air were the same value, for radiocesium with the relaxation mass per unit area (β: g/cm^2) set to 10 (5-20 y) because more than eight years had passed since the FDNPS accident (1.95×10^{-3} (μGy/h)/(kBq/m^2) for ^{134}Cs and 7.55×10^{-4} (μGy/h)/(kBq/m^2) for ^{137}Cs, ICRU 1994) [21], f is the unit conversion coefficient (0.7 Sv/Gy for the effective dose rate in the body per unit absorbed dose rate in air) [22], and s is the decrease in the coefficient by a shielding factor against exposure to gamma rays from a sample at 1 m above the ground (0.7 under the condition of usual land) [23]. These calculations were based on the method described in our previous study [15,16,24].

2.4. Ethics Statement

The present study was approved by the ethics committee of Nagasaki University Graduate School of Biomedical Sciences (project registration number: 17030212), and written informed consent was obtained from the owners of the land containing all sampling points.

3. Results

The air dose rates in Tomioka town are shown in Table 1. In the evacuation order-lifted areas, the median air dose rates inside the homes of the residents who had returned were 0.20 [0.086–0.37] μSv/h indoors, 0.26 [0.088–0.68] μSv/h outdoors (in front of the entrance), and 0.34 [0.14–1.3] μSv/h in the backyard. The annual estimated doses were 1.7 mSv/y indoors, 2.3 mSv/y outdoors, and 3.0 mSv/y in the backyard. Therefore, an additional radiation exposure dose of 1.6 mSv/y was estimated by the formula (1). On the other hand, in the difficult-to-return zone, the median air dose rates were 2.3 [1.1–2.9] μSv/h outdoors and 2.1 [1.8–2.4] μSv/h in the backyard. The annual estimated doses were 20 mSv/y outdoors and 18 mSv/y in the backyard.

Table 1. Air dose rates around residences and assembly halls in Tomioka town, Fukushima Prefecture, during September to October 2017.

Points		Air Dose Rate in μSv/h			External Effective Dose Rate in mSv/y	Shielding Factor
		Average	Range	Median		
Evacuation order-lifted areas (n = 61) [a]	Indoors	0.20 ± 0.058 [c]	0.086–0.37 [d]	0.20 (0.28) [e]	1.7 [f]	0.77 [g]
	Outdoors	0.29 ± 0.12	0.088–0.68	0.26 (0.43)	2.3	
	Backyard	0.40 ± 0.19	0.14–1.34	0.34 (0.63)	3.0	
Difficult-to-return zone (n = 4) [b]	Outdoors	2.2 ± 0.65	1.1–2.9	2.3 (2.7)	20	
	Backyard	2.1 ± 0.23	1.8–2.4	2.1 (2.4)	18	

[a] residences (n = 45) and assembly halls (n = 16). [b] assembly halls (n = 4). [c] mean ± S.D. [d] minimum-maximum. [e] parentheses show 90th percentile. [f] median × 24h × 365d × 0.001. [g] shielding factor of air dose rates ratio (indoors/outdoors).

The distribution of detected artificial radionuclides (radiocesium) and external effective dose rates from the surface soil due to radiocesium and the radionuclide ratios (^{134}Cs/^{137}Cs in Bq/kg [dry]) in Tomioka town are shown in Table 2. The dose-forming artificial radionuclides ^{134}Cs and ^{137}Cs were prevalent in all samples. In the evacuation order-lifted areas, the radiocesium concentrations inside the homes of the residents who had returned were 238 (8.0–6063) (0–5 cm) Bq/kg (dry) and 334 (3.7–5803) (5–10 cm) Bq/kg (dry) for ^{134}Cs, and 1784 (34–45,331) (0–5 cm) Bq/kg (dry) and 2093 (28–48,911) (5–10 cm) Bq/kg (dry) for ^{137}Cs. The external effective dose rates from the surface soil (0–5 cm) were estimated as 0.17 mSv/y. On the other hand, in the difficult-to-return zone, the radiocesium concentrations inside the assembly halls were 8025 (3317–18,552) (0–5 cm) Bq/kg (dry) and 6633 (4654–9034) (5–10 cm) Bq/kg (dry) for ^{134}Cs, and 62,131 (25,559–141,209) (0–5 cm) Bq/kg-dry and 51,840 (36,317–69,377) (5–10 cm) Bq/kg-dry for ^{137}Cs. The external effective dose rates from the surface soil (0–5 cm) were estimated as 6.4 mSv/y. In the evacuation order-lifted areas, the radiocesium concentrations were lower in the surface soil samples (0–5 cm) than in the lower layers (5–10 cm), whereas in the difficult-to-return zone, the radiocesium concentrations were higher in the surface soil samples (0–5 cm) than in the lower layers (5–10 cm). Therefore, in the difficult-to-return zone, there was still an accumulation of radiocesium in the surface layer. In the present study, the concentrations of radiocesium exceeded 8000 Bq/kg (dry), which is the standard value for storing decontamination waste according to the Japanese guidelines, at some (17) sampling points, and the median radiocesium values (^{134}Cs/^{137}Cs ratios) in the soil samples were 0.13 (0.093–0.18) at the time of sampling, regardless of whether they were in the difficult-to-return zone [25]. Moreover, the effective dose rates from the air dose rates in outdoors and soil samples in Tomioka town showed a positive relationship (r = 0.51 and 0.61, Figure 2).

Table 2. Distribution of radiocesium in soil samples in Tomioka town, Fukushima Prefecture.

Points	depth	Radiocesium Concentration in Bq/kg (dry) [a]						External Effective Dose Rate in mSv/y	Radionuclide Ratio in ^{134}Cs/^{137}Cs
		Average		Range		Median			
		^{134}Cs (2.1 y)	^{137}Cs (30 y)	^{134}Cs (2.1 y)	^{137}Cs (30 y)	^{134}Cs (2.1 y)	^{137}Cs (30 y)		
Evacuation-order-lifted areas (n = 61) [a]	0–5 cm	694.3 ± 1137 [c]	4996 ± 8421	8.0–6063 [d]	34–45,331	238 (1950) [e]	1784 (12,966)	0.17 [f]	0.13 (0.14) [g]
	5–10 cm	750.0 ± 1035	5585 ± 8163	3.7–5803	28–48,911	334 (2016)	2093 (15,209)		0.13 (0.14)
Difficult-to-return zone (n = 4) [b]	0–5 cm	9480 ± 5708	72,757 ± 43,211	3317–18,552	25,559–141,209	8025 (15,906)	62,131 (121,336)	6.4	0.13 (0.13)
	5–10 cm	6739 ± 2067	52,343 ± 15,690	4654–9034	36,317–69,377	6633 (8893)	51,840 (68,551)		0.13 (0.14)

[a] Residences (n = 45) and assembly halls (n = 16). [b] Assembly halls (n = 4). [c] mean ± S.D. [d] minimum-maximum. [e] parentheses show 90th percentile. [f] calculated by the formula (2). [g] median (90th percentile).

The effective external doses in the living space of residents within housing sites immediately after the cancellation of the restriction in Tomioka Town (during September to October in 2017) are shown in Figure 3. In the present study, the external exposure doses including radiocesium were mainly higher in the backyard than outdoors in front of the entrance. Naturally, the external exposure doses including radiocesium were higher in outdoors than indoors by the shielding effectiveness of their house. Moreover, the external exposure doses due to radiocesium in soil samples were sufficiently low level.

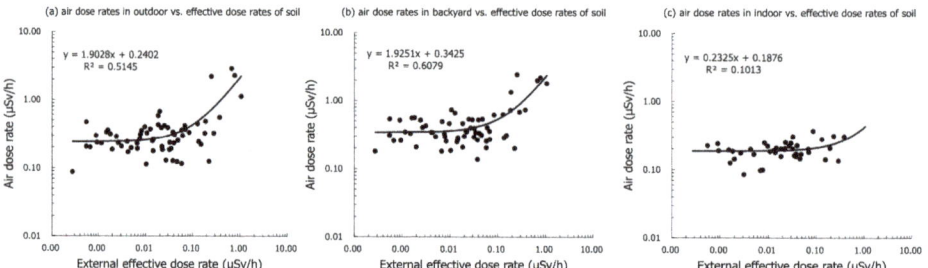

Figure 2. Relationship between estimated external effective dose rates from surface soil and air dose rates in Tomioka town. (**a**) Air dose rates in outdoor (entrance) vs., (**b**) air dose rates in outdoors (backyard) vs. and (**c**) air dose rates in indoor (entrance) vs. effective dose rates of soil samples. The external effective dose rates from soil samples were estimated using a high purity germanium detector (only radiocesium). Air dose rates were measured at the sampling points using a NaI (Tl) scintillation survey meter (natural dose rates including radiocesium).

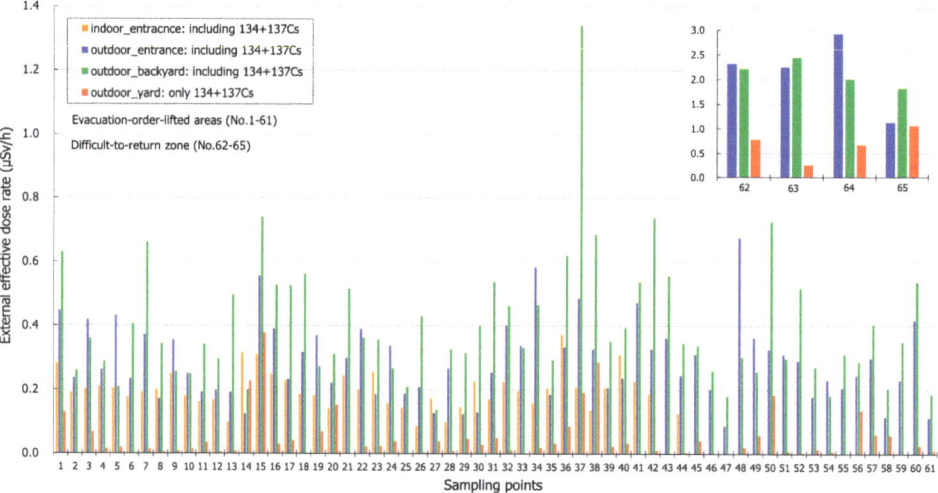

Figure 3. External exposure doses immediately after the cancellation of restriction in Tomioka Town. The effective external doses in residents living space within housing sites during September to October in 2017. Yellow, blue and green squares show the natural dose rates including radiocesium. Red square shows the external effective dose rates from soil samples (only radiocesium).

4. Discussion

In the present study, the artificial radionuclides ^{134}Cs and ^{137}Cs were detected in all samples from Tomioka town by gamma spectrometry, and the ^{134}Cs/^{137}Cs values of these samples were around 0.13, which is thought to be the consequence of the relatively early decay of ^{134}Cs (median: 238 (8.0–6063) Bq/kg (dry) for ^{134}Cs and 1784 (34–45,331) Bq/kg (dry) for ^{137}Cs in the upper layer (0–5 cm); see Table 2). Immediately after the accident, the ^{134}Cs/^{137}Cs values were reported as 0.9 in areas to the south and southwest of the FDNPS, which were higher than those observed around the Chernobyl Nuclear Power Plant [26,27]. Eight years have passed since the FDNPS accident, and it was confirmed that the ^{134}Cs/^{137}Cs values have been decreasing because of the natural decay of ^{134}Cs (half-life: 2.1 y). Therefore, in the present study, the radiocesium (the ^{134}Cs/^{137}Cs values: 0.13 (median)) detected in these samples was obviously derived from the FDNPS accident.

In the present study, air dose rates were higher in the backyard (where trees and plants such as cedar were growing) than outdoors in front of the entrance to homes in evacuation order-lifted areas (0.34 (0.14–1.3) µSv/h in the backyard vs. 0.26 (0.088–0.68) µSv/h outdoors and 0.20 (0.086–0.37) µSv/h indoors; Table 1). In the difficult-to-return zone, the outdoor air dose rates (in the backyard and in front of the entrance) were nearly equivalent, and the samples were still contaminated (2.1 (1.8–2.4) µSv/h in the backyard vs. 2.3 (1.1–2.9) µSv/h outdoors; Table 1). Also, gaps were observed between air dose rates and estimated external effective dose rates. The external effective dose rate in the evacuation-order-lifted areas were estimated at 10 times higher than the external estimated effective dose rates from radiocesium in soil samples (Tables 1 and 2). However, because a positive relationship (r = 0.61) was observed between air dose rates in the backyard and estimated effective dose rates from surface soil samples, the findings of the present study suggest that the environmental radiation dose was mainly derived from surface soil and areas around vegetation, including fallen leaves (Figure 2). Following the FDNPS accident, the residential areas, farmlands, forests (the close to residential areas; <20 m), and roads within the evacuation order areas around the FDNPS were extensively decontaminated by suitable methods, and decontamination of the entire area, excluding the difficult-to-return zones, was completed on 19 March 2018 [25]. However, the decontamination effect of areas around vegetation including fallen leaves may be limited. Some reports have suggested that radiocesium accumulates in various forest environments through the forest biota [24,28–31]. The detection of high ^{137}Cs concentrations in evergreen cedar needles after the accident indicated that the canopy interception of atmospherically deposited ^{137}Cs, and the existence of high ^{137}Cs activity in newly developed foliage during the six years after the accident, particularly in the leaves of Japanese konara oak (*Quercus serrata*) seedlings in an abandoned coppice forest, suggests translocation and efficient recycling of ^{137}Cs within the trees [32]. On the other hand, the effective dose rates from the air dose rates in indoors and soil samples in Tomioka town showed a negative relationship (r = 0.10, Figure 2). The shielding effect by houses was comparatively high because there were a lot of new houses with high airtightness in areas of the cancellation of restriction in the Tomioka Town (shielding factor = 0.77, Table 1) [22,23]. Actually, the additional radiation exposure dose was estimated at low level (1.6 mSv/y) [33].

The Japanese and local government aim to reduce the estimated annual exposure dose rate to 1 mSv/y as early as possible and continue with further reductions in residential areas. In the present study, the current contamination levels due to radiocesium were extremely different in both areas; low (0.17 mSv/y) in the evacuation order-lifted areas and relatively high (6.4 mSv/y) in the difficult-to-return zone in Tomioka town (Table 2). In the eight years that have passed since the FDNPS accident, the estimated external exposure levels in the evacuation order-lifted areas have decreased because of decontamination and the decay of artificial radionuclides; however, further remediation of soil contaminated with artificial radionuclides in the difficult-to-return zone, which is a crucial social responsibility in Japan and internationally, is still needed. Based on the current findings regarding radiocesium concentrations and effective dose rates, decreases in external exposure doses are the evidence that evacuees from the Tomioka town may return (Figure 3). Especially, the concentrations of detected radiocesium in surface soils were low during two layers (0–5 cm and 5–10 cm) in the evacuation order-lifted areas of Tomioka town, and the current levels of environmental contamination around homes in this area of Tomioka town are extremely low. Conversely, in the difficult-to-return zone, the concentrations of detected radiocesium were higher in surface soil samples (0–5 cm) than in lower layers (5–10 cm), because in this area, effective decontamination of the strong absorption of radiocesium by soil particles is not progressing smoothly (Table 2). Most ^{137}Cs accumulated within 1.5 years after the FDNPS accident and ^{137}Cs continued to be retained in the upper mineral soil layer (0–5 cm) [34]. Absorption of ^{137}Cs appears to be the primary process regulating the ^{137}Cs distribution in the soil profiles (vertical distribution) over five years of monitoring after contamination [34]. In other words, these findings suggest that environmental contamination and the effective dose rates on the ground in the evacuation order-lifted areas will be decreased by decontamination procedures, such as the removal of surface soil [35] (Figure 3). In addition, the decontamination of residential areas, farmlands, forests, and roads is being carried out by suitable methods [35]. Reconstruction projects have already started in the area of the difficult-to-return zone in coordination with relevant ministries and agencies such as the Ministry of the Environment and Reconstruction Agency [36]. In Tomioka town, the pre-decontamination of the difficult-to-return zone has been carried out [37]. The investigation of the Ministry of the Environment and our research by the car-survey report the effectiveness of the pre-decontamination in the difficult-to-return zone (data not shown). It is expected that evacuation orders will be lifted for wider areas in the difficult-to-return zone in the near future.

This study did have several limitations. First, the number of soil sampling points were relatively limited, especially in the difficult-to-return zone ($n = 4$), because the size of the sample collection was small under the serious and emergent conditions of the FDNPS accident. Although we researched in the residential area as much as possible for the return to home in the future, further investigation with detailed conditions is needed while confirming the change of radiation doses by the decontamination work.

Second, other types of evidence such as the internal exposure doses, infrastructure repairs and support services also play roles in the decision to return. Especially, agricultural activities and the countryside (*satoyama*) cultural practice of ingesting edible wild plants (*sansai*) and mushrooms are being carried out carefully based on the guidelines by the Nuclear Emergency Response Headquarters of the Japanese government, accompanied by the ongoing decontamination of farmlands and radiation monitoring [5,38]. Edible wild plants and mushrooms are well-known as accumulators of radiocesium [16,18,19,39–42]. Currently, the shipment of agricultural products in Japan is determined based on regulations outlined by the Japanese government [43]. In Tomioka town, the monitoring system for local foods by using the nondestructive equipment for detecting radiocesium such as the NaI spectrometer is an effective tool to avoid unnecessary radiation exposure since February 2018. Further investigations on external and internal effective doses, are needed [44,45].

5. Conclusions

In the present study, we evaluated environmental contamination and contributions from the external exposure due to radiocesium in Tomioka town near the FDNPS. Based on the current findings regarding radiocesium concentrations and effective dose rates, we confirmed that current levels are decreasing sufficiently, especially in the evacuation order-lifted areas located within a 20-km radius from the FDNPS and decontaminated rapidly, even though a certain amount of radiocesium derived from the accident was detected in soil samples in these areas. Thus, decreases in external exposure doses are the evidence that that evacuees from Tomioka town may return with the long-term follow-up, as well as environmental monitoring and countermeasures, such as further decontamination and restrictions on the intake of local foods (edible wild plants and mushrooms) that can cause unnecessary radiation exposure, and physical and mental support [35–37]. The case of Tomioka town is expected to be the first reconstruction model for evaluating environmental contamination and radiation exposure dose rates due to artificial radionuclides, including areas such as the difficult-to-return zone near the FDNPS.

Author Contributions: M.O. and N.T. conceived and designed the framed study; Y.T., M.O. and Y.Y. designed the methodology in this investigation; M.M., Y.T., M.O., Y.Y. and J.I. investigated the environmental radiation in Tomioka town; M.M. analyzed the sample data and wrote our manuscript; Y.T. reviewed and edited the manuscript; N.T. and Y.T. reviewed the sample data; Y.T., M.O., Y.Y. and N.T. administered the project; S.Y. and N.T. supervised the project; N.T. acquired the funding; M.M., Y.T., M.O., Y.Y., J.I. and N.T. contributed to discussing the statistical method and the interpretation of our findings.

Funding: This work was supported by Research on the Health Effects of Radiation organized by the Ministry of the Environment, Japan.

Acknowledgments: We would also like to thank Yoshiyuki Nitta, Tsuyoshi Wakamatsu, and Shinya Kurosawa (Tomioka Municipal Government, Fukushima, Japan) for assistance with our research plan and sample collection.

Conflicts of Interest: The authors declare no conflict of interest.

References

1. International Atomic Energy Agency. The Fukushima Daiichi Accident. In *Technical Volume 1. Description and Context of the Accident*; International Atomic Energy Agency: Vienna, Austria, 2015; pp. 1–225.
2. United Nations Scientific Committee on the Effects of Atomic Radiation. *Report to the General Assembly, Scientific Annex A: Levels and Effects of Radiation Exposure due to the Nuclear Accident after the 2011 Great East-Japan Earthquake and Tsunami*; United Nations: Vienna, Austria, 2013.
3. Hirose, K. Fukushima Daiichi Nuclear Plant accident: Atmospheric and oceanic impacts over the five years. *J. Environ. Radioact.* **2016**, *157*, 113–130. [CrossRef] [PubMed]
4. Fukushima Prefectural Government, Japan. Fukushima Revitalization Station, The Official Website for Fukushima's Restoration. Available online: http://www.pref.fukushima.lg.jp/site/portal-english/list385.html (accessed on 1 April 2019).
5. The Nuclear Regulation Authority, Japan. Monitoring Information of Environmental Radioactivity Level. Available online: http://radioactivity.nsr.go.jp/en/ (accessed on 1 April 2019).
6. Tomioka Town Local Government, Japan. Number of Evacuees in Tomioka Town as of 1 October 2018. Available online: https://www.tomioka-town.jp/oshirase/machi/2029.html (accessed on 1 April 2019). (In Japanese)
7. Japan Atomic Energy Agency. Database for Radioactive Substance Monitoring Data. Available online: https://emdb.jaea.go.jp/emdb/en/ (accessed on 1 April 2019).
8. The Minisiry of the Environment, Japan. Health & Chemicals. Radiation Health Control Measures. Unified Basic Data on Health Effects by Radiation. Available online: http://www.env.go.jp/chemi/rhm/h29kisoshiryo.html (accessed on 1 April 2019). (In Japanese)
9. Naito, W.; Uesaka, M.; Yamada, C.; Kurosawa, T.; Yasutaka, T.; Ishii, H. Relationship between Individual External Doses, Ambient Dose Rates and Individuals' Activity-Patterns in Affected Areas in Fukushima following the Fukushima Daiichi Nuclear Power Plant Accident. *PLoS ONE* **2016**, *11*, e0158879. [CrossRef]
10. The Minisiry of the Environment, Japan. Environmental Remediation in Japan. Available online: http://josen.env.go.jp/en/pdf/progressseet_progress_on_cleanup_efforts.pdf (accessed on 1 April 2019).
11. International Atomic Energy Agency. *The Follow-up IAEA International Mission on Remediation of Large Contaminated Areas Off-Site the Fukushima Daiichi Nuclear Power Plant*; International Atomic Energy Agency: Vienna, Austria, 2013; pp. 1–57.
12. International Commission on Radiological Protection. *The 2007 Recommendations of the International Commission on Radiological Protection*; International Commission on Radiological Protection: Ottawa, Canada, 2007.
13. Reconstruction Agency, Japan. *Basic Guidelines for Reconstruction in Response to the Great East Japan Earthquake in the "Reconstruction and Revitalization Period"*. Available online: http://www.reconstruction.go.jp/english/topics/Laws_etc/index.html (accessed on 1 April 2019).
14. The Consumer Affairs Agency, Government of Japan. White Paper on Consumer Affairs 2017. Available online: http://www.caa.go.jp/en/publication/annual_report/ (accessed on 1 April 2019).
15. Taira, Y.; Hayashida, N.; Yamaguchi, H.; Yamashita, S.; Endo, Y.; Takamura, N. Evaluation of environmental contamination and estimated radiation doses for the return to residents' homes in Kawauchi Village, Fukushima Prefecture. *PLoS ONE* **2012**, *7*, e45816. [CrossRef]
16. Taira, Y.; Hayashida, N.; Orita, M.; Yamaguchi, H.; Ide, J.; Endo, Y.; Yamashita, S.; Takamura, N. Evaluation of environmental contamination and estimated exposure doses after residents return home in Kawauchi Village, Fukushima Prefecture. *Environ. Sci. Technol.* **2014**, *48*, 4556–4563. [CrossRef] [PubMed]
17. Orita, M.; Hayashida, N.; Taira, Y.; Fukushima, Y.; Ide, J.; Endo, Y.; Kudo, T.; Yamashita, S.; Takamura, N. Measurement of individual doses of radiation by personal dosimeter is important for the return of residents from evacuation order areas after nuclear disaster. *PLoS ONE* **2015**, *10*, e0121990. [CrossRef] [PubMed]
18. Nakashima, K.; Orita, M.; Fukuda, N.; Taira, Y.; Hayashida, N.; Matsuda, N.; Takamura, N. Radiocesium concentrations in wild mushrooms collected in Kawauchi Village after the accident at the Fukushima Daiichi Nuclear Power Plant. *PeerJ* **2015**, *3*, e1427. [CrossRef]

19. Orita, M.; Nakashima, K.; Hayashida, N.; Endo, Y.; Yamashita, S.; Takamura, N. Concentrations of Radiocesium in Local Foods Collected in Kawauchi Village after the Accident at the Fukushima Dai-ichi Nuclear Power Station. *Sci. Rep.* **2016**, *6*, 28470. [CrossRef] [PubMed]
20. The Ministry of Education, Culture, Sports, Science, and Technology, Japan. Environmental Radioactivity and Radiation in Japan. Available online: http://www.kankyo-hoshano.go.jp/en/index.html (accessed on 1 April 2019).
21. The International Commission on Radiation Units and Measurements. *Gamma-ray Spectrometry in the Environment*; International Commission on Radiation Units and Measurements: Bethesda, MD, USA, 1994.
22. United Nations Scientific Committee on the Effects of Atomic Radiation. *Sources and Effects of Ionizing Radiation*; UNSCEAR 2000 Report to General Assembly with Scientific Annexes; Annex A: Dose Assessment Methodologies; United Nations: Vienna, Austria, 2000.
23. International Atomic Energy Agency. *Generic Procedures for Assessment and Response during Radiological Emergency*; The International Atomic Energy Agency: Vienna, Austria, 2000.
24. Kanasashi, T.; Sugiura, Y.; Takenaka, C.; Hijii, N.; Umemura, M. Radiocesium distribution in sugi (Cryptomeria japonica) in eastern Japan: Translocation from needles to pollen. *J. Environ. Radioact.* **2015**, *139*, 398–406. [CrossRef]
25. The Ministry of the Environment, Japan. Countermeasures for the Great East Japan Earthquake. Available online: http://www.env.go.jp/en/focus/docs/01_cgeje.html (accessed on 1 April 2019).
26. Tagami, K.; Uchida, S.; Uchihori, Y.; Ishii, N.; Kitamura, H.; Shirakawa, Y. Specific activity and activity ratios of radionuclides in soil collected about 20 km from the Fukushima Daiichi Nuclear Power Plant: Radionuclide release to the south and southwest. *Sci. Total Environ.* **2011**, *409*, 4885–4888. [CrossRef]
27. Mück, K.; Pröhl, G.; Likhtarev, I.; Kovgan, L.; Meckbach, R.; Golikov, V. A consistent radionuclide vector after the Chernobyl accident. *Health Phys.* **2002**, *82*, 141–156. [CrossRef]
28. Akama, A.; Kiyono, Y.; Kanazashi, T.; Shinchi, K. Survey of radioactive contamination of sugi (Cryptomeria japonica D. Don) shoots and male flowers in Fukushima prefectures. *Jpn. J. For. Environ.* **2013**, *55*, 105–111.
29. Koizumi, A.; Niisoe, T.; Harada, K.H.; Fujii, Y.; Adachi, A.; Hitomi, T.; Ishikawa, H. (137)Cs trapped by biomass within 20 km of the Fukushima Daiichi Nuclear Power Plant. *Environ. Sci. Technol.* **2013**, *47*, 9612–9618. [CrossRef]
30. Kuroda, K.; Kagawa, A.; Tonosaki, M. Radiocesium concentrations in the bark, sapwood and heartwood of three tree species collected at Fukushima forests half a year after the Fukushima Dai-ichi nuclear accident. *J. Environ. Radioact.* **2013**, *122*, 37–42. [CrossRef]
31. Ohashi, S.; Okada, N.; Tanaka, A.; Nakai, W.; Takano, S. Radial and vertical distributions of radiocesium in tree stems of Pinus densiflora and Quercus serrata 1.5 y after the Fukushima nuclear disaster. *J. Environ. Radioact.* **2014**, *134*, 54–60. [CrossRef]
32. Kato, H.; Onda, Y.; Saidin, Z.H.; Sakashita, W.; Hisadome, K.; Loffredo, N. Six-year monitoring study of radiocesium transfer in forest environments following the Fukushima nuclear power plant accident. *J. Environ. Radioact* **2018**, in press. [CrossRef]
33. Tsukasaki, A.; Taira, Y.; Orita, M.; Takamura, N. Seven years post-Fukushima: Long-term measurement of exposure doses in Tomioka Town. *J. Radiat. Res.* **2019**, *60*, 159–160. [CrossRef]
34. Fujii, K.; Yamaguchi, N.; Imamura, N.; Kobayashi, M.; Kaneko, S.; Takahashi, M. Effects of radiocesium fixation potentials on 137Cs retention in volcanic soil profiles of Fukushima forests. *J. Environ. Radioact.* **2019**, *198*, 126–134. [CrossRef]
35. The Minisiry of the Environment, Japan. Environmental Remediation. Available online: http://josen.env.go.jp/en/decontamination/ (accessed on 1 April 2019).
36. Reconstruction Agency, Japan. Recovery and Reconstruction from the Great East Japan Earthquake. Available online: http://www.reconstruction.go.jp/english/topics/Progress_to_date/index.html (accessed on 1 April 2019).
37. Reconstruction Agency, Japan. Press Release on March 9, 2018. The Reconstruction Project in the Area where Return is Difficult in Tomioka Town. Available online: http://www.reconstruction.go.jp/topics/main-cat1/sub-cat1-4/saiseikyoten/material/20180309_kouhyou_tomioka_tokuteifukkosaiseikyotenkuikifukkosaiseikeikaku.pdf (accessed on 1 April 2019). (In Japanese)
38. Orita, M.; Fukushima, Y.; Yamashita, S.; Takamura, N. The Need for Forest Decontamination: For the Recovery of Fukushima. *Radiat. Prot. Dosim.* **2016**, *175*, 295–296. [CrossRef]

39. Taira, Y.; Hayashida, N.; Brahmanandhan, G.M.; Nagayama, Y.; Yamashita, S.; Takahashi, J.; Gutevitc, A.; Kazlovsky, A.; Urazalin, M.; Takamura, N. Current concentration of artificial radionuclides and estimated radiation doses from 137Cs around the Chernobyl Nuclear Power Plant, the Semipalatinsk Nuclear Testing Site, and in Nagasaki. *J. Radiat. Res.* **2011**, *52*, 88–95. [CrossRef]
40. The Ministry of Agriculture, Foresty and Fisheres, Japan. The Great East Japan Earthquake. Available online: http://www.maff.go.jp/e/quake/press_110312-1.html (accessed on 1 April 2019).
41. Orita, M.; Nakashima, M.; Taira, Y.; Fukuda, T.; Fukushima, Y.; Kudo, T.; Endo, Y.; Yamashita, S.; Takamura, N. Radiocesium concentrations in wild mushrooms after the accident at the Fukushima Daiichi Nuclear Power Station: Follow-up study in Kawauchi village. *Sci. Rep.* **2017**, *7*, 6744. [CrossRef]
42. Tsuchiya, R.; Taira, Y.; Orita, M.; Fukushima, Y.; Endo, Y.; Yamashita, S.; Takamura, N. Radiocesium contamination and estimated internal exposure doses in edible wild plants in Kawauchi Village following the Fukushima nuclear disaster. *PLoS ONE* **2017**, *12*, e0189398. [CrossRef] [PubMed]
43. The World Health Organization. Global Environment Monitoring System (GEMS/Food). Available online: http://www.who.int/foodsafety/areas_work/chemical-risks/gems-food/en/ (accessed on 1 April 2019).
44. The Ministry of Health, Labour, and Welfare, Japan. New Standard Limits for Radionuclides in Foods (Provisional Translation); Department of Food Safety, Pharmaceutical & Food Safety Bureau, the Ministry of Health Labour and Welfare. Available online: http://www.mhlw.go.jp/english/topics/2011eq/dl/new_standard.pdf (accessed on 1 April 2019).
45. Yoshida, K.; Shinkawa, T.; Urata, H.; Nakashima, K.; Orita, M.; Yasui, K.; Kumagai, A.; Ohtsuru, A.; Yabe, H.; Maeda, M.; et al. Psychological distress of residents in Kawauchi village, Fukushima Prefecture after the accident at Fukushima Daiichi Nuclear Power Station: The Fukushima Health Management Survey. *PeerJ* **2016**, *4*, e2353. [CrossRef] [PubMed]

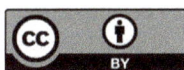

© 2019 by the authors. Licensee MDPI, Basel, Switzerland. This article is an open access article distributed under the terms and conditions of the Creative Commons Attribution (CC BY) license (http://creativecommons.org/licenses/by/4.0/).

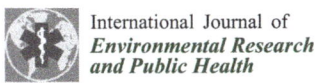 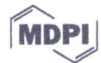

Brief Report

Study of Well Waters from High-Level Natural Radiation Areas in Northern Vietnam

Van-Hao Duong [1], Thanh-Duong Nguyen [1], Miklos Hegedus [2], Erika Kocsis [2] and Tibor Kovacs [2],*

[1] Geophysics Department, Hanoi University of Mining and Geology, No 18, Vien Street, Bac Tu Liem District, Hanoi 100 000, Vietnam; duongvanhao@humg.edu.vn (V.-H.D.); nguyenthanhduong@humg.edu.vn (T.-D.N.)
[2] Institute of Radiochemistry and Radioecology, University of Pannonia, H-8200 Veszprem, Hungary; hegedusm@almos.uni-pannon.hu (M.H.); kocsiserika@almos.uni-pannon.hu (E.K.)
* Correspondence: kt@almos.uni-pannon.hu

Abstract: The determination of natural radionuclide concentrations plays an important role for assuring public health and in the estimation of the radiological hazards. This is especially true for high level radiation areas. In this study, ^{226}Ra, ^{228}Ra and ^{238}U concentrations were measured in well waters surrounding eight of the high-level natural radiation areas in northern Vietnam. The ^{226}Ra, ^{228}Ra and ^{238}U activity concentrations vary from <1.2 × 10^{-3}–2.7 (0.46), <2.6 × 10^{-3}–0.43 (0.07) and <38 × 10^{-3}–5.32 Bq/L (0.50 of median), respectively. ^{226}Ra and ^{238}U isotopes in most areas are in equilibrium, except for the DT-Thai Nguyen area. The calculated radiological hazard indices are generally higher than WHO (World Health Organization) recommendations. Average annual effective dose and excess lifetime cancer risk values due to drinking well water range from to 130 to 540 µSv/year and 7.4 × 10^{-6} to 3.1 × 10^{-5}, respectively.

Keywords: ^{226}Ra; ^{228}Ra; ^{238}U; well water; radiological hazards; REE and uranium mines; northern Vietnam

Citation: Duong, V.-H.; Nguyen, T.-D.; Hegedus, M.; Kocsis, E.; Kovacs, T. Study of Well Waters from High-Level Natural Radiation Areas in Northern Vietnam. *IJERPH* **2021**, *18*, 469. https://doi.org/10.3390/ijerph18020469

Received: 7 December 2020
Accepted: 5 January 2021
Published: 8 January 2021

Publisher's Note: MDPI stays neutral with regard to jurisdictional claims in published maps and institutional affiliations.

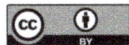

Copyright: © 2021 by the authors. Licensee MDPI, Basel, Switzerland. This article is an open access article distributed under the terms and conditions of the Creative Commons Attribution (CC BY) license (https://creativecommons.org/licenses/by/4.0/).

1. Introduction

Human beings are always exposed to a wide range of natural radionuclides [1]. Natural radionuclides can be present in the whole environment, including soil, water, air, food and even our bodies. Radionuclides in soil, air and water come from different sources, such as the weathering of the earth's crust, mining activities or fertilizer materials [2–7]. The radionuclides in water can enter the food chain, if the water is used for drinking or irrigation purposes. Determination of natural radionuclide concentrations in all the environments plays an important role for public health, because it can be used to assess the population's exposure to radiation and estimate the radiological hazard.

Investigations on natural radiation have received particular attention throughout the world in the last decade, which led to extensive studies in many countries, especially in or surrounding the high-level natural radiation areas. Studies regarding the natural radioactivity in water from different sources were widely conducted [7–15].

Among natural radionuclides, uranium leaches out from the bedrock and is present in water (surface and underground water) in various dissolved and suspended particulate forms. Other sources can be from the dry or wet deposition of aerosol from air. ^{228}Ra originates from the ^{232}Th series, and in contrast to the typically not very soluble of Th element, ^{228}Ra can be partially mobilized in natural waters, giving information on geochemical conditions and enabling contributions to the potential public exposure. ^{226}Ra is a long-lived daughter of the ^{238}U decay series, and it is also found in the water in trace quantities. The concentrations of ^{238}U, ^{228}Ra and ^{226}Ra in the water depend on the lithology, geomorphology and other geological conditions [16]. Thus, the concentration of these radionuclides varies from one site to another. The study concerning ^{226}Ra, ^{228}Ra and ^{238}U concentrations in drinking water allows understanding their distribution and evaluating their impact on human health.

In Northern Vietnam, there are several mines, which contain higher than average concentrations of radioactive elements such as the rare earth mines in NX (Lai Chau), DP (Lai Chau), MH (Lao Cai) and YP (Yen Bai); there is also a polymetallic mine (also containing high uranium concentration) in DT (Thai Nguyen); finally, there is uranium ore in BY (Son La), TS (Phu Tho) and NB (Cao Bang). These mines were recently reported to have a high radioactive background by unpublished data from the Geological Division for Radioactive and Rare Minerals, Hanoi, Vietnam. This presents a possible public health concern. Therefore, in this study, the natural radionuclide concentrations in well water (^{226}Ra, ^{228}Ra ^{238}U) in the area surrounding these mines are investigated. Based on the activity concentrations, the radiological health hazards are also evaluated.

2. Materials and Methods

2.1. Study Areas

The eight areas in Northern Vietnam, including NX-Lai Chau, DP-Lai Chau, MH-Lao Cai, BY-Son La, TS-Phu Tho, YP-Yen Bai, DT-Thai Nguyen and NB-Cao Bang were selected for this study. The location of these areas is presented in Figure 1. The NX mine is one of the largest rare earth element (REE) mines in Vietnam, with probable reserves of about 7.7 million tons. DP mine ranks the second, with probable reserves of about 3.7 million tons and is followed by MH with approximately 400,000 tons and YP with about 5000 tons [17]. BY (Son La), TS (Phu Tho) and NB (Cao Bang) have uranium ore deposits, while DT (Thai Nguyen) is the largest polymetallic mine in Vietnam.

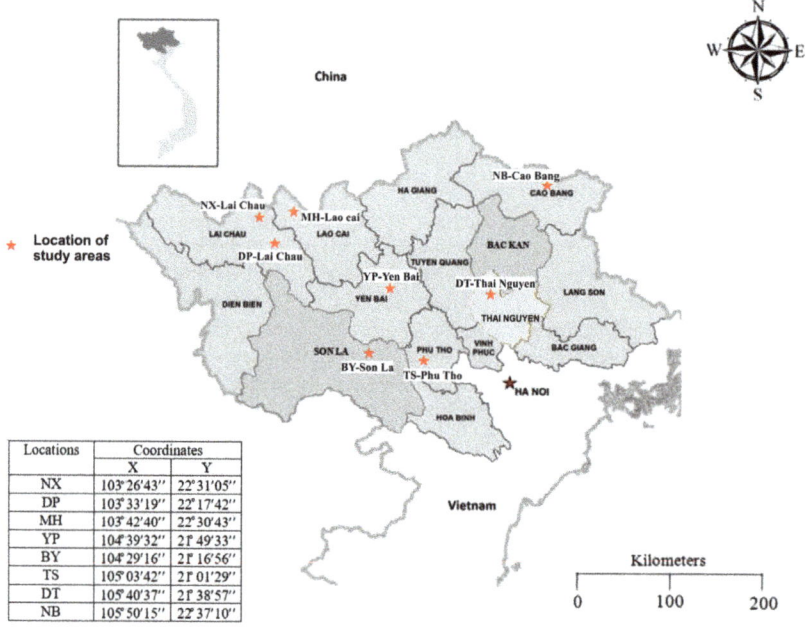

Figure 1. Location of the study areas (map was modified from Hung et al., 2016) [18].

2.2. Sample Collection and Preparation

In each study location, 20 water samples were collected from local wells during 2018–2019. These wells were dug manually in the soil to the depth of about 5 to 10 m, and these wells provide drinking water for the local population. A total of 160 water samples with 50 L for each sample were collected for this study. Each water sample was stored in a big, 50 L plastic container. Each water sample was co-precipitated as Ba(Ra)SO$_4$ for radium isotopes, then the uranium isotopes were subsequently precipitated as (NH$_4$)$_2$U$_2$O$_7$ together with MnO$_2$ [15,19,20]. The solid precipitate was then filtered. Together with study samples, a blank sample was prepared using distilled water in order to determine the background. The obtained precipitated sample was dried and milled to powder, then they were pressed into cylindrical plastic containers, weighted and finally hermetically sealed. The samples were stored for 4 half-lives in order to reach the secular equilibrium (16 days for ^{226}Ra after sealing, and approximately 100 days for ^{238}U after precipitation).

2.3. Methods

2.3.1. Measurements of Activity Concentration of ^{238}U, ^{228}Ra and ^{226}Ra in Water

After the samples reached equilibrium, activity concentration measurements were performed using a high-resolution detector HPGe with a low background made by Ortec™. The analysis was performed using Gamma Vision software. The detector's energy resolution was 1.9 keV at the 1.33 MeV ^{60}Co gamma-ray peak. To reduce the effects of background radiation at the laboratory, the detector was shielded by a 10-cm thick old-lead cylinder with a 1 mm cadmium and 1 mm copper inner lining. The samples were counted for two days to minimize the statistical counting error and activity calculation and calibration were carried out based on standard reference materials (IAEA-375). The level of background radiation present in the laboratory and introduced by the chemical process was determined using the blank sample.

The activity concentration of each sample was determined based on its respective gamma lines. The gamma lines of 609.3 keV, 1120.3 keV and 1764.5 keV of ^{214}Bi were used to determine the activity concentration of ^{226}Ra, the 911.1 keV line of ^{228}Ac was used for ^{228}Ra while the 1001 keV line of ^{234m}Pa was used for ^{238}U (which was verified by ^{235}U measurement using the 186 keV line). The lowest limit detection were 0.0012, 0.0026 and 0.038 Bq/L for ^{226}Ra, ^{228}Ra and ^{238}U, respectively (the values were used for a studied sample volume of 50 L).

The activity concentrations of ^{226}Ra, ^{228}Ra and ^{238}U are calculated based on the following Equation (1) [7]:

$$A_{sp} = \frac{N_{sp} M_{st} A_{st} C_i C_{di}}{N_{st} M_{sp}} \tag{1}$$

where: A_{sp} and A_{st} is activity concentration of studied and standard samples; N_{sp}, M_{sp} and N_{st}, M_{st} are the net measured intensity and mass of the sample and standard sample, respectively; C_i is the correction factor for the differences between the densities of the samples and the standard sample for the i isotope; and C_{di} is the correction fraction for the precipitation efficiency for the i isotope.

2.3.2. Evaluation of Radiological Hazard Indices

- Annual effective dose (AED)

The annual effective dose (AED) due to the ingestion of the drinking well water was estimated to assess the radiological hazards for the local population by using Equation (2) [21]:

$$\text{AED (μSv/year)} = A \text{ (Bq/L)} \times C_w \text{ (L/year)} \times \text{DCF (μSv/Bq)} \tag{2}$$

where AED is the annual effective dose due to ingestion of radionuclides; A is the activity concentration of radionuclides; Cw is the annual water consumption for a person (730 L/year for adults) [22]. DCF is the ingestion dose conversion factor for the corresponding radionuclides (0.28, 0.69 and 0.045 μSv/Bq for ^{226}Ra, ^{228}Ra and ^{238}U, respectively) [21,23]. We all know that there are some other isotopes, like ^{210}Po, which can contribute to a higher annual effective dose caused by drinking well waters, but in this study we only used the ^{226}Ra, ^{228}Ra and ^{238}U values to calculate the AED.

- Excess lifetime cancer risk (ELCR)

Based on the values of AED, excess lifetime cancer risks (ELCR) were calculated using the following Equation (3) [24]:

$$ELCR = AED \times Life\ Expectancy\ (LE) \times Risk\ factor\ (RF) \quad (3)$$

where LE is life expectancy of Vietnamese people in North Vietnam and mountainous areas (71 years) (https://www.gso.gov.vn/default_en.aspx?tabid=774); RF the risk factor associated with radiation, which is equal to 0.057 Sv^{-1} [24].

3. Results and Discussion

3.1. Activity Concentration

The range and average values of activity concentration of ^{226}Ra, ^{228}Ra and ^{238}U measured in the well water samples are given in Table 1. It can be seen that the activity concentration of ^{226}Ra, ^{228}Ra and ^{238}U ranges from <0.0012–2.7, <0.0026–0.43 and <0.038–5.32 Bq/L, respectively. The highest concentrations of all three isotopes are found in DT-Thai Nguyen. This table shows only a slight difference in concentration between ^{226}Ra, ^{228}Ra and ^{238}U in most cases, except for the DT-Thai Nguyen sampling site. ^{226}Ra, ^{228}Ra and ^{238}U ratios near unity indicate recent contact with uranium bearing not yet weathered minerals [25]. The concentrations of ^{226}Ra, ^{228}Ra and ^{238}U are less than 1 Bq/L in most areas, except for DT-Thai Nguyen (Table 1). In the case of DT-Thai Nguyen, the concentrations of ^{226}Ra, ^{228}Ra and ^{238}U are comparatively high and are in the ranges of 0.36–2.70, 0.05–0.43 and 0.33–5.32 Bq/L, respectively. There, the ^{226}Ra concentration can reach levels multiple times higher than the WHO guideline (1 Bq/L) [26]. The high concentrations of ^{226}Ra and ^{238}U in DT-Thai Nguyen can be attributed to the polymetallic mine (which contains high uranium concentration) in this area. There are some activities, such as exploitation and the process of ore sorting going on, which can influence activity concentrations. It should be noted that the water samples in this study were taken from wells with depth of less than 10 m. These type of wells depend on rainfall and surface water as their source of water. Accordingly, they are easily contaminated by surface water and various human activities. Thus, the human activities in the polymetallic mine can lead to a relatively high concentration of ^{226}Ra, ^{228}Ra and ^{238}U in well water.

Table 1. Concentration of natural radionuclides in well water samples in North, Vietnam.

Locations	Type of Mine	Value	Activity Concentration (Bq/L)			$^{226}Ra/^{238}U$
			^{226}Ra	^{228}Ra	^{238}U	
NX-Lai Chau	REE mine	Range (SD)	0.26–0.65 (0.09)	0.04–0.10 (0.01)	0.15–0.72 (0.15)	0.64–1.73
		Average	0.44	0.06	0.50	0.95
DP-Lai Chau	REE mine	Range (SD)	0.35–0.59 (0.08)	0.05–0.15 (0.03)	0.31–0.71 (0.10)	0.60–1.19
		Average	0.47	0.11	0.54	0.90
MH-Lao Cai	REE mine	Range (SD)	0.30–0.78 (0.16)	<0.0026–0.11 (0.02)	0.31–0.87 (0.18)	0.69–1.52
		Average	0.52	0.07 *	0.56	0.96
YP-Yen Bai	REE mine	Range (SD)	<0.0012–0.54 (0.07)	<0.0026–0.12 (0.02)	<0.038–0.70 (0.12)	**
		Average	0.23 *	0.08 *	0.31 *	**
BY-Son La	Uranium mine	Range (SD)	0.25–0.74 (0.11)	<0.0026–0.09 (0.02)	0.27–0.63 (0.08)	0.76–1.44
		Average	0.45	0.06 *	0.41	1.08
TS-Phu Tho	Uranium mine	Range (SD)	0.25–0.97 (0.19)	0.05–0.10 (0.02)	0.27–0.69 (0.11)	0.50–1.76
		Average	0.48	0.07	0.48	1.01
DT-Thai Nguyen	Uranium mine	Range (SD)	0.36–2.70 (0.69)	0.05–0.43 (0.11)	0.33–5.32 (1.46)	0.50–1.42
		Average	1.15	0.18	2.06	0.79

Table 1. Cont.

Locations	Type of Mine	Value	Activity Concentration (Bq/L)			$^{226}Ra/^{238}U$
			^{226}Ra	^{228}Ra	^{238}U	
NB-Cao Bang	Uranium mine	Range (SD)	0.32–0.97 (0.18)	<0.0026–0.13 (0.02)	0.34–0.80 (0.12)	0.53–1.43
		Average	0.53	0.07	0.55	0.97
Overall range		Minimum	<0.0012	<0.0026	<0.038	0.50
		Maximum	2.7	0.43	5.32	1.76

* during averaging values under the detection limit were taken as the detection limit to give a conservative estimate. ** uncalculable values were left out of the ratio calculation.

Table 2 compares the ^{226}Ra, ^{228}Ra and ^{238}U concentrations in the well water samples in this study with that of different water sources in different countries. The concentrations of ^{226}Ra, ^{228}Ra and ^{238}U in well water in the areas observed in this study are significantly higher than those in Hoa Binh, Vietnam. In addition, the observed concentrations are higher than those in reported for many other countries [8–12,16], whereas they are lower than some values reported for tube wells in India. The concentrations observed in well water significantly depend on the type of aquifer rock as well as the chemical and physical characteristics of water [27], thus such differences can be expected. The concentration of studied radionuclides observed in well water in this study is within the worldwide range [28].

Table 2. ^{226}Ra and ^{238}U concentrations in water samples in different areas.

Countries	Samples	Activity concentration (Bq/L)			References
		^{226}Ra	^{228}Ra	^{238}U	
Northern Vietnam	Well water	<0.0012–2.7	<0.0026–0.43	<0.038–5.32	This study
Hoa Binh, Vietnam	Groundwater	0.005–0.029	≤0.020	≤0.0005–0.009	[15]
Italy	Drinking water	0.0050–0.0608	0.00010–0.0257	0.000206–0.103	[12]
Turkey	Drinking water	<0.027–2.431	<0.036–0.270	-	[9]
Jordan	Tap water	0.096	0.170	0.033	[8]
Erbil, Iraq	Surface water	0.274–1.03	0.00676–0.244 *	0.274–1.03 *	[11]
Gogi, India	Tube well	0.0195–10.5	-	0.0123–33.2	[16]
	Open well	0.0366–0.0571	-	0.114–0.160	
Ghana	Groundwater	0.09–0.18	0.22–0.99 *	0.09–0.18 *	[10]
	Surface water	0.08–0.17	0.18–0.74 *	0.08–0.17 *	
World range	Drinking water	0.0002–45	0.0001–7.7	0.000028–150	[28]

* Equilibrium was assumed by the original authors.

Regarding the concentration ratio of $^{226}Ra/^{238}U$ in well water samples, as shown in Table 1, the average value ranges from 0.57 (DT-Thai Nguyen) to 1.09 (BY-Son La). The data presented in Table 1 also shows that on average there is near equilibrium between ^{226}Ra and ^{238}U, except for DT-Thai Nguyen. Kumar et al. (2016) reported that the concentration of $^{226}Ra/^{238}U$ in groundwater in southwestern Punjab in India was varied from 0.08 to 0.22 [29]. In groundwater in Finland, Asikainen (1981) also showed that the ratio of $^{226}Ra/^{238}U$ ranged from 0.05 to 1. By contrast, other previous studies reported the enrichment of ^{226}Ra in groundwater [30]. For examples, Gascoyne (1989) indicated that the $^{226}Ra/^{238}U$ ratios in Canadian groundwater varied from 0.026 to 5300; this ratio in Konnngara Australian groundwater was from 0.02 to 89 [31]. Recently, the research results of Almasoud et al. (2020) indicated that the ratios of $^{226}Ra/^{238}U$ in groundwater samples in Saudi Arabia ranged from 1.25 to 20.4 [32]. The issue is further complicated by the effects of the recoil from the emission of an alpha particle, which can increase the mobility of the daughter nuclide due to the Szilárd–Chalmer effect. On the other hand, the ^{234}Th or ^{234}U can be fixed to more weathering resistant mineral phases, resulting in relatively more

^{238}U dissolving into groundwater [31]. The depletion of ^{234}U in groundwater can also be observed based on the relative abundances of U under various geochemical conditions [30]

The relationship between activity concentrations of ^{238}U and ^{226}Ra in well water samples in this study is shown in Figure 2. A significant positive correlation was found between the two radionuclides with a Pearson correlation coefficient, 0.9402 and a p value < 0.00001 for the overall dataset, due to the influence of the higher values observed at DT-Thai Nguyen. The high value of correlation between ^{238}U and ^{226}Ra shows that these radionuclides have leached from the similar host rock [16]. Excluding DT-Thai Nguyen, there is moderate positive correlation with a Pearson correlation coefficient of 0.6326, and a p value < 0.00001. Similarly, a strong positive correlation was observed both between ^{238}U and ^{228}Ra (Pearson correlation coefficient: 0.8411, with a p value < 0.00001) and ^{226}Ra and ^{228}Ra (Pearson correlation coefficient: 0.7834, with a p value < 0.00001) for the overall dataset, however the effect of the higher values at DT-Thai Nguyen improving the correlation are observable here as well.

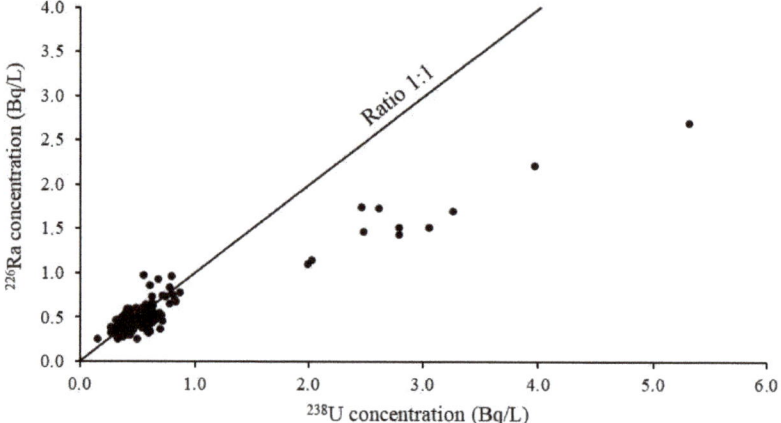

Figure 2. Relationship between ^{238}U and ^{226}Ra concentrations.

3.2. Radiological Hazards

The calculated radiation hazard indices based on the average activity concentrations for some drinking well water in northern Vietnam are listed in Table 3. As shown in this table, the annual effective dose (AED) for ^{226}Ra is significantly higher than that for ^{238}U, while ^{228}Ra is in the middle despite having a higher dose conversion coefficient due to the comparatively low activity concentrations. The average total annual effective dose for adults due to the consumption of water ranges from 130 to 540 µSv/year with the mean value of 240 µSv/year. The average excess life cancer risk (ELCR) due to drinking the investigated well water is from 7.4×10^{-6} to 3.1×10^{-5} (7 to 31 cases per 1 million people) with the average of 1.4×10^{-5} (14 cases per 1 million people). Specific wells can have higher values; the overall maximum activity concentrations were observed in a well in YP-Yen Bai translating to a total annual effective dose of 540 µSv/y for adults and an ELCR of 7.0×10^{-5} (70 cases per 1 million people). As reported by the WHO (2017), the reference values for AED and ELCR due to drinking water are 100 µSv/year and 1.0×10^{-5}, respectively. It can be seen that the results of AED and ELCR due to consumption of well water in this study are higher on average for each area from the observed radionuclides alone than the values suggested by the WHO (2017), with the exception of ELCR for YP-Yen Bai. This indicates that there is a need for defining local policy regarding the wells in high-level natural radiation areas, northern Vietnam (in the observed areas), especially DT-Thai Nguyen.

Table 3. Radiation hazard indices for well water samples in northern Vietnam.

Locations	Type of Mine	AED (µSv/Year)				ELCR
		^{226}Ra	^{228}Ra	^{238}U	Total	
NX-Lai Chau	REE mine	120	40	20	190	1.1×10^{-5}
DP-Lai Chau	REE mine	130	80	20	240	1.3×10^{-5}
MH-Lao Cai	REE mine	150	50	30	220	1.3×10^{-5}
YP-Yen Bai	REE mine	60	50	10	130	7.4×10^{-6}
BY-Son La	U mine	130	40	20	180	1.0×10^{-5}
TS-Phu Tho	U mine	140	50	20	210	1.2×10^{-5}
DT-Thai Nguyen	U mine	320	120	90	540	3.1×10^{-5}
NB-Cao Bang	U mine	150	50	20	220	1.3×10^{-5}
Average		150	60	30	240	1.4×10^{-5}

4. Conclusions

The concentrations of ^{226}Ra, ^{228}Ra and ^{238}U in well waters in different locations surrounding the high-level radiation areas in northern Vietnam were extensively measured and evaluated. The research results show that the concentrations of ^{226}Ra, ^{228}Ra and ^{238}U in well water samples in the observed mining areas of northern Vietnam are comparatively higher than those reported for other areas of Vietnam and other countries. The highest concentrations of ^{226}Ra, ^{228}Ra and ^{238}U are observed in DT-Thai Nguyen. The research also shows that the concentration of ^{226}Ra and ^{238}U for most locations on average are around equilibrium, except for DT-Thai Nguyen. Regarding the radiological hazards assessment, the calculated results of AED and ELCR due to the consumption of well water are often higher, and for DT-Thai Nguyen multiple times higher, than the WHO reference values. The results generated from this study provide important baseline data for the impact assessment of the mining activities in the region in the future.

Author Contributions: Conceptualization, V.-H.D., T.-D.N., and T.K.; methodology, M.H., V.-H.D., and T.K.; formal analysis, M.H., T.-D.N.; investigation, V.-H.D., T.-D.N., E.K., and T.K.; resources, V.-H.D., and T.K.; data curation, T.K. and M.H.; writing—original V.-H.D., and M.H. and T.K. draft preparation, V.-H.D.; writing—review and editing, M.H., E.K., V.-H.D., and T.K.; visualization, V.-H.D. and E.K.; supervision, T.K.; project administration, T.K.; funding acquisition, V.-H.D. and T.K. All authors have read and agreed to the published version of the manuscript.

Funding: The research work is supported by Grant of The National Foundation for Science and Technology Development (NAFOSTED), Vietnam, no 105.05-2019.10. and the TKP2020-IKA-07 project financed under the 2020-4.1.1-TKP2020 Thematic Excellence Programme by the National Research, Development and Innovation Fund of Hungary.

Institutional Review Board Statement: Not applicable for studies not involving humans or animals.

Informed Consent Statement: Not applicable for studies not involving humans.

Data Availability Statement: The data presented in this study are available on request from the corresponding author.

Conflicts of Interest: The authors declare no conflict of interest.

References

1. Sonkawade, R.G.; Kant, K.; Muralithar, S.; Kumar, R.; Ramola, R.C. Natural radioactivity in common building construction and radiation shielding materials. *Atmos. Environ.* **2008**, *42*, 2254–2259. [CrossRef]
2. Azeez, H.H.; Mansour, H.H.; Ahmad, S.T. Transfer of natural radioactive nuclides from soil to plant crops. *Appl. Radiat. Isot.* **2019**, *147*, 152–158. [CrossRef] [PubMed]
3. Cwanek, A.; Mietelski, J.W.; Lokas, E.; Olech, M.A.; Anczkiewicz, R.; Misiak, R. Sources and variation of isotopic ratio of airborne radionuclides in Western Arctic lichens and mosses. *Chemosphere* **2020**, *239*, 124783. [CrossRef] [PubMed]
4. Nguyen, D.C.; Le Khanh, P.; Jodlowski, P.; Pieczonka, J.; Piestrzyński, A.; Van, H.D.; Nowak, J. Natural Radioactivity at the Sin Quyen Iron-Oxide-Copper-Gold Deposit in North Vietnam. *Acta Geophys.* **2016**, *64*, 2305–2321. [CrossRef]

5. Van Hao, D.; Dinh, C.N.; Jodlowski, P.; Kovacs, T. High-level natural radionuclides from the Mandena deposit, South Madagascar. *J. Radioanal. Nucl. Chem.* **2019**, *319*, 1331–1338. [CrossRef]
6. Van, H.D.; Nguyen, T.D.; Peka, A.; Hegedus, M.; Csordas, A.; Kovacs, T. Study of soil to plant transfer factors of 226Ra, 232Th, 40K and 137Cs in Vietnamese crops. *J. Environ. Radioact.* **2020**, *223*, 106416. [CrossRef]
7. Van, H.D.; Lantoarindriaka, A.; Piestrzyński, A.; Trinh, P.T. Fort-Dauphin beach sands, south Madagascar: Natural radionuclides and mineralogical studies. *Viet. J. Earth Sci.* **2020**, *42*, 118–129. [CrossRef]
8. Al-Amir, S.M.; Al-Hamarneh, I.F.; Al-Abed, T.; Awadallah, M. Natural radioactivity in tap water and associated age-dependent dose and lifetime risk assessment in Amman, Jordan. *Appl. Radiat. Isot.* **2012**, *70*, 692–698. [CrossRef]
9. Altıkulaç, A.; Turhan, Ş.; Gümüş, H. The natural and artificial radionuclides in drinking water samples and consequent population doses. *J. Radiat. Res. Appl. Sci.* **2015**, *8*, 578–582. [CrossRef]
10. Awudu, A.R.; Darko, E.O.; Schandorf, C.; Hayford, E.K.; Abekoe, M.K.; Ofori-Danson, P.K. Determination of Activity Concentration Levels of 238U, 232Th, and 40K in Drinking Water in a Gold Mine in Ghana. *Health Phys.* **2010**, *99*, S149–S153. [CrossRef]
11. Ezzlddin, S.K.; Aziz, H.H. An Investigation of Activity Concentration of 238U, 232Th, 137Cs and 40K Radionuclides in Drinking Water Resources in Iraqi Kurdistan Region-Erbil. *ZANCO J. Pure Appl. Sci.* **2017**, *28*, 32–40. [CrossRef]
12. Jia, G.; Torri, G.; Magro, L. Concentrations of 238U, 234U, 235U, 232Th, 230Th, 228Th, 226Ra, 228Ra, 224Ra, 210Po, 210Pb and 212Pb in drinking water in Italy: Reconciling safety standards based on measurements of gross α and β. *J. Environ. Radioact.* **2009**, *100*, 941–949. [CrossRef] [PubMed]
13. Landsberger, S.G.; George, G. An evaluation of 226Ra and 228Ra in drinking water in several counties in Texas, USA. *J. Environ. Radioact.* **2013**, *125*, 2–5. [CrossRef] [PubMed]
14. Yalcin, P.; Taskin, H.; Kam, E.; Taskin, H.; Terzi, M.; Varinlioglu, A.; Bozkurt, A.; Bastug, A.; Tasdelen, B. Investigation of radioactivity level in soil and drinking water samples collected from the city of Erzincan, Turkey. *J. Radioanal. Nucl. Chem.* **2012**, *292*, 999–1006. [CrossRef]
15. Van Hao, D.; Nguyen, C.D.; Nowak, J.; Kovacs, T.; Hoang, Q.A. Uranium and radium isotopes in some selected thermal, surface and bottled waters in Vietnam. *J. Radioanal. Nucl. Chem.* **2019**, *319*, 1345–1349. [CrossRef]
16. Yashodhara, I.; Kumara, S.; Karunakara, N. Activity concentrations of 226Ra and 238U in water samples and estimation of radiation dose around the proposed uranium mining region in Gogi. In Proceedings of the Proceedings NSRP, Mamallapuram, India, 12–14 December 2012; Volume II, pp. 525–528.
17. Moody, M.D. Mother Lode: The Untapped Rare Earth Mineral Resources of Vietnam. Department of Joint Military Operations, Naval War College, Newport, USA, 2013. Available online: https://www.google.com.hk/url?sa=t&rct=j&q=&esrc=s&source=web&cd=&ved=2ahUKEwjkj7KtuIvuAhWBbN4KHQvIBMYQFjAAegQIAxAC&url=https%3A%2F%2Fapps.dtic.mil%2Fdtic%2Ftr%2Ffulltext%2Fu2%2Fa594225.pdf&usg=AOvVaw2ILnJx__vGU5DFZKIMd7J- (accessed on 7 December 2020).
18. Hung, T.Q.; Thu, T.T.N. Utilization of maize animal feeds in northern upland region of Vietnam. *AGRIS* **2016**, *32*, 283–298.
19. Nguyen, C.D.; Rajchel, L.; Van Duong, H.; Nowak, J. 224Ra and the 224Ra/228Ra activity ratio in selected mineral waters from the Polish Carpathians. *Geol. Q.* **2017**, *61*, 771–778. [CrossRef]
20. Nguyen, D.C.; Niewodniczański, J.; Dorda, J.; Ochoński, A.; Chrusciel, E.; Tomza, I. Determination of radium isotopes in mine waters through alpha-and beta-activities measured by liquid scintillation spectrometry. *J. Radioanal. Nucl. Chem.* **1997**, *222*, 69–74. [CrossRef]
21. ICRP. Publication 73. Radiological protection and safety in Medicine. *Ann. ICRP* **1996**, *26*. [CrossRef]
22. WHO. *Guidelines for Drinking-Water Quality*; WHO Library Cataloguing-in-Publication Data-NLM classification: WA 675; World Health Organization: Geneva, Switzerland, 2011.
23. UNSCEAR. *Sources and Effects of Lonizing Radiation. Report to the General Assembly with Scientific Annexes*; United Nations: New York, NY, USA, 2000.
24. ICRP. Publication 60. Recommendations of the International Commission on Radiological Protection. *Ann. ICRP* **1990**, *21*. Available online: https://www.icrp.org/publication.asp?id=icrp%20publication%2060 (accessed on 7 December 2020).
25. Alvarado, J.C.; Balsiger, B.; Röllin, S.; Jakob, A.; Burger, M. Radioactive and chemical contamination of the water resources in the former uranium mining and milling sites of Mailuu Suu (Kyrgyzstan). *J. Environ. Radioact.* **2014**, *138*, 1–10. [CrossRef] [PubMed]
26. WHO. *Guidelines for Drinking-Water Quality*; WHO Library Cataloguing in Publication Data; Licence: CC BY-Nc-SA 3.0 IGO.; World Health Organization: Geneva, Switzerland, 2017.
27. Gascoyne, M. High levels of uranium and radium in groundwaters at Canada's Underground Research Laboratory, Lac du Bonnet, Manitoba, Canada. *Appl. Geochem.* **1989**, *4*, 577–591. [CrossRef]
28. UNSCEAR. *Sources and Effects of Lonizing Radiation. Report to the General Assembly Scientific Annexes A and B*; United Nations: New York, NY, USA, 2008.
29. Kumar, A.; Karpe, R.K.; Rout, S.; Gautam, Y.P.; Mishra, M.K.; Ravi, P.M.; Tripathi, R.M. Activity ratios of 234U/238U and 226Ra/228Ra for transport mechanisms of elevated uranium in alluvial aquifers of groundwater in south-western (SW) Punjab, India. *J. Environ. Radioact.* **2016**, *151*, 311–320. [CrossRef] [PubMed]
30. Asikainen, M. State of disequilibrium between 238U, 234U, 226Ra and 222Rn in groundwater from bedrock. *Geochim. Cosmochim. Acta* **1981**, *45*, 201–206. [CrossRef]

31. Yanase, N.; Payne, T.E.; Sekine, K. Groundwater geochemistry in the Koongarra ore deposit, Australia (I): Implications for uranium migration. *Geochem. J.* **1995**, *29*, 1–29. [CrossRef]
32. Almasoud, F.I.; Ababneh, Z.Q.; Alanazi, Y.J.; Khandaker, M.U.; Sayyed, M.I. Assessment of radioactivity contents in bedrock groundwater samples from the northern region of Saudi Arabia. *Chemosphere* **2020**, *242*, 125181. [CrossRef]

MDPI
St. Alban-Anlage 66
4052 Basel
Switzerland
Tel. +41 61 683 77 34
Fax +41 61 302 89 18
www.mdpi.com

International Journal of Environmental Research and Public Health Editorial Office
E-mail: ijerph@mdpi.com
www.mdpi.com/journal/ijerph

www.ingramcontent.com/pod-product-compliance
Lightning Source LLC
LaVergne TN
LVHW070426100526
838202LV00014B/1536